D0555141

Final Acts

Final Acts

Death, Dying, and the Choices We Make

EDITED BY

NAN BAUER-MAGLIN AND DONNA PERRY

RUTGERS UNIVERSITY PRESS

NEW BRUNSWICK, NEW JERSEY, AND LONDON

LIBRARY OF CONGRESS CATALOGING-IN-PUBLICATION DATA

Final acts : death, dying, and the choices we make / edited by Nan Bauer-Maglin and Donna Perry.

p. cm.

Includes bibliographical references and index.

ISBN 978–0–8135–4627–8 (hardcover : alk. paper) —

ISBN 978–0–8135–4628–5 (pbk. : alk. paper)

I. Death.   I. Maglin, Nan Bauer   II. Perry, Donna Marie, 1946–

HQ1073.F557   2009

306.9—dc22   2009000773

A British Cataloging-in-Publication record for this book is available from the British Library.

Ruthann Robson's "Notes on My Dying" was originally published in *Creative Nonfiction* 18, 8 (2001).

June Bingham's "Live Better or Live Longer?" appeared as an op-ed article in *The Riverdale Press*, July 5, 2007, 1, A9.

Stephen P. Kiernan's "The Transformation of Death in America" combines material from throughout his book *Last Rights: Rescuing the End of Life from the Medical System*. Copyright © 2006 by the author and reprinted by permission of St. Martin's Press, LLC.

Marge Piercy's "End of days" appeared in *Rattle* 14, no. 2. Copyright © 2006 Marge Piercy, Box 1473, Wellfleet, MA 02667. Used by permission of Wallace Literary Agency, Inc.

Visit our Web site: http://rutgerspress.rutgers.edu

Manufactured in the United States of America

CONTENTS

PREFACE

When we issued a call for contributions to a book on death and choice, we hoped for strong, convincing essays: personal stories, professional analysis, some historical background, political and social contexts. We wanted essays that would explore how complicated it is to put death and choice in the same sentence, particularly when one is talking about terminal illness. Given a death sentence, what kind of choice or agency does one have?

With that common purpose, we also came to the project for different reasons and out of different life circumstances.

Nan

I have been interested in the subject of death and choice for some time—way before I turned sixty-five. I have taken care to do the "normal" things like write out an extensive living will, draw up a power of attorney and do-not-resuscitate instructions; before I travel on an airplane I tend to look at my living will and update it with yet another procedure or mechanical device I do not want inflicted on me. Before almost every departure, I write a note to my daughter (there are years of them sitting in sealed envelopes waiting for her to read after I have died) and now I have decided to write an ethical will for my grandchildren.

I have always been a strong defender of death by choice, of self-suicide and assisted suicide, telling my friends and relatives that I plan to take my own life at some point if and when I am incapacitated or no longer feel I am able to have the quality of life I want for myself. I have even advocated for suicide when you are not incapacitated—before you get to that point—and I have argued against those who say that people who do that are depressed. Like so many people, I watched my mother spend her last years lying, unaware, unable to communicate, and maybe in pain, in a nursing home. While my concern about dying and taking control preceded this experience, my mother's dying certainly convinced me that I needed to take action on some level about my own death.

However, recently I have been somewhat taken aback by reading some feminist gerontologists who argue that we are aged by culture and that my unease (to the point of planning suicide) about my aging, my fear of becoming ill, of not being able or of being in debilitating pain, is "caused" by ageism. I have to think more about this. While I want to take this in, I do not want to forget or ignore the material nature of our bodies and the arc the body follows from birth to death. I want to look at the D word, as Nora Ephron calls it, straight on: "I am dancing around the D word, but I don't mean to be coy. When you cross into your sixties, your odds of dying—spike. Death is a sniper. It strikes people you love, people you like, people you know, it's everywhere. You could be next."[1]

Meanwhile, I am aging—moving into my late sixties—as are so many millions of other people, so I thought it would be useful to collect a number of voices who speak to these complicated issues of dying, death, choice, aging, and living. Eugene O'Kelly, who was told at age fifty-three that he would die in three months, suggests that "we should all spend time thinking about our death [and not wait until we are old or given a death sentence], and what we want to do with our final days, insofar as it's within our control." He wonders "if how we die is one of the most important decisions we can make," then, "why do most people abrogate responsibility?"[2] This collection is helping me think hard and long on the subject.

Donna

When Nan approached me about co-editing a collection of essays on death and choice, I was enthusiastic. I did have one concern, though, and a request: I didn't want to work on a suicide book and I wanted to contribute an essay on former Columbia University professor and feminist author Carolyn Heilbrun, my former mentor, who committed suicide at the age of seventy-seven. As we talked, I realized that Nan didn't envision a book that would focus exclusively on suicide, so my concern was met. And since she welcomed the idea that I would write about this influential teacher and scholar who chose to die on her own terms in her own time, the deal was struck.

I didn't feel that I could do justice to a collection on suicide because I've always been ambivalent about it. In most cases, I support an adult's right to choose to die. I also consider Oregon's Death with Dignity Act, which allows for physician-assisted suicide under certain prescribed circumstances, an important and humane piece of legislation that should be replicated throughout the country. Nevertheless, although I know it is my right, I also know that it is extremely unlikely that I would ever take my own life. If I had a terminal illness and were in excruciating pain, perhaps. But, even then, I'm not so sure.

My attitude toward life and death probably has something to do with my personal history.

I never expected to live into old age. My father died ten days after having a massive heart attack when he was forty-seven, and my mother suffered a fatal cerebral hemorrhage at sixty-two. Four of their six siblings were also dead of natural causes by sixty-two, the age I am now. An only child, I have no brothers or sisters to compare myself to, but I consider myself lucky to have made it this far. Especially after a bout with breast cancer when I was thirty-five.

I was also raised Catholic, which has undoubtedly contributed to a strong sense of life as sacred. Although I've left the Church (or "lapsed," as my high school nuns would say), that feeling persists.

When I tell my husband that I feel like I am living on borrowed time, he says I am being maudlin. He reminds me that I have excellent health. But I can't shake the feeling, and it doesn't get me depressed. Instead, it gives me a *carpe diem* approach to life which is strangely liberating. I don't put off pleasures (trips, visits with friends, good food and drink), hardly ever worry about money (although I don't spend it lavishly), and try not to take myself too seriously. Ultimately, I feel that each day is a gift I didn't really expect.

I don't want to be kept alive at any cost and through artificial means, however. If I have lost brain function—as my mother had after her stroke—I want to die, as she did, quickly and painlessly. I've prepared the necessary documents—a living will, do-not-resuscitate order, and power of attorney—to indicate my wishes; although I now realize, as some contributors indicate, that sometimes even these preparations don't guarantee that a patient's intentions are followed.

My ambivalence about suicide may have kept me from writing that essay on Carolyn Heilbrun. Although she had written and talked about her intention to kill herself when she no longer considered her life useful, when Carolyn finally did it she left most of us who loved and admired her stunned.

She wasn't ill or depressed; by all accounts, she just chose to die. I couldn't understand why Carolyn, who seemed to take such pleasure in life, chose to leave it. I could write about the way her death was being read in various ways by others—as feminist victory, personal choice, depressive act, sign of internalized ageism, and so on—but I found all of these interpretations, ultimately, inadequate. For me her choice to die remained a mystery she might have written herself, under her pseudonym, Amanda Cross.

These essays have helped me think about life, death, dying, agency, and choice in new ways. They have unsettled some of my previous assumptions and shown me how powerful it is when we, like Carolyn Heilbrun, write our own lives and deaths.

Our Thanks

Nan sends particular thanks to Xiaoxi (Susan) Chen, The Transition Network literary gerontology book group and my thirty-plus-year-old women's group, Susanne Paul of Global Action on Aging, and to my friends and family (husband, children, grandchildren) who have stood witness as I have delved into this heavy and very personal subject in the making of this book.

Donna particularly thanks Sharon Dennihy-Bailey, Penny Dugan, and Joan Harden for reminding me of what I still believe, William Paterson University for providing release time from teaching, my friends and family for their patience and support, and my husband for being a mensch.

We both thank everyone who contributed a prospectus or draft essay for the collection. We regret that we couldn't include everyone's good work.

Special thanks goes to Neill Rosenfeld, who was enormously helpful as we wrote and rewrote our introductions, and to Leslie Mitchner, Associate Director/Editor in Chief at Rutgers University Press, who welcomed our idea and asked the right (if tough) questions; to the other RUP staff members for their efficiency and assistance; and to Susannah Driver-Barstow for her close and careful copyediting.

NOTES

1. Nora Ephron, *I Feel Bad About My Neck: And Other Thoughts On Being a Woman* (New York: Knopf, 2006), 131.

2. Eugene O'Kelly (with Andrew Postman), *Chasing Daylight: How My Forthcoming Death Transformed My Life* (New York: McGraw-Hill, 2006), 14.

Final Acts

Introduction

"Dealing with death is a third rail issue in the United States. We don't talk about death and dying as a societal problem, but it's going to become more and more so."

−Dr. Joseph Messer to Studs Terkel, *Will the Circle Be Unbroken? Reflections on Death, Rebirth, and Hunger for a Faith*

Most of us don't want to think about death and dying. We know that someday we may have to be caretakers to the terminally or chronically ill, and we may have strong opinions about issues like suicide or aid in dying or the government's role in end-of-life decision making. But, generally, we choose to avoid what we consider a depressing subject. Feeling powerless to control our deaths, we shrug our shoulders, go on with our lives, and hope to die peacefully in our sleep of natural causes at ninety.

The writers whose essays are gathered in *Final Acts* provide us with a reality check and wake-up call. For most of us, death won't be quick. Although we may be lucky enough to reach ninety, we probably won't die at home in our own beds. And, unless we do some advance planning, our deaths may be prolonged and/or painful. In addition, most of us (particularly women) will end up caring for elderly parents, relatives, friends, or partners before we die. And they won't die in their sleep either.

By demystifying the process, these writers deactivate death and dying as a "third rail issue" and demonstrate how the dying—and those who care for them—can make informed and loving end-of-life choices. And what can happen if they don't.

We hear from patients, caretakers, physicians, journalists, lawyers, social workers, educators, hospital administrators, academics, lawyers, psychologists, and a poet. There are ethicists, religious believers, and nonbelievers. They discuss intensely personal issues, like choosing or rejecting medical interventions, deciding among options for pain relief, calling or not calling

911, selecting the amount and type of end-of-life care (such as hospice or palliative care), accepting or challenging the wishes of loved ones, and, most importantly, deciding who should control the overall process.

They consider broader questions, including: where we die (for example, home, hospital, nursing home, hospice); the role of doctors, technology, law, and the state; the personal and societal costs of death and dying; and the documents one should have in place (health proxy, do-not-resuscitate order, living will, and power of attorney). They discuss death from natural causes (slow or sudden), suicide, and aid in dying (which some offer as an alternative term for *assisted suicide*).

Unlike previous books on death and dying, *Final Acts* isn't designed to advance a cause or explore, in depth, a hot topic (suicide, aid in dying, the hospice movement, escalating end-of-life care costs, or the nursing home industry, for example). It examines these and other issues—from many perspectives—but the collection's strength lies in its attempt to address broader questions: What characterizes the good or bad death? What role does individual agency or choice play at the end of life? What role do other factors—beliefs, customs, values, family situation, money, location, class, race, ethnicity, and gender—play? What final acts will smooth our passage or the passage of those we love?

Final Acts begins a conversation long overdue.

Death and dying, arguably the most private human experiences, are also public events. More than ever before, an individual's dying directly involves others—not just family members, friends, neighbors, and coworkers, but also teams of medical professionals, like doctors, nurses, social workers, and hospice workers, as well as health aides and attendants. Medical facilities (hospitals, hospices, nursing homes) and health-care programs (Medicare, Medicaid, private health insurance) become involved, as do religious institutions, a multimillion-dollar funeral industry, and occasionally even politicians and the courts. So, while we may die alone, these days we die intimately connected.

As journalist Stephen Kiernan points out in his essay in this collection, the American way of death has changed: today most people die gradually, from incremental illnesses, rather than from heart attacks or the fast-moving illnesses that killed earlier generations. Life expectancy has reached record highs: 80.7 years for women and 75.4 years for men, according to 2006 data from the National Center for Health Statistics. The number of Americans aged sixty-five and over increased ten times and those over 85 increased more than thirtyfold during the twentieth century. By 2020 there will be 53.2 million Americans older than age 65—forming 15.8 percent of the population—and 6.5 million of them will be over 85, according to the Census Bureau. And, as Kiernan writes, most of us will experience a slow death.[1]

Nonetheless, while late-life aging and death are so public and, in most cases, prolonged, we do not talk openly or fully about them. We avoid the ill and old, writes Dr. Ira Byock, participating in a "collective psychological avoidance of illness, physical dependence, dying, death and grief."

In the article "The Way We Age Now," Dr. Atul Gawande, associate director at Brigham and Women's Hospital's Center for Surgery and Public Health, says that "people naturally prefer to avoid the subject of their decrepitude. There have been dozens of best-selling books on aging, but they tend to have titles like 'Younger Next Year,' 'The Fountain of Age,' 'Ageless,' 'The Sexy Years.'" Gawande adds that avoiding reality has serious consequences: "For one thing, we put off changes that we need to make as a society. For another, we deprive ourselves of opportunities to change the individual experience of aging for the better."[2]

It takes a particularly dramatic situation or individual to break our national silence around death and dying.

In 1975, for example, British journalist Derek Humphry caused a sensation with the publication of *Jean's Way*, a book in which he detailed his forty-two-year-old wife's battle with terminal cancer and his own part in assisting her to commit suicide. Five years later, relocated to the United States and working with like-minded people, he founded the Hemlock Society, which became the most powerful right-to-die organization in the United States in the 1980s. Although the group dropped the name in 2003 and merged into Compassion and Choices, Humphry's best-selling *Final Exit: The Practicalities of Self-Deliverance and Assisted Suicide for the Dying*, published in 1991, remains the self-help bible for terminally ill people wanting to commit suicide.[3]

Another right-to-die advocate, Dr. Jack Kevorkian, a Michigan pathologist, thrust physician-assisted suicide into the news, claiming to have assisted in the deaths of nearly one hundred terminally ill people between 1990 and 1998. Tried numerous times for assisting in suicides, Kevorkian was convicted in 1999 and served eight years of a ten-to-twenty-five-year term for the second-degree murder of Thomas Youk, fifty-two, who was in the final stages of ALS (amyotrophic lateral sclerosis, or Lou Gehrig's disease). Kevorkian videotaped himself administering a lethal injection to Youk, who had given his fully informed consent. When *60 Minutes* broadcast the tape, Michigan filed charges.[4]

Kevorkian's contention that laws restricting the assisted suicide of fully informed, competent adults were inherently unjust sparked a national debate that continues to resonate. But other cases over more than thirty years raise the equally controversial question of euthanasia, or a right to die, for those who cannot make the decision themselves. Every day, countless ordinary people make decisions involving life support and feeding tubes for their loved ones; only occasionally do their decisions make news—and when they do, there's often high drama on the national stage.

In 1975 the parents of twenty-one-year-old Karen Ann Quinlan asked a hospital to remove the ventilator that had been keeping her alive, but in a persistent vegetative state, for several months. When hospital officials refused, her father sued and eventually brought the case to the New Jersey Supreme Court, which ruled in their favor. Ironically, when the ventilator was removed, Quinlan was able to breathe on her own. She lived on, fed by artificial nutrition, until she died of pneumonia in 1985.

The right-to-die case of Nancy Cruzan made headlines in 1987 when her family waged a legal battle to remove her feeding tube. Cruzan had been diagnosed as being in a persistent vegetative state four years earlier, following an automobile accident. Their petition lasted for three years, going as far as the United States Supreme Court. The feeding tube was finally removed on December 15, 1990, and Cruzan died eleven days later.

Most recently, the case of a comatose Florida woman, Terri Schiavo, galvanized public opinion. At issue was her husband's attempt to remove her feeding tube in 1998, a decision opposed by her parents. Schiavo had been in a persistent vegetative state for eight years. Religious and advocacy groups entered the controversy, stoking what became a political wildfire. After appeals, motions, petitions, and hearings, after the Senate majority leader (a thoracic surgeon) diagnosed Schiavo as conscious based on a videotape, after President George W. Bush flew across the country to sign a special law that shifted jurisdiction in the case from the state to the federal courts, the U.S. Supreme Court refused to hear the case. The state court's ruling held. Schiavo was disconnected from her feeding tube and died in 2005.[5]

Equally controversial was the state of Oregon's vote to legalize physician-assisted suicide in 1994. Despite safeguards including age (at least eighteen), Oregon residency, a confirmed diagnosis of a terminal illness with less than six months to live, and confirmation by two physicians that the patient is capable and acting voluntarily, the Death with Dignity Act, enacted in 1997, garnered fierce opposition by some disability and religious groups (notably the Roman Catholic Church). They charged that it devalues human life and can result in pressure on people with disabilities to end their lives. In 1999 Illinois Representative Henry Hyde and Oklahoma Senator Don Nickles moved the debate to the national stage when they tried to nullify the act by making it a federal crime to use scheduled drugs to assist in hastening a death.

Their attempt was unsuccessful, and in 2006 the U.S. Supreme Court sided with Oregon in upholding the law, a decision that represented a stinging rebuke to the Bush administration. Public support for physician-assisted suicide has spread to the neighboring state of Washington, where voters in 2008 approved a law allowing doctors to prescribe lethal medication to terminally ill patients. But the issue is far from settled. Voters in California, Michigan, and Maine have defeated similar measures in the past, suggesting that the debate stirs strong—and important—arguments on both sides.

The terminally ill, themselves, sometimes break the code of silence around death and dying, often with great impact. Four recent examples that captured national attention tell us more about how to live than about death or the dying process.

Mitch Albom's best-selling *Tuesdays with Morrie* (1997) chronicled the author's meetings with his terminally ill college professor from twenty years earlier, Morrie Schwartz. Later made into a stage play and movie, the book stresses Schwartz's optimism and refusal to be defeated by ALS.[6]

By the time Associate Professor of Computer Science Randy Pausch delivered his now-famous "Last Lecture" at Carnegie Mellon University in 2007, his doctors had said he had "three to six months of good health left" after a grueling bout with terminal pancreatic cancer. The title of the annual lecture series was ironic. Speakers were supposed to give a hypothetically final talk answering the question, "What wisdom would you try to impart to the world if you knew it was your last chance?" Pausch died ten months later, on July 25, 2008. Millions have seen Pausch's inspirational lecture, "Really Achieving Your Childhood Dreams," on YouTube or bought his "Last Lecture" book, coauthored with Jeffrey Zaslow. Like Schwartz, Pausch is concerned with living well and fully, not dying.[7]

In *Chasing Daylight*, Eugene O'Kelly, who was told at age fifty-three that he would die in three-and-a-half months, describes the process of saying good-bye to family, friends, business associates, and acquaintances. Trying to come to terms with his death, he asks a fundamental question: "Who teaches you to embrace it?" The subtitle of the book, *How My Forthcoming Death Transformed My Life*, indicates that, in light of this ultimate loss, he made important discoveries about living.[8]

On National Public Radio, listeners got an inside look at life with a terminal cancer diagnosis over a span of two years. Leroy Sievers, a broadcast journalist and executive producer of *Nightline*, charted his life and battle with colorectal cancer. For two years, in daily blog entries published on www.npr.org, weekly podcasts, and occasional commentaries on NPR's *Morning Edition*, Sievers wrote with startling honesty about his life and the various painful and experimental treatments he underwent after being told that he had six months to live. Each blog entry began with the same message: "After that day, your life is never the same. 'That day' is the day the doctor tells you, 'you have cancer.' Every one of us knows someone who's had to face that news. It's scary, it's sad. But it's still life, and it's a life worth living." Sievers died in August 2008 at age fifty-three.[9]

Many Americans face long-term deterioration from Alzheimer's disease. In fact, Kiernan informs us, deaths from Alzheimer's have doubled since 1980. Some 24.3 million people have the illness today, with an average life expectancy of eight years. By 2020 the number is expected to climb to 43.3 million. Alzheimer's and similar debilitating conditions have become the topics of provocative and sometimes popular films.

Two movies, *Iris* (based on the memoir about British writer and philosopher Iris Murdoch by her husband, John Bayley) and *Away from Her* (adapted from the Alice Munro story "The Bear Came Over the Mountain"), depict the progression of Alzheimer's disease and the consequences for the victims and their husbands. Until her death, Iris (played by Judi Dench) was cared for at home by her husband (Jim Broadbent). When Fiona (Julie Christie), in *Away from Her*, realizes she is forgetting things and wandering off, she asks to go into a nursing home. We watch as her husband Grant (Gordon Pinsent) comes to terms with the multiple losses: "He could not demand of her whether she did or did not remember him as her husband of nearly fifty years."[10]

Movies have treated more controversial end-of-life issues. *The Sea Inside* movingly captures the situation of a terminally ill patient who chooses to die. It chronicles the real-life story of Spaniard Ramón Sampedro, who fought to be allowed to die with dignity after twenty-seven years living as a quadriplegic due to a diving accident. While his father says that his son's condition is God's will, Sampedro (Javier Bardem) asserts that living is a right, not an obligation. Sampedro's petitions to the Spanish courts to commit suicide legally are denied. Despite its illegality, he convinces Rosa (Lola Dueñas), with whom he has made friends, to help him die.[11]

While *The Sea Inside* shows us the fight for the right to die by aid in dying, *Igby Goes Down* and *Million Dollar Baby* actually depict the act. *Igby Goes Down*—a dark comedy critiquing the teenaged protagonist's privileged world—opens and closes with a scene in which Igby (Kieran Culkin) and his older brother, Oliver (Ryan Phillippe), put their heavily sedated mother (Susan Sarandon) out of her misery by feeding her a mixture of pills and sauce, then putting a plastic bag over her head. While their relationship has not been a good one, the sons' action is done in neither rancor nor vengeance, but with her consent. To the viewer this presentation of assisted suicide is new and shocking.[12]

In *Million Dollar Baby* (2004) the young working-class boxer (Hilary Swank) becomes paralyzed as the result of a fall in a fight. Maggie asks her trainer, Frank Dunn (Clint Eastwood), for help to die. After speaking to his priest about his dilemma, Frank refuses, so Maggie attempts suicide by biting her tongue multiple times in an attempt to bleed to death. The hospital staff prevents her further attempts. After much internal struggle, Dunn decides that Maggie's suffering should not continue, and he injects her with an overdose of adrenaline.[13]

And in what is said to be "the first broadcast on British television of the moment of death in a voluntary euthanasia case," on December 10, 2008, the video *Right to Die?* was shown. It follows fifty-nine-year-old Craig Ewert, almost completely incapacitated with a motor neuron disease, to Dignitas, a clinic in Zurich, where he took a fatal dose of barbiturates. Ewert's wife described his deliberations: "Craig talks at length about all of this, he talks about his situation being one where his choice is between death and between suffering and death, and so, given those two choices, if he were to make a decision, he had to make a decision on which of those it would be for him." She supported him in his decision to *publicly* take his life: "For Craig . . .

allowing the cameras to film his last moments . . . was about facing the end honestly. . . . He was keen to have it shown because when death is hidden and private, people don't face their fears about it."[14]

Television took on the subject of death with the darkly comic, popular HBO show *Six Feet Under*. Running for five seasons from 2001 to 2005, the show was set in a funeral parlor in Los Angeles. While death was the context, the real focus of the show was the relationships among the family members who ran this undertaking business. Jessica Mitford's 1963 exposé of the American funeral industry, *The American Way of Death*, is the progenitor of *Six Feet Under*. And before Mitford's book, in 1948 Evelyn Waugh's novel *The Loved One* bitingly exposed the L.A. funeral industry.[15]

Dealing with death has become a central theme in recent memoirs. In 2005 Joan Didion described the unexpected and instantaneous death of her husband of forty years, novelist John Gregory Dunne, due to a massive heart attack suffered at the dining room table. He died five days after their only child had lapsed into septic shock and a coma from which she would not awake for a month. In *The Year of Magical Thinking*, later turned into a play starring Vanessa Redgrave, Didion describes her first year of widowhood. In thinking about the message to her husband several years before about the dangerous condition of his arteries, she says, "As I recall this I realize how open we are to the persistent message that we can avert death. And to its punitive correlative, the message that if death catches us we have only our-selves to blame."[16]

Fiction writer and critic Susan Sontag's slow, painful death from cancer is told in words by her son, David Rieff, and in photographs by her partner, Annie Liebovitz.[17] In *Swimming in a Sea of Death* (2008), Rieff angrily and sadly describes his mother's "positive denial" that she was going to die: "She was no more reconciled to extinction at 71 than she had been at 42 [when she was diagnosed with stage 4 breast cancer]." Liebovitz includes many pictures of Sontag in her retrospective, *Annie Liebovitz: A Photographer's Life, 1990–2005* (2006). Included are earlier photographs, but also a memento mori image of the writer's body on a table in a funeral home and images of her as she was a patient at the Fred Hutchinson Cancer Research Center in Seattle, obviously dying. Unsettling in their intimacy, the photographs nevertheless make death and dying brutally real.

If Liebovitz's photographs reveal an attempt to capture a moment, Didion's and Rieff's complex memoirs suggest the ways in which we try to both avoid and control death, the limits of these attempts, and the pain of loss and guilt for those who remain behind.

This question of control lies behind many, though not all, of the headline-grabbing controversies, legal disputes, best-selling books, and powerful, if rare, media treatments of death and dying. This isn't surprising. In *Last Rights: Rescuing the End of Life from the Medical System,* Stephen P. Kiernan (see his chapter in Part Two) reminds us that "[w]hen dying is a process, the manner and meaning of a person's final days are not left to chance. There are options and opportunities; there are choices."[18]

Writers throughout this collection stress the importance of last options, including the "occasional need for an assisted death," an option now available legally in the United States only in Oregon and Washington. Quoting Dr. Timothy Quill of the University of Rochester School of Medicine, *New York Times* columnist Jane E. Brody writes that "knowing last-resort options are available 'is very important to those who fear being trapped in a life filled with suffering without the prospect of a timely escape.'"[19] This holds whether people choose to exercise this option or not.

Does a measure of autonomy contribute to a good death? The term itself can be problematic since everyone may not have the same criteria for what is "good." Our definitions are shaped by our culture, our religion or lack of religion, and our value system, among many other factors. Jane Brody says that coming to an acceptance of one's death is often defined as necessary for a good death (certainly by those in the hospice movement). But this may not always be true. She adds that those who never achieve acceptance, remaining in denial and/or fighting to the end by "leaving no therapeutic stone unturned," can also have a good death.[20]

Robin Marantz Henig, in the *New York Times* article "Will We Ever Arrive at the Good Death?" warns that "we're addicted to the belief that we can micromanage death. We tend to think of a 'good death' as one that we can control, making decisions about how much intervention we want, how much pain relief, whether it's in the home or the hospital, whom will be by our sides. We even sometimes try to make decisions about what we will die from." This effort is unrealistic, she adds, since "dying is awfully hard to choreograph."[21]

The essays in *Final Acts: Death, Dying and the Choices We Make* aren't about choreographing death, but about learning how to dance with it as a full partner, with dignity, without letting it lead your every move.

Sherwin B. Nuland, writing in *How We Die*, says that there isn't really such a thing as a good death, but there are right and wrong deaths, over which we should have some control.[22] Death with dignity is thus about understanding the dying process and lethal illness and not having unrealistic expectations. "It is also the recognition that the *real* event taking place at the end of our life is our death, not the attempts to prevent it."[23]

NOTES

1. The United States ranks second among nations of the world in the number of people eighty and over. (China ranks first.) Although the United States contains less than 5 percent of the world's population, it has 13 percent of its people eighty and over (http://www.census.gov/Press-Release/www/2002/cb02cn173.html). A good source on aging is the monthly electronic newsletter edited by H. R. Moody, *Teaching Gerontology* (AARP Office of Academic Affairs), available at http://www.aarp.org/research/academic/teaching_gerontology.html.

2. Dr. Atul Gawande, "The Way We Age Now," *The New Yorker*, April 30, 2007, 50–59.

3. The most recent editions are: Derek Humphry, *Jean's Way* (Junction City, OR: Norris Lane Press, 2003) and *Final Exit: The Practicalities of Self-Deliverance and Assisted Suicide for the Dying*, 3rd ed. (New York: Dell, 2003). In a 2005 letter available at www.assistedsuicide.org/farewell-to-hemlock.html, Humphry explains how the organization's name changed. It has merged into Compassion and Choices (www.compassionandchoices.org).

4. See Caryn James's review of the *60 Minutes* episode, "'60 Minutes,' Kevorkian and a Death for the Cameras," *New York Times*, November 23, 1998.

5. An Italian case similar to Schiavo's is that of Eluana Englaro, age 38, who had been in a persistent vegetative state since a 1992 car accident. Opposed by the Catholic Church, her father repeatedly fought in court for the right to remove her feeding tube. A private clinic finally agreed to remove the tube, after public clinics refused. Prime Minister Silvio Berlusconi then introduced an emergency measure forbidding the removal, but President Giorgi Napolitan refused to sign it, so it was drafted into a bill for Senate consideration. Ms. Englaro died during the emergency session of the Senate. "Death Ends Coma Case That Set Off Furor in Italy," *New York Times*, February 10, 2009.

6. Mitch Albom, *Sundays with Morrie: An Old Man, a Young Man, and Life's Greatest Lesson* (New York: Doubleday, 1997).

7. See Pausch's Web site, http://download.srv.cs.cmu.edu/~pausch/, to download "Last Lecture" and for further information on him. Randy Pausch with Jeffrey Zaslow, *The Last Lecture* (New York: Hyperion, 2008).

8. Eugene O'Kelly (with Andrew Postman), *Chasing Daylight: How My Forthcoming Death Transformed My Life* (New York: McGraw-Hill, 2006), 134.

9. For information on Leroy Sievers, see National Public Radio's Web site: http://www.npr.org/templates/story/story.php?storyId=5503400.

10. *Iris*, directed by Richard Eyre (Miramax Films, 2001), was based on John Bayley's *Elegy for Iris* (New York: Picador, 1999). *Away from Her*, directed by Sarah Polley (Lions Gate Films, 2007), was adapted from Alice Munro's short story "The Bear Came Over the Mountain," in her *Hateship, Friendship, Courtship, Marriage* (New York: Vintage, 2002).

11. *The Sea Inside*, directed by Alejandro Amenábar (Fine Line Features, 2004). The director was influenced by Sampedro's best-selling collection, *Cartas desde el infierno* (*Letters from Hell*) (Barcelona: Planeta, 2005). See also the documentary *Exit: The Right to Die*, directed by Fernand Melgar (First Run/Icarus Films, 2006). Another award-winning film, *The Diving Bell and the Butterfly*, directed by Julian Schnabel (Miramax Films, 2007), based on Jean-Dominique Bauby's memoir, depicts a debilitating condition known as locked-in syndrome, which the writer had after suffering a massive stroke at the age of forty-three. Totally paralyzed, Bauby could communicate only by blinking his left eyelid. When his speech therapist and later his friends would read him an alphabet, Bauby (Mathieu Amalric) would blink at the letter he wanted; over the course of two months, he completed a memoir, only to die of pneumonia ten days after its publication. While his first words, when he learned to communicate, were "I want to die," Bauby, in contrast to Sampedro in *The Sea Inside*, never pursued that impulse. Instead, he put all his energy into writing his memoir. He was not locked in for as long as Sampedro, who lived for twenty-seven years in his paralyzed state. In an interview in the *Guardian* (as quoted in *Salon*, as well as in an interview on *Charlie Rose*), Schnabel says that he was terrified of death his whole life. "I made this movie, and I'm not scared to die," he says. (From Beth Arnold, "The Truth about 'The Diving Bell and the Butterfly,'" http://www.salon.com/ent/feature/2008/02/23/diving_bell/print.html, and an interview on the DVD).

12. *Igby Goes Down*, directed by Burr Steers (United Artists, 2002).

13. Narrated by Morgan Freeman, playing a long-time employee of the gym, *Million Dollar Baby* (Lakeshore Entertainment and Warner Bros. Pictures, 2004) was directed by Clint Eastwood; the screenplay is by Paul Haggis. Some disability rights activists protested the ending, in which Frank carries out Maggie's wish to die after she becomes a quadriplegic as a result of a spinal cord injury. Disability rights activists believed that the ending supported the euthanasia of disabled people. For a discussion see, for example, Mary Johnson, "'Million Dollar Baby' Cheap Shot at Disabled," February 24, 2005, http://seattlepi.nwsource.com/opinion/213287_disability24.html; and "Million Dollar Baby Built on Prejudice about People with Disabilities,' February 2005, http://www.dredf.org/archives/mdb.shtml.

14. See http://news.sky.com/skynews/Home/UK-News/Sky-Real-Lives-Shows-Craig-Ewert-Suicide-Death-On-Day-Daniel-James-Assisted-Suicide-Inquest-Opens/Article/20081221517602I and Sarah Lyall, "TV Broadcast of an Assisted Suicide Intensifies a Contentious Debate in Britain," *New York Times*, December 11, 2008.

15. Just before her death in 1996, Mitford revised and updated her best-selling study with *The American Way of Death Revisited*, looking at new trends, such as inflated cremation costs, pay-in-advance funerals, and the domination of the death-care industry by multinational corporations. The film *The Loved One* was directed Tony Richardson and written by Terry Southern and Christopher Isherwood.

16. Joan Didion, *The Year of Magical Thinking* (New York: Knopf, 2005), 206.

17. David Rieff writes about his mother, Susan Sontag, in "Illness as More Than Metaphor," *New York Times*, December 4, 2005, and *Swimming in a Sea of Death: A Son's Memoir* (New York: Simon & Schuster, 2008). Liebovitz includes photographs of the ill and dying Sontag in *Annie Liebovitz: A Photographer's Life* (New York: Random House, 2006).

18. Stephen P. Kiernan, *Last Rights: Rescuing the End of Life from the Medical System* (New York: St Martin's Griffin, 2006), 13.

19. Jane Brody, "A Heartfelt Appeal for a Graceful Exit," *New York Times,* February 5, 2008. She quotes Quill from the May 2004 issue of *New England Journal of Medicine*.

20. Jane Brody, "World Enough and Time for 'a Good Death,'" *New York Times*, October 31, 2006.

21. Robin Marantz Henig, "Will We Ever Arrive at the Good Death?" *New York Times*, August 7, 2005.

22. In *How We Die: Reflections on Life's Final Chapter* (New York: Vintage Books, 1995), Nuland traces the concept of the good death and then the beautiful death, saying that the good death has always been for the most part a myth, but "never nearly as much as today" (XVI). Nuland explains that "too often, patients and their families cherish expectations that cannot be met," causing the death process to be frustrating and disappointing (142). "For each of us," he writes, "there may be a death that is the right death, and we should strive to find it, while accepting that it may prove ultimately to be beyond our grasp" (264).

23. Ibid., 258.

PART ONE

Personal Stories

Part One contains personal stories about death and dying. Individuals with terminal illnesses write in strikingly different voices about their uneasy standoff with death. Daughters (and a daughter-in-law), sons, and nieces write about their struggles as caretakers of and/or witnesses to the death and dying of family members. Their experiences differ—in significant ways—in these accounts of loss and gain, of bad and good deaths, of acts neglected and taken. And, like all stories worth reading, these stories make us think about our own lives and most intimate relationships.[1]

We open this section with two very different, deeply personal accounts of living with terminal illnesses. Diagnosed at forty-two with a rare sarcoma, Ruthann Robson—writing ten years later—is ferocious in her fight against that diagnosis. At ninety-two, June Bingham approaches her impending death from metastasized cancer with equanimity and humor. Yet both women recognize their isolation. Robson writes, "I cannot bridge the distance between my self and everyone else, including the ones I love most," a sentiment Bingham shares.

"I do not want your good death," says Robson. Railing against the understanding of caregivers and theorists from Elisabeth Kübler-Ross on down, she does not want understanding, either.[2] She wants possibility; she wants to live. Writing with dark humor, she imagines taking someone with her, if she has to die. Perhaps she could assassinate someone she considers politically evil; as a lawyer, she considers a Supreme Court justice. Above all, she does not want to be taken in by lady death's seductions; she does not want to go gently into that good night. And she does not.

Bingham's clear-eyed approach to her forthcoming death includes humor and gratitude. She writes about being freed to eat all those foods that are no good for you "and still lose weight," for example. She appreciates the time for "closure," telling friends and family about her situation, even though she often comforts them, rather than being comforted. And she is thankful for hospice's "fine work." Before this book was completed, Bingham died, at home, surrounded by family.

In other essays, caretakers get a crash course in slow dying. Nancy Barnes and Susan Perlstein write honestly and movingly about the challenges they faced when their strong-willed mothers—at eighty-four and ninety, respectively—began to fail.

Barnes is up-front about her resentment at having to take on the demanding role of caretaker to her mother. She is frustrated about the conversations they never had in light of her mother's growing frailty and refusal to acknowledge it: "We never talked about how she would cope if she had disabilities as she grew older; we never talked about nursing homes or paid companions; we never talked about death, or any arrangements she might have wanted." Barnes adds, "We certainly never talked about the possibility of her suicide," although earlier her mother had signed a living will, in which she expressed her unwillingness to be kept alive in a number of circumstances. Because that living will was never mentioned by mother or daughter, Barnes was surprised when she found a copy of one of Derek Humphry's books by the bedside after her mother's death.[3]

Barnes admits wishing for her mother's end "in the face of her anguish, and the anguish she caused me." Susan Perlstein also feels frustrated by her mother's desire to seek every consultation and care possible, including the decision to go to the hospital's emergency room despite previous agreements with her doctor and hospice worker not to do so. Once a decision was made, for example, to move to assisted living, Perlstein's mother "seemed to forget the long process of choice and announced to all that I had forced her to move." Yet the daughter respects her mother's autonomy: "For my mother and me, this meant that, as long as she had her mental wits about her, I would respect her decisions and help to negotiate her choices with the health-care system—doctors, nurses, social workers, hospitals, hospice, and home health-care workers."

Both daughters, writing in appreciation of their mothers, share lessons learned. Barnes says she learned truths that speak to the themes of this book: "that whatever happens at the time of my death may well involve others I love as deeply as it does me, and that the possibilities of choice about one's own death can silently and swiftly slip away. . . . I . . . have loosened my grip on the certainties of choice." As a social worker, with extensive experience working with the elderly, Perlstein admits that she was still unprepared for her mother's decline. She concludes her essay by acknowledging "great comfort and pride that I was able to help create a way for my mother to live until the end of her life as she wished. In return, she gave me insight into human willpower as I witnessed her indomitable spirit and eternal passion for life."

Sara Evans chronicled the last three years of her parents' lives in a series of e-mails to family and friends. These accounts of days the couple spent together and with friends and family, days relatively free from pain, suggest that Claude and Maxilla's deaths were as close to "good deaths" as any in this collection. Their daughter's narrative suggests some reasons why.

Besides a strong and sustaining religious faith, the certainty that they had lived long and fruitful lives, the love of family and friends, and excellent medical care, Claude and Maxilla felt—and were—in control of their own lives, as much as possible.

In both cases, they chose to stop treatment. With Claude's eventual dementia, the family came to believe that, as Evans explains, "it is time to let him go, to stop whatever medications he is on that have the purpose of prolonging life, and to pay attention to his comfort on every level." Maxilla refused drugs for her cancer and invasive treatment for her heart because she did not want a prolonged decline. Their daughter's e-mails trace their twisting paths to death, bittersweet, with grief and losses as well as moments of enjoyment and intense communication.

Jean Levitan tells the story of the deaths of her aunt and uncle: "two people, from different sides of the family, who each ended their lives when they chose to. Perhaps it is more accurate to say: they ended their lives when they couldn't stand to live any longer with their illness and pain." Her aunt's death was a violent one; her uncle, age eighty-seven, unable to get pills, stopped eating. He made sure his wife did not call 911 and left her with notarized paperwork so that no charges would be levied against her.

These deaths lead Levitan to explore the meaning of death with dignity for herself, but more immediately for her father, ill and diagnosed with dementia. She wonders how much of her own—and her family's—experiences to share with the university students she teaches in classes on death and dying. Yet into the somber dialogue that *Final Acts* weaves, Levitan offers humor. After reading the book *Exit Strategy: Thinking Outside the Box* by Michelle Cromer, she says that of all the options for one's cremains—aka ashes—"I think I'd like to become a diamond."[4]

At age seventy-six, with a terminal cancer diagnosis, Carol Oyster's father also decided to stop eating and drinking, against the wishes of most family members. This was a very deliberate decision: "After his death, we found that around this time Dad had created a stack of folders for Mom to examine after his death. They included, in the order they should be handled, all the information about his cremation, interment, insurance, and annuities—complete with contact names and phone numbers. He also purged all of his work-related files and his closet. He had come to terms with his death and done everything he could to make it easier for the family after he was gone. And perhaps these were some of his final opportunities to exert control."

A social psychologist by training, Oyster traces how the various family members reacted to her father's dying (by experiencing, at various times, the "stages" outlined by Kübler-Ross, for example) and how she, personally, came to accept his "courageous, difficult" choice. She reveals how her father's death has led her to rethink her own and "to believe in the cliché that exhorts us to live every day as if it were our last."

Alan Pope and Mary Jumbelic process their mothers' deaths through the prisms of their own experiences and beliefs. Fascinated by death since he was a child, Pope suffered a debilitating illness that drove him inward and led him, ultimately, to the spiritual path of Tibetan Buddhism. In his revealing essay he charts his movement from judgment to acceptance of his mother's final acts and choices and offers an intriguing interpretation of her decision to discontinue dialysis treatments, an act, he says, of "passive suicide." Through Tolstoy's nineteenth-century novel *The Death of Ivan Ilyich*, and Tibetan Buddhist teachings, he eventually understands her passing and his "own inevitable death."

As a medical examiner, Mary Jumbelic is on intimate terms with death, whom she calls her "colleague." She knows death's physicality: "The majority of my professional life has been consumed with trying to explain death—the etiology of the injuries and diseases responsible for that physical moment when the heart stops beating. I live with death in the background of my day, watching me as I try to replay in my mind the last few moments of a person's life. . . . I am the deceased's advocate and their final voice. Their damaged organs, skin wounds, stomach contents, and drug tests all speak to me and provide me salient details of their last few hours. I am the modern sleuth of forensic medicine."

But when her mother becomes terminally ill, Jumbelic's balance of empathy and distance is challenged: physician and daughter, she experiences personally what she knew only professionally. What had struck Jumbelic the forensic pathologist about the dying process of the chronically ill was that there often emerges a recurring story (from the next of kin) "of physical and emotional alienation at the time of the patient's last breath. This isolation is universally experienced by each of the patient's loved ones and, saddest of all, by the patient, especially when there are emergency medical lifesaving measures administered."

As a consequence, Jumbelic recommends that we embrace the natural process of death, hoping that "when we can approach the acceptance of disease with a realistic consideration of our alternatives, we may be able to choose our end in a way that is more dignified and peaceful than many of the deaths I have evaluated."

Watching her mother die, however, Jumbelic is aware that this embrace of the natural process is not easy. She asks herself, "What if death had been unkind, slower and more cruel in its approach with my mother? Would we have done anything differently?" In this case, the family had been able to adhere to her mother's wishes for no interventional therapy, no hospitalization, no treatment, and no invasive tube. What if the situation had been otherwise?

Like Jumbelic, Mimi Schwartz wonders about alternatives. What if her optimistic eighty-four-year-old father-in-law hadn't chosen aggressive, debilitating treatment for his advanced stomach cancer—treatment that, in the end, led him to whisper, "If I had known I'd end in here, like this, I would have put a gun to my head." Instead of the confirming enthusiasm of nurses and doctors who suggested that he might beat his disease, a dose of realism would have better served him,

Schwartz suggests. Then, instead of debilitating artificial feeding, chemotherapy, radiation, blood transfusions, and the eventual nursing home, her father-in-law might have chosen to die at home with hospice care.

The essays in this section reveal the paths the terminally ill and their caretakers or loved ones follow: often parallel or crossing, but inevitably divergent. Historian Gerda Lerner describes this dual journey beautifully in *A Death of One's Own*. During the almost yearlong dying process of her husband of thirty-three years, Lerner imagines the oncoming role of widow. She describes their separate paths: "We battled on separate battlefields, each very much alone. Mine to prepare myself for his death, to help him die a good death. His: to live."[5]

NOTES

1. See Sandra M. Gilbert, *Death's Door: Modern Dying and the Ways We Grieve* (New York: W. W. Norton, 2006). Writing about her husband's sudden death, Gilbert looks at dying and grieving through the lenses of autobiographical narrative, cultural studies, and literary history.

2. Elisabeth Kübler-Ross, *On Death and Dying* (New York: Macmillan, 1969).

3. Derek Humphry, *Let Me Die Before I Wake: Hemlock's Book of Self-Deliverance for the Dying* (New York: Grove Press, 1986).

4. Michelle Cromer, *Exit Strategy: Thinking Outside the Box* (New York: Jeremy P. Tarcher/Penguin, 2006).

5. Gerda Lerner, *A Death of One's Own* (Madison: University of Wisconsin Press, 1985), 49.

Notes on My Dying

RUTHANN ROBSON

I believe in death with dignity, don't you? At least in the abstract.

Grace. Nobility. Even beauty.

As abstract as that.

As abstract as other people.

As abstract as characters in fiction.

"All anyone wants is a good death," I read. This is in a short story. It's a prize-winning story, a story about a nurse who is dying of cancer. She is graceful, noble, and even beautiful.

I hate the story. I hate stories about people dying of cancer, no matter how graceful, noble, or beautiful.

When I read the author's note, I learn that he is an administrator in the famous cancer center where I am enduring chemotherapy and the news that I am going to die very shortly.

This is what I say to his story: I do not want your good death.

This is what I say to his biography: You make your living off other people's deaths.

This is what I insist: I am not your story.

If I were constructing this as a story, with myself as the protagonist, I would not only be dignified, I would be brave and beautiful, courageous and kind, humorous and honorable.

I would enshrine myself in narrative.

But this cannot be a success because the elements of narrative are corrupted.

There is no beginning. The beginning is not diagnosis. The beginning is before that. Before the suspicions, before the reconstructed past when one began to feel this or that, before everything except a tiny cell that got twisted and frisky. The absence of the beginning is compounded by the middle collapsing into the past.

Everything is end.

Some endings are longer than others.

I am trying to act as if I have a future. When I'm not too weak, I go to work. I go to the library and the post office. I go for walks. And when I am too weak, I go anyway. The worst that could happen to me is already happening.

I cannot pretend I am who I was a few months before, so I pretend I am a fashion model. I am a Buddhist nun with a shaved head. I am anorexic. I have a lovely pallor. I have a noble beauty, a beautiful nobility.

I am not interested in fooling anyone except myself.

I call it survival.

I survived a dangerous adolescence.

In school, the sentiments of "Death Be Not Proud" belied its title. On the large and small screens, *Love Story* jerked tears, and the body bags and the immolated monks screamed for my attention. In the streets and bathrooms, needles in the arm and suicide sang their romantic dirges.

Not all of us made it.

When I made it to twenty-one, I assumed I would live until eighty-seven.

Death was for the young. And the old.

At twenty-six, I was hospitalized intermittently for six weeks with a strange malady that spiked my temperature to 107 degrees.

"You should be dead," the doctor said, confirming my temperature.

"I'm not," I replied, thinking myself witty.

The year was 1984.

I was sure I had AIDS.

Instead, I was diagnosed with pesticide poisoning, contracted from the sugarcane fields where the migrant farm workers who were my clients worked.

A nurse told me I should be grateful for the advancement of antibiotics.

No one told me I should be irate about the development of agribusiness.

I knew I had almost died.

I thought I was cured.

There are those who argue that cancer is ancient, prevalent now because other diseases have been cured and humans live longer, and unconnected to environmental degradation.

My body knows differently.

But who is there to blame? Industrialization? Capitalism? Corporate greed?

Anger is the second stage of dying in the classic work of Elisabeth Kübler-Ross. She notes that dying can cause a "usually dignified" person to act "furious," but with a bit of tolerance by the caregivers, the patient's anger can be soothed. Dying people, above all, want to be heard.

I do not want to be heard.

I do not want to talk.

I want to live.

My first decision about dying is that I will die at home. I will have the control and comfort I would not have in a hospital. The winter sun will be weak but brilliant, sifting through my window, refracting through a prism I have had since I was young. Then the light will fade, leaving only a slat of brilliant pink. Twilight was once my favorite time of day.

My second decision about dying is that I won't. Like all my most outrageous ambitions, it first appears on my horizon as a question: "what if?" What if I refused to die? I am neither stupid nor naive and know that it isn't a simple matter of choice. Nevertheless, my aspiration persists.

The first stage of dying is denial.

Ask anyone who has read Elisabeth Kübler-Ross.

Or who has not.

Still, what if I refused to cooperate?

The manifestations of my resistance are illogical and small. I refuse Ensure, Ativan, a port, a wig. I refuse to talk to my oncologist, who warns me about depression. Depression, the fourth stage of dying, is the "preparatory grief that the terminally ill patient has to undergo in order to prepare himself for his final separation from this world."

If I were talking to her, I would tell her I am not depressed, although I may seem defeated, decimated.

I am simply deep.

I am inside myself so deeply the world is an abstraction. I cannot bridge the distance between my self and everyone else, including the ones I love most. The ones I said I loved more than life itself. Now, this is no longer true.

My death is only my own. No matter the connection, no matter the love. No matter that I came from the bodies of my parents or that my child came from my body or that my lover and I have joined as if we inhabit one body without boundaries. Each body lives separately. And dies separately. Perhaps I knew this before. In the abstract.

I think about taking someone with me.

If I'm going to die anyway, shouldn't I kill someone? Shouldn't my death be useful? I scan my personal life but find no one evil enough to deserve to die. My passions are faded. I concentrate on the person I once hated most, but cannot seem to despise him enough to deprive him of his narrow miserable life.

Assassination is a possibility. I imagine buying a semi-automatic weapon. I have enough time for the license waiting period, to learn how to shoot, to do the legwork necessary to find a gap in the security. I think it would be relatively easy, since I'm not worried about getting caught. I would prefer not to die in prison, so I guess I'd kill myself as soon as my deed is done. I settle on a certain Supreme Court justice. But I find I don't care enough to kill him. Or even to think about it more than once.

Dying is lonely.

I am popular in my dying: People I have not heard from in several years call me.

"Is there anything you want to say to me?" she asks. She is crying.

"My mother died of cancer," he says to me. He must think this is an expression of empathy.

"You have always meant so much to me," she blurts. She does not stumble over the past tense.

I never respond.

They must think I am being dignified.

Someone actually tells me this: "I really admire the way you are conducting yourself with such dignity," she says to me.

"I'm not."

"Well, it seems like that to us," she persists. She is a colleague and has always been comfortable speaking for everyone at work.

"That's not the way it seems to me." I prove I can still argue.

She smiles as if she thinks I am being modest.

I am not.

I am trying to be honest: I am all claws and sobs and vomit. I am small and getting smaller. I am bereft and bald. I am more tired than tired.

How could she not see that when she looks at me?

But she does see that. Despite the dignity, when she looks at me she sees I am dying.

And when I look at her, I see my dying reflected back to me, a shiny silvery object without form or function, an abyss of pity.

I am grateful for the people who do not pity me. Or at least who do not show their pity.

We have written letters for almost twenty years. When I write to tell her the news that I am dying, I ask her to try to write to me as she always has, to write to me about her life and what she is reading. She writes me every day. Every single fucking day. Beautiful exquisitely boring letters about her job or what she ate for breakfast or something she hopes will be amusing. I live for her letters.

We have written letters for eight years. I fudge the fact that I am dying, but also ask her to keep writing to me as she always has. Her letters get longer. Pages and pages that require extra postage, pages filled with assessments of novels, pages brimming with struggles about her own writing, pages of poetry. I reread every page until I believe that I am strong enough to write back.

We have never written letters. She sends me a card. "Here's a second opinion: You're the greatest." It's in a package of gourmet food that once would have been appetizing.

We have lived together for more years than I can count. She was once my lover, now she is my caretaker. She tries not to cry in my presence. I am not so considerate.

She brings me books from the library when I can't get there myself. "Novels," I tell her, "from the new fiction section." Sometimes she brings me the same book twice. Three times. Sometimes I recognize when this has happened.

Maybe I believe I can save myself through reading. Or at least escape. Or maybe it is that I have always read. Books were my first acquaintance with grace.

Although soon I stop reading fiction. I know she is screening the selections, but death penetrates the pages. Sometimes it is in the prize-winning story. Sometimes it is there casually and without warning. It seems there is always a convenient cancer death in the background somewhere, even if only in a character's memory.

In novels, they never recover.

Loss. Grieving. But life goes on.

I close the book and reach for the next one.

Soon, I am requesting biographies. As if I have forgotten that the person in the biography is going to die. As if I didn't know somehow that Rachel Carson died, at fifty-seven, of cancer. She hid it from the world, as if her dying was a recrimination of her work linking the toxins with tumors in humans, an irrefutable rebuke that she was less than objective. Or perhaps she was trying to be dignified.

Desperation is not dignified.

Perhaps that is why Kübler-Ross does not name desperation as a stage. There is "bargaining," the third stage, but she gives it short shrift. She theorizes it as a belief in a reward for good behavior. She doesn't seem to understand the will to live.

It allows the decision to be strapped into a chair and poison injected into my veins to seem rational.

It propels me into the alleys of alternative healing, alternative theories, alternative alternatives. I visualize and vitaminize. I spread myself on the floor of an apartment in Chinatown so that a man can bruise my flesh as a way of clearing my meridians. I ingest herbs from different continents, animal parts pressed into pill form, teas that smell like mentholated piss.

I meditate.

There are those who argue that cancer is a message: "Appreciate the beauty of each moment."

The moments most often invoked are populated with children. What could be more precious than the kiss of a toddler?

Other moments to be cherished occur in nature: oceans, sunsets, trees and their turning leaves.

Even a circumscribed life has its moments to be appreciated. The soft sheets of the bed, the taste of a strawberry, the flames in the fireplace.

Never mentioned are the moments in which I am managing to live. The moments, long and slow, during which I am dizzy and puking red on the bathroom floor, trying to appreciate the texture and temperature of the tile against my cheek. (How smooth! How cool!) The moments, as panic-filled as a fire, when I can feel the chemical burn in my veins and watch the skin on my arm lose all its color. The moments, shallow and distant, when I try to think about anything other than what is happening to me.

Acceptance is the fifth and final stage of dying, according to Kübler-Ross. She warns that the harder the struggle to avoid the inevitable death and the more denial, the more difficult it will be to reach acceptance with peace and dignity. In her examples, the patient wants to die, but the medical professionals believe it is better to prolong life.

This is not my experience.

My medical professionals are very accepting of my death. They proclaim it inevitable and do not deny or struggle. They do not seem to believe it is better to prolong my life. They are very noble.

Perhaps they read Kübler-Ross in medical school.

Or perhaps they're simply burnt out.

Or they know the grim statistics for my rare cancer and see no reason why I should be in the smallest of minorities who might survive.

I loot the world for survival stories. Not the narratives of Himalayan treks or being lost at sea, but illness. The bookstore has an entire section on diseases and five shelves on cancer. I inspect every title, except the "prevention" ones, looking for possibilities. I buy a book by a Christian fundamentalist woman who attributes her survival to prayer and coffee enemas. I buy a book by a scientist who attributes his survival to vitamins. I buy books on healing by popular writers who intersperse their homilies with anecdotes of people given "six months to live" but who are alive ten years later.

Possibilities.

I do not want nobility or beauty.

I do not want a good death.

I want possibility.

I am in my office, looking at the diplomas on my wall and sobbing over all that accomplishment, now utterly worthless. The skills I had mastered are the wrong skills for my situation. I know no medicine; my last biology class was in the ninth grade. I can't even cope: my degrees are not in psychology or divinity. I learned how to think, how to read, how to argue.

My faith—in hard work, in intellectual pursuits, in books—has been misplaced. Nothing I know could save me. I want to rip my diplomas from the wall.

With dignity.

But I don't have the strength to carry a single book down the hall to the classroom. I can't stand up more than three and a half minutes. I no longer have the ability to assassinate that Supreme Court justice or to recall which one I had singled out as especially dastardly.

Still, I refuse to accept I am dying. I prefer denial, anger, and even desperation.

When I can sit up, I spend hours at the computer, leaving no Web site unturned. I become an expert in my rare type of cancer. A medical dictionary replaces my thesaurus.

I read books, articles, pamphlets. I have begun to eschew fiction. I want true stories of survival. I relish attacks on statistics and science. I avoid all eulogies, all obituaries. I do not update my will or think about the existence of my property without me. I don't care what happens to those hundreds of letters, the ones I have written or the ones I have read. I don't worry about my office and its diplomas. I am not interested in any legacy.

I try to think. To argue.

There are those who argue that cancer is an infectious disease, like
tuberculosis, because a gene-based disease would have been
eliminated through natural selection. Cancer could be cured by
the correct antibiotic.

I would like this to be true.

Now.

I had thought I had looked at death before. I had seen her dance with
the ones I loved who have died. I had suffered my own flirtations.
This time, though, death is gazing back. Not just a glance, but a
full seductive stare. As if we are in a bar and I am dressed in black
leather, ready for adventure tinged with danger.

How alluring to be chosen.

This is what she whispers: I can follow her with grace and dignity. Or
I can resist and it can get ugly. Either way, she will win, she promises me.

That is her story.

If she writes my story, I will be brave, beautiful, and dignified. The
word *struggle* will be used, but with no incidents of sweating or
cursing or thrashing. In her story, it will be as if I have fallen into
a deep sleep.

As long as I am still able to write, this is my story: I resist the lure of
dignity; I refuse to be graceful, beautiful, and beloved. I am not
going to sleep with her. I'm going home, alone.

Back to my books, my computer, my Australian herb and shark car-
tilage, my visualizations, meditations, and bruised meridians.
Back to my bedroom with the prism at twilight. Back to my office
and its useless diplomas.

Back to my life.

NOTE

For references to and quotations from the classic work of Dr. Kübler-Ross, see
Elisabeth Kübler-Ross, *On Death and Dying* (New York: Macmillan, 1969).

Live Longer or Live Better?

JUNE BINGHAM

When my doctor told me I have metastasized cancer, my first reaction was: "Hey, this isn't as bad as I thought it would be." Why not? Well, one reason is being really old, eighty-eight, as is my husband, ninety-two. Recently we've been forced to take note of the fact that we absolutely have to die of something pretty soon. Another reason is that for me the prospect of being the first to sneak off rather than be the one left behind feels like a major relief. Having once been widowed (after a marriage of forty-six years), I have no desire for a second round (after a further marriage of twenty years). On the other hand, I hate to load this burden on my husband and I hope he'll forgive me.

A third reason is that cancer is a physical ailment, not a mental or emotional one. My greatest fear has concerned the loss of mind, as with my pals with Alzheimer's, or, even worse, the loss of lifelong personality. One warm-hearted, gentle soul I knew ended up biting her nurse the day before the Grim Reaper, mercifully, put an end to her disease's typical tangling of the brain's neurons.

Furthermore, even within the category of physical, a metastasized cancer is, relatively speaking, a quickie, as against, say, the long-term crippling that can result from a bad stroke or ALS (Lou Gehrig's disease) which forces the person to drag along in radical helplessness for years, even decades.

A fourth reason is that I can retain some control over what happens to my deteriorating body, like trying to keep it at home with hospice care, and thus avoid any well-meant but to me unwelcome curative treatment at the hospital.

As I foresee the coming months, there will be two stages. The first is the current one in which I can function in limited fashion. For my husband and me, who lived through those long years of World War II, the emotions are familiar: a poignant treasuring of each day that we can still be together and a determination to put a brave face on whatever is coming next.

The second stage is being bedridden and in pain. Although the oncologist has recommended surgery, radiation, and chemotherapy, I turned down all of them.

Five years ago I had abdominal surgery and took six months to recover. Today I don't want to lose even one month of first-stage living. As for radiation, I still suffer from its aftereffects. As for chemo, its side effects would remove days from my first stage and likely addle my already addled pate. Besides, I would lose the hair that I rely on to camouflage my vanity-secret, namely, the ugliness of my ears.

What I feel especially grateful for is the time that will allow closure with my beloved family members and friends. The process of reporting my ailment to them has been far more tiring than I had expected because I am often forced into the role of comforter rather than comfortee. At the same time, it has also brought times of unprecedented closeness.

I asked my oncologist why a patient like me is forced into the comforter role. He said, "People are scared to death of cancer." (I thought of adding, "People are also scared to death of death.") He and I agreed that many people, especially the young and middle-aged, have avoided coming to terms with their own mortality, and therefore to face the mortal illness of someone they love makes them squirm for themselves. Another doctor warned me that some people's reluctance to face their own mortality may cause them to stop wanting to see me while I undergo this process.

As of now, my descendants and the few friends I have told about my ailment cannot help knowing that I love them, and I, in turn, know that they love me. Yet I also feel grief for their grief, which will last so much longer than mine. I lunched with a woman who cried all through the meal, yet she also used an expression that made us both laugh: "I'm emotionally incontinent," she said.

In trying to comfort her and other recipients of my bad news, I find that humor is a real help. In reporting to my erstwhile Flower Child, I mentioned that because my husband and I are living so much in the present (the present is our "present"), we consider ourselves "now" people—and might plan to start wearing headbands and beads.

Our dog senses that something is awry and follows me from room to room. When I lie down, she burrows her head between my shoulder and my jaw and squeaks gently to the effect that her love is far greater than her ability to express it. My husband and I agree with her in regard to one another.

Some of my pals report that they are putting me on their prayer list. One says that my name is now in **bold type**. I am grateful at many levels for this attention, but I also want to hear from them what the news is in their lives. If it is bad, I can try to suggest ways of getting around it; if it is good, I can genuinely rejoice. One of the ancient saws was "You can forgive your friends anything but their success." But, when you're not far from death, that no longer applies. Having basically stopped being competitive, you can welcome another person's success with wholehearted exultation.

Not infrequently I find myself asked for advice. Sometimes I know what to say; other times I haven't a clue. Even while speaking, I can't judge whether what I am dispensing is wisdom or nonsense. Yet I enjoy being questioned, and afterward may check the substance of my response with my peers. Most times they agree, and when they do not I can still amend my advice for the original questioner.

Several unexpected forms of relief have emerged recently. One is a dieter's paradise: I can eat everything I want and still lose weight. My husband and I have thrown caution to the winds and now buy 2-percent milk instead of the boring 1-percent. We also make club sandwiches with white bread. Nor need I do any more shopping beyond the daily fundamentals. We are also freed from much of the hard work of decision making: most things, like taking a trip or even going into town to the theater, are now simply impossible, so we don't need to concern ourselves with them. I also don't need to choose and order new notepaper.

A further unexpected relief is canceling my annual checkup with the eye doctor and the skin doctor and the ear doctor. Yet I haven't yet reached the point mentioned by my friend who, when asked what she would do if told she had only six months to live, said, "I'd stop flossing." I still go for tooth cleaning because I like the feel of a fresh mouth and I don't want to be caught by a toothache during stage two. As for the uglification that may accompany that stage, my resolve is never to have a mirror near my bed. I yearn to be able to exhibit a bit of style at the end, although I can no longer follow my father's sound advice: "Always leave while the party is good."

The main thing is to convey my blessing as the party goes on and to thank hospice for the fine work they do for the guests who are forced to drop out.

"Life which is ours to know just once"

NANCY BARNES

I will never know whether my mother wished, when the time came, that she had been able to end her own life. Everything I know about this woman—her personality, her biography, and her politics—would have predicted that she would be the one to decide, by herself, as she did most things. But it's not surprising that she never said anything about the possibility. My mother, who relished serious conversation the way other people relish gossip, almost never spoke about her own feelings. All I know is that she had made certain preparations.

It is easy to say that old age and illness overtook my mother. Some of the most devastating losses she suffered were induced by high-dose steroids administered over more than two years. But this is too simple. When a terrible, long illness struck her in her mid-eighties, she fought valiantly not just to survive but also to be independent. I am the person who attempted to take care of her, as she insisted that she was perfectly able to take care of herself. And I am the person who remembers that as a healthy, forceful woman in full command of her faculties, my mother signed a living will that indicated she would not want any of what, in the end, happened.

My mother died of a pulmonary embolism when she was living in a nursing home in Florida. Her death was a long time coming; the time it took cost her, and me, too much suffering. But once she was failing, there was no way in which I could have honored my mother's legally stated desire not to continue beyond a certain point. I've had to accept that. It haunts me, however, that I will never know whether that remained a meaningful wish. What I lived through with her, during years that forever changed me, was her passionate intention to continue her life as she had known it.

Entering my sixties, I feel quite sure that there are conditions in which I myself would no longer want to live. I believe that I could act on that knowledge. I have discussed this with several carefully chosen people and taken what few legal steps we have available to us in this country. They are the same steps my mother took before she became ill. I am acutely aware, however, of two truths that I witnessed emerging as my mother declined. The first is that this decision which seems so solitary may well involve others I love just as deeply as it does me. The second is that this seemingly most deliberate decision may turn out to be quite elusive. These truths weave throughout the story I want to tell, a story of how swiftly and silently the possibilities of choice about one's death can slip away.

The phone rang as I lay reading in bed, a little after eleven, when my mother was often in her deepest sleep of the night. All she said when I picked up the phone was, "I think I may be a person in the early stages of having a stroke." My mother's pattern had always been to fall asleep around ten, waken at three or four in the morning, read for several hours in a long book such as *The Voyage of the Beagle* or *War and Peace*, then doze again. That night, it frightened me just to know that she was awake. When I got to her apartment I found her stretched out flat on the white couch in the living room, unable to sit up, extremely dizzy.

I'm not sure, now, whether I had any warning of what was to come. M (as my mother signed her notes and letters to her children) was eighty-four. She had stopped dyeing her hair so that it was almost completely white, but her face had the same wonderful high color it always had. Visiting with her the summer before she became ill, I scrolled forward into old age a thousand times a day. One afternoon M's friend Loretta called. Loretta was a retired nurse in her seventies who had gone to Spain with the Lincoln Brigade. She lived downstairs in my mother's building. "Is your mother all right?" Loretta asked hesitantly. We were awkward with each other but she managed to say, "It's alarming that your mother charges so aggressively down the street when we go out together." When Loretta cautioned her that a light was about to change, my mother turned on her and snapped, "I am a driver, you know."

This was it—the stage of my mother's life that I had been dreading since my father's death more than twenty years earlier. I had been aware that my mother's frailty was increasing. Old age both softened her character, some-how, and intensified it. M asked me to do certain things for her, which she almost never had. But her need to be in charge was unchanged.

I drove my mother to Vermont for a friend's memorial service that July. On the long trip back we approached the tollbooths as we headed south on the Saw Mill River Parkway. "If you want, I'll tell you a secret," M said. "If you stay to the far left, of course you must have the correct change, but if you stay to the far left and have your money ready, there is almost never anyone else in that lane." I swung left, pricked by the annoyances of a lifetime, wonder-ing if I could stand another half hour of her bossiness until we got home. Pulling away from the tollgate I commented how fortunate it was that youngest children (of which I am one) are often compliant. "Yes," M said with acerbity, "and well rewarded for it, too."

My mother had handled many aspects of her increasing age admirably; independence and a lack of self-pity stood her in good stead. I had done well, too, in my role as the closest child, the unmarried youngest daughter. I had lived in the same city as my mother for most of my life. We also shared our family's house in the country, a lovely plain farmhouse my parents called Freewind because it sat on a high, open hilltop; the breezes were strong even on the hottest days of August. Surrounded by woodlands and fields in north-western Connecticut, Freewind was the heart of our family life although we lived in New York City during the week.

Nearing eighty, my mother sold the house. It was a hard decision, about which she must have been sad. She never said. By the time she talked with us, her grown children, the decision had been made. Some months before the sale, M had asked me to accompany her to her lawyer's office. I had no idea why, but assumed it had to do with Freewind; she deflected the question when I asked. We met at a Wall Street firm on a high floor. The lawyer was a pleasant, reticent fellow who had a weekend home not far from Freewind. The two of them chatted about our respective towns as I waited, admiring his spectacular view of the New York harbor.

Then the lawyer slid some papers across his huge polished desk and showed us each where to sign. "Do you have any questions about what you are signing?" he said to me. I must have looked confused—the papers had nothing to do with Freewind. The lawyer explained that one document gave me M's power of attorney; a second was her living will, in which M expressed her desire not to be kept alive in quite a number of circumstances. I have reflected on those documents a number of times since then, but I have no memory of what I thought as I signed my name that afternoon. Perhaps it seemed obvious that this woman who valued self-control so highly would not want to have her life prolonged. That choice would have been consistent with all the ways I knew her. But it is odd to realize that my mother never said a word, then or later, about the contents of the legal documents—and I never asked.

My mother kept acres of land when she sold the house in Connecticut; I go there whenever I can. The fields at Freewind have comforted me since I was a child. They fall softly away from the brow of the hill, stubbly at the end of the summer, the hay cropped as though by many horses. I'm not even sure how much I like this landscape now. I've filled my eyes with much more spectacular colors, the light in the village in Tunisia where Paul Klee painted, the ocean at Anahola, Kauai, as the sun goes down, and my nose with many more amazing smells. These fields smell of grass and leaves in the weeks before autumn settles into winter. But whether I like them doesn't matter. They hold my childhood; they hold me. I longed for them as I understood that my mother was failing.

At the end of August my mother had a fall in the shower of a motel where she was staying on a weekend excursion. She cracked her face, which left a black eye, and wrenched her back. Home in New York, she did nothing for several weeks. My mother was a person who did not complain. I could tell, though, that the pain in her back was severe. She finally went to an orthopedist who said she had fractured several vertebrae. She mentioned that her head hurt, that she felt terrible fatigue in her neck, her jaw. M, who had always had the sharpest powers of observation, described her ailments in a frustratingly diffuse way. She refused to see any more doctors.

That weird combination of precise observation and disconnection was something I had worried at for years, trying to figure out why this person I knew so well was incapable of saying she felt sick, or was afraid, or needed anything. The morning after the episode of vertigo when M thought she was having a stroke, a doctor at New York University's Tisch Hospital sent us traipsing around the hospital for hours of tests. A week later, we sat in his office again. The doctor spoke only to me even though M sat at my side. "That was no stroke," he said. "Where we are today is that she probably has a disease called polymyalgia rheumatica which I have to tell you has a dire complication, temporal arteritis. Temporal arteritis can cause sudden blindness."

When my father had become ill I had simply refused to admit it. I loved him, with none of the complexity that surrounded my feelings for my mother. I just loved him. Not long after the surgeon told us that his cancer had spread so widely that he just took a look and sewed him up, I made a trip to Freewind. I walked alone, taking refuge in that familiar place. All the leaves were off the trees, revealing the stone walls that border the fields. The next thing I remember I was stretched out on the ground, twenty-two years old, sobbing, my face pressed against the dry grass as though it were a pillow, sobbing and sobbing.

For the longest time I couldn't say the words "my father died," or before that, "my father has cancer." The loss was unspeakable. But I wasn't responsible then; my mother cared for him, by herself and with great tenderness. His illness was short and I was barely adult. It never occurred to me to wonder whether he thought about ending his life.

I'm not sure that my mother was intimate, as I understand intimacy, with anyone except my father. Her isolation once she was sick did not surprise me. She was an intensely private person despite her big family, which included eight grandchildren, who were themselves having children, and a wide net of devoted friends and other relatives. Shortly after M's diagnosis I went over to drop off some groceries and cash. She instructed me to "leave the money on the desk, please." I saw a tiny blue spiral notebook in which she made entries about her health. That day, she had left the notebook open on her desk: "Seven AM. Sharp pains in left eye, vision much diminished." I read from the page that was exposed, decided not to read any more.

We had tea that afternoon, as we had done for as long as I could remember. I waited while my mother criticized the television coverage of the approaching election, the commentary sometimes irritating now that her mental territory, once so broad and variegated, was shrinking. She was entitled to her opinions. The news was, after all, the life's work of her son, a newspaper publisher, as it had been of her husband, my father, a newspaper editor and foreign correspondent. Those grooves were worn deep. Finally I asked, "How are you feeling today?" She just gave me a look. I asked again, "How are your eyes?" "Fine," she said, annoyed.

I was on sabbatical that fall, excited and nervous about the plans I had for my research and writing. M's situation filled me with dread. I knew I would have to take care of my mother before I could go ahead with my projects; the attachment sucked at me like a terrifying undertow. Friends counseled me to back off, thinking my mother would acknowledge that she couldn't manage by herself and, luckily, could afford help. I was anxious all the time; I knew she would never admit that she needed anything. Of course I knew she had to have help; she knew she had me.

The doctors doubled the dose of the steroids my mother was taking. The drugs had already made her quite sick; she admitted that she felt "very rocky." M dealt with her increasing neediness with a weird combination of denial and surrender. I'd known the denial all my life. Denial was what made her launch into discussing the day's news whenever a friend asked how she was feeling. Denial was what made M insist, even as she became increasingly unsteady on her feet, that she would fold her laundry the way she wanted it. She carefully refolded the towels in thirds when they came back, neatly folded in half, from the place on Ninth Avenue. She refolded the sheets too, to expose the bits of red yarn she had sewn onto the ends of the doubles to separate them from the twins.

The surrender was unfamiliar. Lying flat on the bed, fully dressed but unable to sit up, M asked me, "Would you mind very much picking something up at the drugstore?" This was harder to bear.

M's behavior around food had become odd. I brought her egg custard, which she had always loved, from Jefferson Market. After we'd finished supper she sidled into the kitchen mentioning that she had to get something. When I stepped into the kitchen I saw her dipping big spoonfuls of the sweet yellow stuff out of the container, gulping it down. Another evening she stood leaning against the doorjamb between the living room and the kitchen, tottery from the drugs, and gnawed on a wing of the roasted chicken we'd just finished, working it over as though she hadn't eaten for weeks. Was food the only pleasure left in her life? M had always been reserved, sometimes maddeningly so; I did not want this new intimacy.

My mother's life had been filled with pleasures: her relationship with my father, travel, swimming, conversation, gardening, politics. M was quick to sense when someone she cared about needed something and it gave her great satisfaction to be able to respond. But if I were to pick her greatest pleasure, it would be reading. Whenever she began to read on a new subject my mother said that she was furnishing her mind. She busied herself lending and culling her books almost as fast as she acquired them. When she sold the house in the country, M gave away hundreds of volumes, one by one, to carefully chosen recipients.

Later, when we were clearing out my mother's apartment in Chelsea, Claire, my partner, said that she would pack the remaining books while I worked on the unsorted piles of letters and bills and miscellaneous stuff. Lifting the dusty volumes, many of them tagged with the unused Kleenex that M favored for bookmarks, Claire, herself a voracious reader, said, "Your mother had such a wide-ranging intellectual life."

Who my mother was washed over me as we handled the books. She had sustained so many passionate interests, Mary Kingsley and Freya Stark, and, more than anything, Mary Sheldon, an early feminist and teacher who had been my paternal grandfather's first wife. A shelf of the choicest readings, fiction and nonfiction, on postcolonial Africa. Many volumes on China, spanning from the reissue of Owen Lattimore's books on Mongolia in the 1930s (Owen and his wife, Eleanor, were among my parents' closest friends, my father's summons before Congress linked to Owen's persecution by the House Un-American Activities Committee), to the most contemporary voices exposing the Cultural Revolution. There was a Fowler's, almost as tattered as *The New York Times Cookbook* M had favored. A Hammond's world atlas and a State Department book of maps of China from the seventies. Darwin, so many volumes of Darwin.

I believe my mother prized her place in my family's plan for women. The plan, familiar to everyone who grew up in the upper middle class during the fifties and sixties, read: get married young (each of my three siblings married before the end of college or immediately after graduation), get an interesting job but never let it conflict with the work of the man you are marrying (for my mother and my sisters), have children and devote yourself to their development and well-being. Most of all, never neglect the needs of everyone else in the family: to be driven to music lessons and doctors' appointments, accompanied on trips and to professional meetings, tended when they were sick, painstakingly well educated and, without fail, enticed and directed to become serious readers.

I escaped the family plan by not marrying. Some of my oldest friends might even say that I became a lesbian as I turned thirty in order to escape that plan. It hadn't been easy for me to come out to my mother, to feel comfortable in my skin as I made an independent life with Claire. Now, as my mother's illness worsened, I found myself doing the things that women in my family had always done. Exactly the same things: shopping for special foods that M might enjoy, arranging countless doctors' appointments, selecting books-on-tape at the library as her vision dimmed, bringing fresh flowers, managing the bills and other banking, running her household. How had this happened?

It happened for many reasons, which belong in other stories. The point is, my mother and I never spoke about it—just as we never mentioned the documents we both signed at the lawyer's office. We saw each other often throughout my adult life and discussed so many things. But we had never talked about how she would cope if she had disabilities as she grew older; we never talked about nursing homes or paid companions; we never talked about death or any arrangements she might have wanted. We certainly never talked about the possibility of her suicide. M had been a supporter of Concern for Dying, an organization that promoted euthanasia, and admired my aunt who worked for them. Yet my mother, who had taken care of a close handful of other people through the last chapters of their lives, who was a principled woman and a realist, had never spoken to me about the end of her life at all.

The phone rang very early on a Sunday morning in November. My mother was in the hospital. I witnessed many terrible things during the two months that followed. I saw my mother who had managed to climb out of the high hospital bed, over the rails, and had a terrible fall. "I can't imagine why I was so disoriented," she said, while the hospital lawyers hovered around us. I saw my mother, wearing a huge crinkly adult diaper, the blue tissue paper edge showing through her nightie, who sat as still as a stone against the back of the bed raised to its full upright position, waiting to see whether or not she would throw up from the massive doses of antibiotics they were giving her. I saw my mother sprawled on top of the sheets as though she had been washed up by the waves, her legs spindly thin and her hospital gown hiked up too high.

After the fifth week of her hospital stay M's physician pulled strings to get her admitted to a renowned rehabilitation center. M was so weak that she couldn't sit up without help, her muscles eaten away by the drugs even before the pneumonia and the long weeks in bed. At first she flatly refused the idea of rehab. "There is absolutely no reason for me to go there," she said, sounding almost like herself. Then she gave up, too sick to resist.

Nothing had weakened the powers of her tongue, however, not yet. My mother had especially enjoyed her shower every morning. Now she referred to the women who got her out of bed at five AM and wheeled her to the communal shower as "the harridans." Whenever she had felt cornered by the suggestion that she might not be able to live forever in her apartment on Twenty-first Street between Ninth and Tenth Avenues, M had always said, "I suppose I can consider almost anything, as long as it is on a good bus line. Of course, Tenth Avenue has an excellent bus line." I couldn't imagine how she would manage once she was home. She was unable to get out of bed by herself. She barely tolerated a wheelchair, acting as though it were some novel conveyance that we would all adopt shortly. Nurses and residents pulled me aside to say that I really should not consider letting my mother live independently again.

My brother, who lives in Florida, came to the city. M told Andy that I had become manipulative because I was so concerned about her living arrangements (which affected my getting back to work). "I feel this is a failure of our entire relationship," she said. The three of us assembled in the Family Room, a dim interior cavern at the rehabilitation center. Four televisions blared on different channels in the four corners of the room; stroked-out people were parked in wheelchairs all around us. My mother sat in a wheelchair too, enraged that we were not willing to take her to her apartment for the day "so that we can have this discussion in private." I was bolstered by the dismay I read on my brother's face; I must have believed that taking her home would have been the right thing to do.

M's need to be right lay at the core of her personality. I've read only one love letter from my mother to my father. The letter was written in pencil, dated when she was still officially married to her first husband. I assume my parents had begun their love affair, because M wrote, "I feel I am married to you." It must have been one of those moments when all the fixed points in one's life are turning and thumping like clothes in the washing machine. Yet my mother's voice was unmistakable: "Joe, sweetheart, you were absolutely wrong," she announced in the opening paragraph, "about the weather here."

My mother's will prevailed; she was not moved to a nursing home. She returned to her apartment at the end of January. An agency sent home health aides. A number of them were unable to cope; my mother dismissed others by saying, "Thank you, but we won't need you to come again." I didn't know what to do. I especially hated it that I no longer slept well. Sleep was a particular pleasure for me, tied in subterranean ways to swimming and sex, my

other immeasurable physical pleasures. I lived from day to day, poised for the
next crisis.

Someone gave M a pamphlet about lupus, an autoimmune disease with
some similarities to her original illness. The pamphlet said that people with
lupus are often "extremely fatigued and vulnerable and need help with routine living." "If only I had had that booklet," M said, "we would have avoided
our family conflict." "That's one way of describing it," I thought, remembering the Family Room. "I would have known that I would need help when I
came home," M continued, "though I certainly don't need anything now."

Finally I found Clarissa, a beautiful, tall, dignified Jamaican woman who
was in her mid-forties, like me. I asked her to tell me how she would describe
her job, having learned that home health care consisted not just of nurses
and aides and housekeepers and physical therapists, but of people who will
vacuum and people who won't, people who will answer a ringing telephone
and people who won't. Clarissa said simply, "I work with the elderly." As
things began to settle down, my mother fussed endlessly that the job was not
good for Clarissa. "There is absolutely nothing for her to do here," M said.

Ellen, my mother's most congenial friend in her apartment building, was one
of several women who lived there who had devoted their entire careers to the
New York Public Library. The summer that marked the first year of my
mother's illness Ellen told M that she had been diagnosed with Alzheimer's.
My mother reported to Claire and me that she had been talking with Ellen,
looking out the living-room windows, which had a wonderful view of the
Hudson River, and Ellen had said, "The river is the answer."

Towards the end of the summer Ellen vanished. "She's walked into the
river," M said. After weeks of desultory searching by the police, it turned out
that Ellen had indeed chosen the river. Everyone who had known her was dis-
turbed; some people were angry at her. My mother was the only person who
defended Ellen's right to end her life as she chose.

M, exquisitely sensitive to the needs of others, seemed to have no capacity to
see herself in the fabric of the family, to see how her feelings and actions
affected us. I needed Clarissa to be there so that I could resume my life.
Looking back, I suspect that my mother never had an inkling of how powerful she seemed to her grown children. All her life M had done things because
other people needed her to. My uncle Dick, M's only sibling, was left in her

care when she was scarcely a teenager. He was a handsome, funny man with red hair who became an alcoholic. He died in an accident that involved a gun when he was in young middle age and I was in high school. Somehow, everyone sensed that he had probably committed suicide. Much later, when I asked my mother how she had felt about his death, she replied with a startling directness: "I loved him very much, but he always made me feel a terrible, impotent anxiety. I no longer have to feel that." I loved my mother too—and I recognized the terrible, impotent anxiety that might be relieved by another's death.

Even as Clarissa skillfully made a place for herself, M refused the idea that Clarissa should accompany her when she went out. Instead, she requested that I go with her to an appointment across town at the New York Eye and Ear Infirmary. When we started home my mother, exhausted from the stress and exertion, nearly blinded by a long series of eye drops and high intensity lights, teetered on the edge of the curb, facing into the heavy traffic on Fourteenth Street. I searched frantically for a cab, trying to keep her from stepping into the street to help. My eye caught sight of an elderly black woman toting a huge plastic bag full of empty soda cans, perhaps fifty yards from where we stood. Just at that moment the old lady with the bag of cans suddenly fell backward onto the sidewalk. It was such a straight fall that I knew she must have cracked her head on the pavement. I started to go to her, then stopped. What would I do with the frail, imperious, white woman I was responsible for? How could I help this stranger when I had to help my mother?

One Tuesday morning, late for class as I tried to resume my teaching, I rushed for the bus stop on Sixteenth Street. Exiting the passageway under the Fulton Houses and starting across the street I suddenly saw my mother, standing with the other people who were waiting for the bus. My mother! Waiting to take the bus—by herself! A surge of incredulous anger welled up in me. My mother, who still couldn't get to her feet from the chair where she sat to watch television! My mother, with whom I pleaded not to go out by herself!

I couldn't bring myself to greet her. M had her red raincoat on, no glasses, no cane, black old lady's walking shoes with laces. My imagination flooded, my heart beat faster as it did every time I saw her teetering, in danger of losing her balance and falling. I was unable to go up to her and say, "How nice to see you, now we can take the bus together." I ducked between two parked trucks on Sixteenth Street, craning my head toward Tenth

Avenue to see whether the bus was coming. Then, embarrassed and a little bit ashamed, I pulled myself together. I walked toward the bus stop. M was looking right at me—less than fifty feet away. Nothing. She didn't recognize me. I didn't want to see my mother; she couldn't see me.

I was so worn out that Claire and I fled to the beach on the Caribbean side of Puerto Rico. Crabs, clear-colored as though they wore camouflage in the powdered white sand, skittered in and out of their holes as I rested by the rippling water. I found myself thinking about the scale of a person's life, her desires and ambitions. I had staked my claim to an independent, professional life. Now, it felt as though everything I did revolved around taking care of my mother. M had devoted herself to many people, never asking anything in return. But was this what she wanted? M had been active in left-wing politics in the thirties. She supported my radical politics in the sixties; she too went to Mississippi during the civil rights movement. M was always a feminist, albeit of a certain time and place. Where was the person who had insisted in word and deed that she never wanted to burden anyone? What had happened to her choices?

And why hadn't she talked to me about what we would do, if she became ill or infirm? I sat watching the ruby glow of sea urchins in the underwater sun. Paddling through the thick mangroves that flanked the canal where we swam, schools of yellow fish flickered through the water with us; the bottom was littered with chunks of coral like the shit of some giant fish. The green overhanging banks closed in on us like a tunnel, shadow and light bouncing everywhere. Gigantic leaves grew and fell, trash from the lush vegetation. Each individual plant grew entwined with three or four others; that was just the way it was.

The night of my birthday, early in December of the year after my mother's long hospitalization, my sister Lila was in New York. Lila cooked a special supper for the three of us. M sat in her usual place at the table but she kept nodding off, unable even to make the gestures of family conversation. It was alarming. Two days later I sat in the lobby of the emergency room at the hospital.

Visitors were allowed in for fifteen minutes of every hour. Finally, the officious young security guard let me pass. I made out my mother's figure, draped with sheets on a high narrow gurney at the back of the emergency room, which was a few hundred feet from the doors. She was enraged. Her voice carried down the hall long before she could possibly have seen me. She was chastising my sister and me for having been out on a binge the night before. "You have good color," she declared as I drew near, "but Lila's wan face was the final proof!" (I had almost stopped drinking because a friend had said that alcohol might make my insomnia worse. My sister, who has never been on a binge in her life, was home in Minneapolis.)

After four days in the hall they finally moved M to a proper hospital room. I got back to my apartment after nine that night. Close to midnight, as I began to feel relaxed enough to fall asleep, the phone rang. When I answered a woman's voice barked at me, "Your mother says she is dying and you should come at once." "Who is this?" I asked. "A nurse at the hospital," she said as though I were slow, or stupid. "What's wrong, what happened?" I asked. She just repeated herself. I said I needed to talk to my mother.

Someone managed to get M to the phone and she said in a strong voice, "I know that I am dying and you should come right away." My mother, who never complained about any physical distress? Who said, whenever I mentioned her long stays in the hospital, "Really? I don't remember a thing about that!" I couldn't take it in; I just kept pressing her with questions: "What makes you say that? What do you think is wrong?" "You should come," M replied, "for the same reasons that I would expect any member of my family to come if I were dying!"

The minute we hung up I called Minneapolis. My brother-in-law, who is a professor of medicine, answered the phone. I spilled it all out, almost breaking down with this man I have loved since I was a little girl. Harry told me to call the hospital again. "Why?" I asked, dreading the mean nurse. "It's been five minutes," he said. I didn't know what he was talking about, but I was so relieved to have him tell me what do that it didn't matter. The person who answered the phone at the nurses' station, a stranger, said, "Your mother is sound asleep."

I called Harry again to report that M was sleeping. I couldn't stop fretting about why the mean nurse hadn't bothered to let me know that she was okay. Harry talked on and on too, frustrated that the doctors couldn't reach a diagnosis. Neither of us mentioned that my mother seemed to be out of her mind. As we were hanging up Harry said, "I'm going to get a plane to New York in the morning," and I began to cry, cradled by his recognition that I was too alone with her, this was too hard.

Claire and I spent our second Christmas at the hospital. My mother was tied into a chair in something called a Posey restraint, a canvas and nylon contraption that looked exactly the way a straitjacket should look. Parked in the hall outside her room, M barely made contact with us. She didn't speak at all. "Is it that you can't speak, or you just don't want to?" I asked, hearing myself honor her formidable will even in the face of such distress.

The end of the afternoon was the time of day when M became most agitated; the winter light went early. The nurses called this sun-downing, a period of acute disorientation at the fall of dusk. M lost her ability to eat by herself, plucked and fussed with the bedclothes in a way that the nurses said was typical. She insisted that a pea she had lost in the folds of the sheets was a bug, then reached out in the middle of an exchange about something else to scratch at my glasses. "You have a cornflake stuck right there," she said in a disapproving tone of voice.

Lila came to New York again after the holidays. My mother had long, loopy conversations as we sat at her bedside. Sometimes they were about Lila's father, her first husband. They had been married in the early thirties and had an apartment on Eleventh Street in the Village. "I saw Fred last night," she reported one morning. "We went dancing and had such a wonderful evening! And we ended up staying someplace much nicer than this."

I tried to explain to M that she couldn't go home because the doctors couldn't figure out what was wrong with her. She refused to believe me. "I feel you have become perfidious," she said. When Clarissa came to stay with her so that I could teach my classes, M insisted that Clarissa did not want to work for us anymore. "What are you talking about?" I said crossly. "You know, I believe she may have taken a job at this same hospital," M said. I must have looked skeptical. "Why else would she be here?" M countered. "She just may not be available now," my mother cautioned, never looking at Clarissa, who sat two feet away.

To escape the hospital vigil I took the train to Connecticut where Claire worked and we spent many weekends. By the time I got there, a blizzard had begun. I wanted to feel the air, to be out in the snowfall, so I said I would take the dog for her last walk of the evening. Daisy whoofled the drifts with her nose, sneezing with delight. It was so beautiful, so still, the flakes driven against the pools of light made by the streetlamps, no cars, the snow a squeaky light powder underfoot.

Everything fell quiet as I walked alone with the dog: medical decisions in the face of such vast uncertainties, sickening cab rides as I bounced over the same potholes going to the hospital day after day, hours of rounding up M's mail and laundry and phone messages from worried friends, bouts of terrified wakefulness in the middle of the night when I tried to determine what my mother would have wanted, dread glimpses of my own neglected, disorganized life as I taught my classes on the fly week after week. Walking through the silent dense snowfall, I suddenly understood that my mother would never walk in the snow again. The realization blanketed me like the cold falling snow: how she had loved being out in a snowstorm. Bit by bit, my mother was losing everything. Snowflakes pelted against my face; my cheeks ran with icy drops of water.

That spring, loss grew on top of loss like the scales of lichen on the stone walls that edged the fields at Freewind. I brought my mother home from the hospital again, feeling as though I had a second job. She seemed to think that this was just what you did for your family. "I'm the one," I announced to myself as I would never have done out loud. "I am the one of all your children who chose not to have a family." When we sat visiting over tea M would start to speak and then interrupt her own sentence, a thought floating away like a butterfly, hovering and darting off. I told her a story about the president of my university, a dreadful man I'd worked with and complained about for years. M listened closely as she always had. Then she said apologetically, "Who are you talking about? I'm afraid I missed that."

Memory was a theme in the books I clung to during those months. Philip Roth comes to the end of his account of his father's harrowing final illness and says, "You must not forget anything."[1] My mother had always been the one to listen and remember, attending to the words of others. Now I was the one listening, remembering for her, forgetting nothing.

Snow fell hard outside the big window in our city apartment. There hadn't been so many heavy snowstorms for years. The phone rang. "Is this Nancy Barnes?" my mother asked, her voice vigorous and strong. We had a short, hearty exchange. "I just hope that the train is running," she said, "and that you have good galoshes and your friend will be able to get out to meet you." It was a fine conversation except that it was Tuesday and I wouldn't be going to the country for three days and my mother had forgotten the name of the woman with whom I had lived for more than ten years. No one wore galoshes anymore, either.

Clarissa called before seven one morning. She had stayed with M the night before. Either she couldn't hear M calling or my mother forgot that there was anyone with her. "Anyway," Clarissa said, "around three AM she had to use the commode. When I went in to check on her she is lying on the floor." "You can't possibly get me up," my mother had informed her. "You will have to go out in the street and get a man to help you." "At three AM!" Clarissa exclaimed, as though that were the shocking part of the story. I couldn't bear the physical intimacy of these details—my mother got up in the darkest hours to relieve herself, she fell on her way back to bed and lay on the floor, unable or unwilling to call for help.

Was this a life my mother wanted? "Please let someone else do this," I begged when I found M squirreling through piles of bills and letters strewn across her desk, looking for a check. "That would just be extravagant," M said. "Don't you realize how expensive that would be, especially when we just need someone to tide us over?" All I could think was, "Don't you realize that this is the end of your life? That we are not just tiding things over?" I said nothing, still able to feel it was merciful that my mother didn't remember how sick she had been, the indignities she had endured. Clarissa told me that my mother had taken everything out of the fridge, vegetables, little half-sticks of butter wrapped in foil, jars of somebody's homemade jelly that had been in there for ages. When Clarissa asked her what she was doing M said scornfully, as though it should be obvious, "I'm looking for my check."

We went to see a neurologist at the hospital. The doctor stayed with M in the examining room for some time. When he came back to his office where I waited, he handed me a breadstick like the one he was crunching. "This is not Alzheimer's," he said, "but there is no way of knowing what she has. My mother-in-law was going strong in her mid-eighties, going to concerts and movies and running around town. Then she had a rather routine operation. Since then her brain hasn't quite come back. Your mother," he said to me, "has had a number of terrible, terrible insults to her brain."

Before we left, the neurologist spoke directly to M. Not one of her many other doctors had done that. He told her that the CT scan showed signs of stroke, and that she had something that was benign and senescent. (When I looked it up at home, I learned that senescence is the state or process of becoming old. In plants, it is a growth phase, from maturity to death.) After he had finished speaking the doctor said gently, "What has been bothering you?" He sat quietly waiting, which made me like him even more. M didn't say anything for the longest time. Finally she spoke: "I'm afraid I'm losing my mind."

I hadn't been to Freewind for months. I needed to go, as Terry Tempest Williams had needed to go to the Great Salt Lake which rose and rose to terrifying, record heights during the many months that her mother was dying of cancer. "I go to the lake for a compass reading," Williams writes in *Refuge*, "to orient myself once again in midst of change. Each trip is unique. The lake is different. I am different."[2]

The fields were clouded with beds of violet-blue Quaker ladies and plump handfuls of fuzzy purple clover. Claire and I walked across the hilltop to have a look at our old house, which was being remodeled by a wealthy New Yorker. We held hands, watching the dog race ahead. The maples had the unmistakable red glow of spring, each branch festooned with tiny pendant parachutes waiting to release. I wondered if my mother knew how much these fields comforted me, how much I had loved growing up here, having her teach me the wonderful names of plants like vetch and where to find wild iris hiding in the tall grass.

The first thing we saw was the slope where my eye used to fall when I did the dishes at the kitchen sink. It was raw, scraped down to the dirt. No more beauty bush, the slatternly wash of light pink blossoms that my parents had brought from my grandmother's garden in New Hartford before I was born. No more of the pine trees my father had planted so that they grew along with me, each one a mere stalk of a tree as he heeled it into the ground, grown to more than the height of the house. We peered in the windows; the inside appeared to be gutted. My eyes glistened with tears. Claire, who is a historian, just kept repeating, "That beautiful old farmhouse is gone."

It was the end of an era.

My mother, too, was living the last chapter of her life. She was determined to maintain her independence, to act as though she were in control, even as everything was slowly being stripped away. Had she ever imagined that it would come to this, that day we sat together in the lawyer's office? I said to my friends that I was living out a script that had been written long ago, as though that made it okay. I hated to hear myself sounding harsh with her. This was my mother, who had filled our rooms with flowers every single summer's day, whose gardens at Freewind made visitors draw in their breath: brilliant curves of scarlet poppies and dark purple Japanese iris splashing color in June, magnificent stands of delphinium a few weeks later. Gardening, like reading, must have been how my mother, a woman of a certain generation, class, and race, made time for herself, time to create something beautiful and undemanding, essentially without purpose, quite unlike meals or checkbooks or children.

I went to Philadelphia to give a talk at a conference not long after the trip to the neurologist. It was the first time in ages that I had left town for work. When I got back to my room at the Sheraton, tired and exhilarated, a green message light was blinking wildly in a panel on the wall. Apparently my mother had called the police the night before. She was alarmed by the aide, who was sitting in the second bedroom in order to stay out of M's way. M said that there was "an intruder, who had a whole group of rowdy people in there." Several of my relatives said in their messages that they had no way of knowing, when they got calls from a New York City cop, whether there really had been an intruder. All I could think was, "This woman's powers are simply fantastic, right to the end."

Later, when M was gone, I carried boxes of stuff from her apartment to the stairwell so that I could cram it, handful by handful, down the infuriatingly small incinerator chute. My hands filled with precariously balanced trash, I turned and pushed the door open with my shoulder. Across the small landing my eyes lit on the crazy lady who lived directly above my mother. This was the lady who cruised their Chelsea neighborhood in her bedroom slippers, her long, straight white hair flying around an oddly unlined pink face, sorting through rubbish for things that she placed in a wire shopping cart, scavenging everywhere. "Oh no," I thought to myself. "I should've known she would show up." She stood above me on the stairs, waiting while I unloaded things into the tiny porcelain sink. The crazy lady was watching for the good stuff as I dismantled my mother's last home. What good stuff?

I greeted her politely, as I always had, and continued making my trips. Then, thinking that the coast was clear, I heard her creeping down the steps again to see what choice items I might have brought. I whirled to face her, "Look, you can have anything you want, but please just wait until I'm finished, okay?" She nodded her head frantically and slipped back up the stairs to where I couldn't see her. I made several more trips in privacy. Suddenly she was there again. "Does your mother have Alzheimer's?" she asked. "No," I said, biting my tongue on all the other retorts that flooded my mind. She looked at me suspiciously. "The other lady did, you know," she said, referring to Ellen, my mother's friend who had walked into the Hudson River. "She did—the other lady had Alzheimer's—and you know I live right on top of both of them!"

When I had begun to realize that my mother's illness did not mean she was going to die, not immediately, anyway, I had contacted a gerontologist in Brooklyn. She started to walk me through the intricacies of home care for the elderly. At the end of our conversation, she gave me an assignment: "Go visit half a dozen nursing homes," she said. "Not that your mother is ready for a nursing home yet, I know, but you need to see them. Go soon." My mother? My mother would never permit herself to enter a nursing home. M had been shipped off to boarding school when her father died suddenly in his forties; her mother had been hospitalized before that, when M was nine or ten. M never talked about her childhood, but I knew she had no intention of being abandoned to an institution. The gerontologist wasn't wrong, but I didn't go to see the nursing homes, not then, not yet.

"Was there some talk about swimming, or was I dreaming?" This was the first glimmering that my mother had indeed heard us when my siblings and I assembled once again to talk with her about moving to an assisted living facility near my brother's home in Florida, almost five years after she fell ill. M even said that in such a place she "might make a few new acquaintances." I held my breath, longing for her to say that this move was all right, that we were somehow honoring her wishes. But then she reversed herself and announced in one long breath, "All my friends are in New York; my whole life is in the city. I don't know a single soul in Florida. The Florida heat is brutal for months out of every year. And," she said, delivering the coup de grâce, "I don't know if you realize this, but my Florida family is very busy."

I fully believed that the move to Florida would not happen, that my mother would somehow outfox us. But I had been convinced that this entire journey would not happen, that my mother would not allow it. I had witnessed the documents in which she said that she did not wish to live with irreversible mental impairment. And, I had always known that she considered the ending of one's own life a choice that belonged to each of us. Perhaps the last years had simply outfoxed her. M called the police again.

First she yelled "Thief, thief!" out the window on the tenth floor. Someone called the Ecuadoran super, a particular friend of hers. Gregorio came immediately to see if he could help. M did not recognize him and dialed 911 to report that there was a strange man in her apartment.

Clarissa met me at the door with this whole story. When I asked M what had happened, she rebuked me for interfering. Then she began to cry. Had I seen my mother cry a half dozen times in almost fifty years? She lay on her bed where I sat next to her, a light smell of urine everywhere, her body turned away so that her feet pressed against me; she was crying and gasping. Her skinny calves made me think of Daisy, our old dog whose legs were like sticks.

We moved my mother to Florida. Coming into the city from Newark Airport after the trip I heard myself tell the cabbie to take me to Twenty-first Street. It was close to midnight. For some reason, I needed to go to M's apartment before I could go home. I had grown to hate that building. I hated the heavy front door, so cumbersome that an able-bodied person had difficulty with it. I never opened that door, even years before M started to go downhill, without thinking how easily it could crush a hand, or an ankle. I hated the elevator, out of order so frequently that I worried about what would happen if my mother had ventured out alone on one of her errands and couldn't get back up. I hated the smell in the hallway, a foul sweet odor that must have had to do with the cleaning products or the floor wax. I hated how poorly lit the hall was, which meant that M had to fumble to get the door open. I fumbled with the keys that night.

The apartment was stripped almost bare. The furniture was gone, the lovely pictures down. All that remained was the stuff in her bedroom. I roamed around, almost the way she had been doing for the last sad, anxious weeks, touching things, running my hands over the surfaces. School pictures of M's great-grandchildren; the announcement of a New School concert series that she and I had attended; random loose pages of my father's writings from his travels in Russia in 1927 that my mother had been assembling into notebooks ever since he died; dozens of envelopes from the left-wing political and environmental organizations to which she contributed every year, $100 checks as important to her as though they were $1,000; scraps of paper with her shaky handwriting recording my phone numbers in New York and Connecticut over and over again.

I was too worn out to be there. The memories overwhelmed me. A plastic bag crammed with postcards from our trips to Israel and Greece when I was thirteen, to Africa when I was seventeen. I glanced at a photo of a huge herd of goats moving down a dirt road in Senegal, blocking a car's passage. Those were the travels that had turned me into an anthropologist. Buried in a box full of dried-out drugs and toiletries, there was a large untouched bottle of Seconal. The prescription was signed by a doctor whose name I barely recognized. I did recall my mother's having said, years earlier, "I'm very glad to have found her." There was a card from a well known Marxist, a wealthy man who had supported causes that were vital to my mother as well, in which he addressed her as "Beautiful lady, beloved friend." And, risen to the top like the bubbles released by plant life deep underwater among the mangroves, there was a copy of one of Derek Humphry's books, sent by the Hemlock Society to people who wanted to know how to end their own lives.[3]

The gerontologist I had consulted had observed that doing this with my mother would teach me a lot about myself. That was the only suggestion that the ordeal might prove valuable to me, somehow apart from my feelings for my mother, my loyalties as her daughter. I said at the outset of this essay that I had gleaned two truths from the experience: that whatever happens at the time of my death may well involve others I love as deeply as it does me, and that the possibilities of choice about one's own death can silently and swiftly slip away. Now, I would also say that I have loosened my grip on the certainties of choice. It means as much to me as ever that I lead a largely chosen life as a college teacher, a lesbian who does not have children, a life that is profoundly different from my mother's. How could I have dreamt that my life would encompass years of taking care of my mother, a commitment that I both resisted and chose?

I know I have loosened my grip on the certainties of choice. I was the witness to my mother's life, so much life—why couldn't she acknowledge that it was ending? Perhaps it was grief that brought me to her apartment in the middle of the night after the move to assisted living. I ached to remember all the other ways I had known her, been shaped by her, loved her, before this struggle.

But my mother wasn't dead, not yet. Several times I had wished her dead in the face of her anguish, and the anguish she caused me. But then I thought of Philip Roth, confronting his father's deterioration from a brain tumor. Roth too yearned for relief, even as he asked, "How could I take it on myself to decide that my father should be finished with life, life which is ours to know just once?"[4]

I was the witness to the woman who walked into her room in assisted living in St. Petersburg, Florida, sat down on the ugly green couch that came with the rental furniture and spoke to her grown children, who were gathered around her. "I can't imagine," M said in her firmest, most righteous voice, "whatever made you think that I could live here. I don't know a soul in Florida, not a single soul, and I need to see about my reservations to go home to New York."

NOTES

The title of this essay is a quotation from Philip Roth's *Patrimony*, page 232.

1. Philip Roth, *Patrimony* (New York: Vintage Books, 1996), 238.

2. Terry Tempest Williams, *Refuge: An Unnatural History of Family and Place* (New York: Vintage Books, 2001), 75.

3. Derek Humphry, *Let Me Die Before I Wake: Hemlock's Book of Self-Deliverance for the Dying* (New York: Grove Press, 1986).

4. Roth, *Patrimony*, 232.

Caregiving Beulah

A Relentless Challenge

SUSAN PERLSTEIN

I have spent my entire working life dedicated to improving the quality of life for older people; however, nothing prepared me for my mother's final journey. I have sat by the side of the dying, sharing their last wishes and stories. I have worked in long-term care, hospice, and assisted-living facilities and in many capacities—as a teaching artist, program developer, social worker, educator, and administrator. I have developed programs for caregivers and trained staff to run creative programs for caregivers and their loved ones.

So I expected to be prepared when my mother—in her nineties—began to fail. As a social worker, I had practiced the discipline of listening to what people need and want. For my mother and me, this meant that, as long as she had her mental wits about her, I would respect her decisions and help to negotiate her choices with the health-care system—doctors, nurses, social workers, hospitals, hospice, and home health-care workers. As the oldest daughter and the one living closest to her, I would be the primary caregiver, although I would always inform and engage our immediate family in caregiving decisions. Together we would wend our way through my mom's last years.

My mother, Beulah Hoskwith Warshall-Cohn, was a second-generation daughter of poor Eastern European Jewish immigrants escaping persecution to find a better life in America. Success meant that Beulah married a doctor, a dream come true. Beulah birthed three children: first me, then my brother, and last my sister. Beulah, the matriarch of the large extended family, would do anything for her children and her sister's children. All my cousins loved her. She was the family social worker who, without a degree, listened to and encouraged them.

She deeply wanted to be a successful American, to assimilate into the American way of life. Her children had to do it for her; they had to be the best and that meant that nothing her children did was good enough. As her oldest daughter, I was held responsible for everything and anything. My younger brother and sister left New York City in part to avoid her constant advice. Somehow she could always get under your skin. For example, when I was just about to get married, she informed me that I could do better. I should be marrying a doctor. I said, "But Mom, he is a PhD." She replied, "You know what I mean, a real doctor." Although we fought, I knew she loved her children and she meant well—as she would often remind me.

If she decided she wanted something, there was no stopping her. Her endless energy, strong opinions, fierce determination, and intelligence contributed to her many successes. When my father was dying, she notified the U.S. government in Puerto Rico and had my brother flown back to the United States from his research project. Following my sister's bitter divorce, her husband kidnapped their daughter to his country, India. All efforts to return her failed. Consequently, Beulah took the extreme step of selling her house to raise required funds and hired an international detective to rescue her granddaughter. The rescue was successful and, again, Beulah succeeded—on an international scale.

Beulah married my father, Hyman Beryl Warshall, a pediatrician. Hyman dedicated his life to providing good medicine for working people in New York City and was one of the founders of the Health Insurance Plan of New York. He was an idealistic workaholic and one of the last of the doctors who would do home visits to sick children in the middle of the night and on weekends. Beulah enabled my father's progressive politics by working as his nurse and secretary, preparing dinners for his friends and colleagues, and running the family affairs while he worked. She joined Women Strike for Peace and worked on the board of a local community center for youth at risk.

Because she loved gardening, all her children belonged to the Brooklyn Botanic Gardens Children's Garden, where we planted vegetables. After my father passed away, Beulah became an active volunteer for the garden, teaching young students about plants. I am not sure where she developed her love of classical music, especially opera. When we were young, she took my brother and me to the opera. She often listened to *La Traviata, La Bohème,* and *Rigoletto.* She especially loved Pavarotti's singing.

As she aged, my mother became more and more religious. When she was married to my father, an atheist, she claimed she, too, did not believe. In her nineties, she went to Friday night services at the assisted-living facility. I think what was really important to her was to be part of a close cultural community and to celebrate together with them. With my father, she was an atheist, and in her old age, she embraced her Judaism.

My sister became an orthodox Jew and moved to the West Bank in Israel. Her second husband was a well-known singing rabbi in the Jewish renewal movement. Both my sister and mother believed that the family should be the center of a woman's life. Beulah had always celebrated the Jewish holidays with as many family members as possible. After my father died, my mother married my father's dear friend. She included all the members of this second family in holiday celebrations at Rosh Hashanah, Hanukah, and Passover, which she held in her home. On her deathbed, she asked me to carry on these Jewish traditions. I will need to address this request at some later time, since my generation lives across continents, both literally and figuratively.

My mother also believed in science and medicine. She loved the medical world and I believe that, had she been born at a different time, she would have become a doctor. She praised the miracle of modern drugs to cure ills, and she also loved to take medicine. In fact, as a doctor's wife, she would prescribe medicines for all her children, nieces, and nephews. To my surprise, my cousin became a doctor, and none of us became drug addicts. Beulah truly wished that all her children would become doctors. Since none of us did, that became a great and continual disappointment to her.

At ninety years of age, the beginning of the end of her life, my mother wished to be taken to see doctors as frequently as possible for her ills, but also because she enjoyed the visits. As a result, I spent hundreds of hours in doctors' waiting rooms during the last three years of her life. In her mid-eighties, her decline began when she fell and damaged her ankle. The tendons in her foot never healed well and she needed a walker after the accident. From that time on, she was in constant danger of falling. Too often I would get a call at work that Beulah had fallen and needed to go to the hospital. She was admitted for falls that caused a head injury, a hand injury, a hip injury, and more. Each fall required a hospital stay and rehab, followed by the need for home health care. She developed spinal stenosis of her neck and back that caused constant pain. In addition, she was diagnosed with COPD (chronic obstructive pulmonary disease). Each winter, she developed bronchitis and often needed hospitalization.

Each time she returned from a hospital stay, a home health aide would be assigned. I would be at her home until she felt comfortable with the necessary care. She constantly complained that she did not like the aide's cooking or cleaning. Sometimes she couldn't understand the person's accent. Mostly, she did not like someone in her home who wasn't family. Over the two years before she moved into an assisted-living facility, she fired thirteen home health aides.

While my mother was still living at home, I continually spoke with her about home safety and suggested she might be better off moving. Her walker could not easily turn from the hallway into the kitchen. She would lean against the wall, drag the walker into the kitchen sideways, and then try to straighten out the walker and rebalance herself. She often left the stove on and burned food. She was notorious for arbitrarily deciding which pill she would take on a given day. She was totally housebound, because she lived in a second-floor walk-up. Many years before, we had had escalator stairs installed, but at this time she could no longer manage to get into the seat to go down or up. She needed constant guidance not to fall. Yet, she carried on, complaining, "You want to put me away. What kind of daughter are you? If you were a good daughter, I would move in with you and you would take care of me."

I would calmly explain that I did not have the room in my apartment, and that I worked full time, but she refused to speak with me about the situation. When Beulah was at Coney Island Geriatric Center for rehab after one of her falls, I called my brother and sister to carefully prepare our discussion with her. We took her in a wheelchair to the Coney Island boardwalk, looked out at the sand, sea, and sky, and suggested that while she was in the geriatric rehab center, Beulah seriously needed to think about moving to a safer environment, either an assisted-living facility or a nursing home. She qualified for both. We reminded her how she complained that no one came to visit anymore, that she felt lonely, that her friends could not get around and so did not come to see her. We reminded her that she could no longer cook or clean. We also reminded her about the hours of care that were now necessary. We thought her life would be easier if she were safer and able to have a better social life. She protested that she did not want to live with old people. We reminded her that she was ninety and had already lived longer than the average life expectancy.

After hours of discussion and negotiations, Beulah agreed to move to an assisted-living facility and she signed the contract for Prospect Park Residence. She told us that her greatest fear was the move itself. Since the residence was a block from my home, I promised to help her with the move. I also promised to visit with her every Saturday and stop by when I could during the week.

We set the date for the move and began packing. My mother was overwhelmed with the sadness of the move. It was certainly more of a challenge than I had expected. When I came on weekends, I would help her pack. She needed to decide what she would give away, to whom, and what she would take with her. So, we would pack a box, and I would return the following weekend to find the box unpacked and things put back in her bureau. I needed to figure out a way to make the move happen.

Focusing on the details of the move, I forgot what I had learned from my professional experience with older people. For years, I had conducted reminiscence groups for older people in senior centers. It is important to older people to make sense of their lives and reflect on what has given their lives a sense of meaning and purpose. In the sharing of life histories, listeners learn about the speaker's family as well as cultural history. Older people share the time-honored role of the keepers of culture. After all, we are our stories and that is how we are remembered.

So I made a deal with my mother. I asked her to tell me the stories of her clothing and suggested that we have a fashion show. Once she decided where the item would go, then she could no longer unpack it. So she tried on the pink organza dress that she wore to my wedding, the zipper straining to close. We shared stories about the wedding ceremony at the neighborhood temple and the home reception, and spoke about her wedding to my father and how she loved him. The packing strife was eased through this story sharing, and we were able to pack and make the move. This experience with my mother reminded me that we need to share stories, especially during transitions.

Once Beulah arrived at the assisted-living facility, she seemed to forget the long process of choice and announced to all that I had forced her to move. When she met a new person, she never failed to inform them that her family had put her away. What can I say? She was a drama queen. And yes, this was a difficult and challenging transition: coming to terms with leaving home and facing the end of life is hard.

I thought it would be easier for us with Beulah at the assisted-living facility. I never expected the relentless, thankless challenges that I would face. First the practical work. Each weekend, I would shop for her, do her finances, write letters for her, and try to do something special. Her list of needs incrementally increased: Depends diapers, medications, Ensure, vitamins, nail polish, lipstick, et cetera. She would say, "I do not want to be a burden to my family. Please get me . . ." I was trying my best and it was not good enough for her. The emotional toll began impacting my life. I had no time for friends, for other family, for my artwork. I was constantly being interrupted at work. I had no time for myself. I was having trouble setting limits and felt both physically and mentally rundown.

Friends suggested that I join a caregivers' support group, but I protested that I did not have the time. Fortunately I had friends who understood the situation. Many were taking care of their aging parents and we could support each other with telephone conversations and an occasional cup of tea at a café. My son helped out by visiting when he could and by listening to me when we got together. I could never have handled the daily stresses without my life partner. His generous loving support made it possible for me to both work and to care for Beulah. He put himself on the back burner and helped out, knowing we would have more time for each other in the future.

Finances became an important issue. Once in assisted living, my mother was spending her savings at a rapid rate. She could no longer manage her finances and turned them over to me and my brother. I was shocked at the exorbitant costs of her doctors, office visits, medications, and medical equipment as well as the residence—room, food, and aides. She was spending over $5,000 a month, and we understood that it would only get worse.

Soon we might be caught in the dilemma of Medicare/Medicaid.[1] The way her money was disappearing, she would soon need Medicaid, but would she be eligible for Medicaid and when would it be? And would the residence accept Medicaid? I checked to see if Beulah could live in the facility on Medicaid. She could not. It was a private-pay institution. We closed our eyes and hoped for the best.

After a few months, Beulah reported to me that something was wrong. She was losing weight and having trouble holding down food. At first we thought she was having trouble adjusting to the assisted-living facility; however, a doctor diagnosed stomach cancer and she was given about six months to live. I discussed with my siblings the possibility of home hospice care.

Beulah wished to learn all her options and then to make a decision. Believing in medical solutions, her doctor did not approve of hospice. This doctor thought that not responding with the most advanced medical interventions was bad medicine. So the medical doctor, chief of geriatric medicine at a large metropolitan hospital, suggested that she see an oncologist. The oncologist offered her an experimental drug, Glevac, which had never been tried on anyone her age.

Beulah liked the idea of being an experiment. I continued to discuss the possibility of not taking chemotherapy and joining hospice care, suggesting that her quality of life might be greatly diminished by the treatment and perhaps she would be happier with comfort and care. She replied that she would consider that option later, but for the present she wanted whatever medical intervention she could get. She wanted to live even if she suffered.

Meanwhile, I was feeling a mixture of guilt and anger. Guilt because I really did not want to watch her suffer and complain, even though I respected her choice. Anger because I anticipated the heavy burden that the family and I would bear as we went down the medical road. It is difficult to reveal these uncomfortable feelings now because I fear being judged, even though I understand from my social work training that these are normal feelings.

So chemotherapy began. Choosing an aggressive intervention was a difficult adjustment for me. This meant for both of us at least a day a week in the hospital because my mother also needed Procrit, a treatment for anemia (a lack of red blood cells in the body), a side effect from chemotherapy. The upside of these hospital visits was the attention she received from the young, male, Chinese doctor, speaking to him about her late husband, the doctor. Since she wanted to speak to him daily, I had to help her understand that she was not his only patient. Until we could get her on the Elderly Pharmaceutical Insurance Coverage Program, we also needed to pay $600 a week for the medication.[2]

At this point, my dual role of geriatric social worker and daughter started to become a great strain. Personally, I needed relief and none was in sight. Tasks piled up. I needed to find the resources for the many levels of support for her. She now needed twenty-four-hour home health care to monitor her many medications and her ADL (Activities of Daily Living). First we tried using the cluster care offered by the assisted-living facility, but my mother objected to the constant turnover of different home health aides. She spared no words and let each know her mind. She would lecture them on the downfall of the medical system and the glory of her husband and "good" medicine. I agreed with her that the current system was not working well and that we could try a very expensive alternative, private home health care. Since she was given a short period of time to live, the family agreed.

Again, the geriatric social worker in me went to work in hiring home care. Fortunately, I found Brenda, a wonderful, experienced, Panamanian home-care worker who soon became my right hand. I came to think of Brenda as an earth angel. All decisions for Beulah's well-being were now made by Beulah first, then Brenda and me, as well as family, doctors and nurses, and social workers. Once Beulah was on chemotherapy, she had a daily central support team of ten people. The oncologist and medical doctor would call me to ask how she was doing and to try to figure out dosage adjustment. Friends and family called regularly. Beulah had more visitors than any other resident at the assisted-living facility.

After a year of intense care, and to everyone's amazement, Beulah began to improve and the stomach cancer began to shrink. She was still plagued with falls and breathing problems. In this remission period, my mother and Brenda attended every program offered at the residence: trips, card games, music programs, art, Jewish services, exercise, and gardening on the roof. Beulah won the resident-of-the-month award for helping to plant the roof garden. She befriended residents and found new friends.

This respite gave us quality time. Together Beulah and I looked over picture albums. We created a family tree and hung it on the wall by her bed. We found photos of the living relatives and created a collage. We shared many stories about my growing up in Flatbush, Brooklyn, in the 1950s. I asked her for a springtime highlight. She described the daffodil hill in the Brooklyn Botanic Gardens. Together we painted the hill—splendid with bright yellow blossoms. On Saturdays, Brenda held a beauty salon, washing and combing my mom's hair and doing her nails in her favorite fire-engine-red color. We all shared dress-up stories in her room at the assisted-living facility.

The respite did not last long. Old problems worsened. Each time she returned from the hospital, her overall health declined and she would plateau at a lower level. The COPD needed more attention, and so we added visits to a pulmonologist. An oxygen tank was attached to Beulah's wheelchair. When bronchitis sent her to the hospital, the prognosis was not good. In fact, her doctors said she was actively dying. Preparing for the worst, I informed friends and relatives. A steady stream of visitors came to pay their last respects. Surprisingly, when my sister arrived from Israel, my mother perked up and came back to life. When she returned to assisted living, she said that she never wanted to go to a hospital again. This seemed to us like the right time to have another discussion about hospice care and dying with dignity, not plugged into machines.

We explained to Mother what was involved in home hospice. She could have more personal care. A hospice doctor could actually come to the home and she would not have to go to the hospital. The hospice team (nurse, social worker, rabbi, and volunteer) would regularly come to visit her. Beulah accepted hospice comfort care and understood the meaning of "no extra-ordinary measures." Of course, she had signed the health-care proxy form, do-not-resuscitate order, and power of attorney. We children were all now prepared for what we expected would be the last phase of her journey.

One evening I got an emergency call from Brenda. "Susan, I think this is it. Get over here. She is having trouble breathing."

I ran down the block as fast as I could. "When I arrived, Beulah was slouched in her wheelchair by an open window, sweating, and gasping for breath." I hugged her and said "Mom, I love you. I think it is time for you to go to bed."

Brenda called hospice and they approved morphine to ease the breath-ing. Hospice had prepared us for the use of their emergency pack, which lay ready for use in the bureau.[3] They said they would be sending a nurse immediately.

Beulah looked at me and Brenda as if we were crazy.

"911, 911," she gasped.

"Mom, I thought that you never wanted to go to the hospital and you hated the emergency room."

"911, 911." She grasped my arm.

My heart raced, sweat began to pour down my back. What do we do? Brenda looked at me, confused. Beulah did not want to go to bed. Brenda and I conferred, agreeing that Beulah knew her mind. We tried again to remind her of her past decision. She loved her hospice doctor. The nurse would be with us soon.

"911, 911," she insisted. And so we called the ambulance to take her to Maimonides Hospital, packed our overnight cases, and waited.

Brenda and I spent another horrific night in the emergency room, while they hooked my mother up to an antibiotic drip and a breathing ventilator,

and began a long process of draining her lungs. She was diagnosed with sep-
ticemia as well as bronchitis. She spent two weeks in the hospital—against
her earlier wishes never to return—under emergency care with round-the-
clock antibiotics and the draining of her lungs. Most of the time she was not
conscious of her surroundings.

I started thinking about health-care priorities and whether the government should set limits on costs for various procedures. The hospitalization
cost to Medicare was $80,000. I wondered if these measures we were paying
for were extraordinary and unjustified, given my mother's situation.

Again, the family vigil began, with my brother coming in from Tucson,
my sister flying in from Israel, and the parade of visitors. My small apartment
became a hotel. By now, I was living from day to day.

When my mother was brought home to the assisted-living facility, she
was bedridden, but glad to be alive. And once more she said that she never
wanted to see a hospital room again and that she wanted to return to hospice
care. So I reopened her account with the hospice care. Both the hospice doctor and the medical doctor were angry with this change in plans and blamed
me for taking her to the hospital, instead of waiting for the hospice nurse. As
a geriatric social worker, I reminded both that, for better or worse, Beulah
had her mental faculties with her and she would be making the decisions. As
her daughter, I shared their frustration and, in my exhaustion, I seriously
thought that Beulah would outlive me.

In the meantime, Beulah's poor health had created a financial crisis in
the family. She had already spent down most of her money and we had no
idea how we could afford to keep Brenda. At a family meeting, my cousin
offered to contribute to Beulah's care. It was with his help that my brother
and I managed her continued quality care.

Another year passed with the usual complications—doctor's visits, hospice, and hospital stays. Brenda, now a family friend, thought that my mother
wanted to live to see her great-grandchild born. She wagered that Beulah
would pass soon after that visit. My mother, bed bound, no longer left her
room. She and Brenda played cards, listened to opera, and talked about my
father and grandfather and her mother's childhood. When Beulah halluci-
nated that her mother and father were with her, Brenda simply asked how
they were.

My mother was wasting away and eating little. She had little energy and
spoke in a whisper. She slept much of the time, but she held on with the

strength of her extraordinary willpower. When Beulah's grandchild from Israel showed up with the new baby, Beulah opened her eyes—and smiled with such joy, giggled, and tickled the baby.

After my niece and her baby left, Beulah began to let go. First, she stopped eating and only drank. Her systems were shutting down. Then she could no longer swallow and stopped drinking. Hospice said it would be a few days, maybe a week. The rabbi visited. The hospice social worker helped us prepare for the end. My mother would open her eyes and smile for each visitor. If you put your ear to her mouth, you could hear her thanking the visitors and saying good-bye.

After she stopped drinking, I called the family, even though I could not promise that my mother would not sit up and start eating the moment one of her other children arrived. My sister arrived with prayers for the dying. We made all the funeral arrangements and drew up a list of people who needed to be notified. Everything was in place for her passing.

Another week went by and my mother was still smiling. She also said she was hungry and wanted ice cream. We tried to feed her, but she could not swallow.

During the day, my sister prayed by her side. At night, Brenda and I tried to figure out how to make her passing more comfortable. Brenda moved the bed so Beulah's feet would face the window, thinking that a new position might help her soul in passing. Brenda brought in holy water to wash my mother's body. We played her favorite Pavarotti recordings. I sang peace songs such as "Down By the Riverside," and "Last Night I Had the Strangest Dream." Brenda sang "Besame Mucho."

Days passed . . . day fourteen without food or water. Brenda planned to leave on vacation. I thought mother would not stay long without Brenda. The day after Brenda left, Beulah's death rattle began. My sister prayed, my brother arrived, and my mother passed peacefully and gently in her home as she wished.

Looking back, I believe that my mother made the very best of her last three years, demanding great support from many. From the window of her room, she looked out on the trees of Prospect Park. Her family called and visited daily. She came to enjoy the activities and people at the residence. She had home health care. Fortunately, she stayed mentally aware and had the pleasure of Brenda's sensitive care. Her strong determination and the support of those around her enabled her to do it her way. She chose life with daily pain and discomfort. Beulah chose hospice care, but every time a breathing crisis arose, she would change her mind and, by any means necessary, fight for her life, at any cost to the medical system and to the family. This came to about $100,000 in the last year of her life. I sometimes ask myself whether the last three years were an act of love and kindness or a waste of time and resources.

What did I learn about death and choice? I have seen many older people give up or not know how to find the resources they need. I have seen bitterness, loneliness, quiet despair, and depression. I have seen older people let things take their course without wishing to fight and others finding acceptance and peace. Some do not feel deserving of the care and attention that my mother expected and demanded. I know very few people able to experience the amount of choice in dying that Beulah experienced.

Mother-and-daughter relationships are at best complex. Mine was so often challenging due to my mother's demanding and critical nature, and my deeply felt sense of family responsibility. While still in recovery, in the end, I feel great comfort and pride that I was able to help create a way for my mother to live until the end of her life as she wished. In return, she gave me insight into human willpower as I witnessed her indomitable spirit and eternal passion for life.

NOTES

1. Although their names are similar, Medicaid and Medicare are very different programs. Medicare is an entitlement program funded entirely at the federal level, a social insurance focusing primarily on the older population. The Medicare Program provides Part A, which covers hospital bills, Part B, for medical insurance coverage, and Part D, which covers prescription drugs. Medicaid, on the other hand, is a needs-based social welfare program. Eligibility is determined by income. States provide up to half of the funding for the Medicaid program. In some states, counties also contribute funds and the rest is funded by the federal government. The main criterion for Medicaid eligibility is limited income; requirements differ from state to state.

2. The Elderly Pharmaceutical Insurance Coverage Program is a New York State–sponsored plan for senior citizens who need help paying for their prescriptions.

3. An emergency pack contains drugs that may be needed in the dying process. The hospice nurse trains the family in their use, and they are used by the family or caregiver with approval from hospice. Some medications in the pack are morphine drops, a morphine suppository, colace for easing the bowels, and epinephrine for easing the breathing.

E-mails to Family and Friends

Claude and Maxilla–Declining Gently

SARA M. EVANS

Introduction

From the summer of 2005 until the end of 2008, I stayed in touch with a growing list of family and friends as my parents weathered a series of health crises. At the time this chain of messages picks up, in October 2006, they shared a room in the nursing home at Givens Retirement Community in Asheville, North Carolina. Having arrived at different times, they were not in the same room initially. Their declines were a study in contrasts as my father (Daddy/Claude) slid gently into dementia, a state he was aware of and open about for several years before he lost the ability to communicate deeply. The mental faculties of my mother (Mama/Mackie/Maxilla) remained incredibly sharp while her body succumbed to lymphoma and heart disease (the latter probably caused by chemotherapy). Maxilla's story is in the foreground here as she accompanied Claude through his final months and learned to live with her own impending death by focusing on the joys of the present and making her own, clear choices. She had already declined further chemo and any invasive procedures related to her heart, but the need for decisions, as you will see, presented itself continually.

Maxilla's passion for the natural world was rooted in her childhood on a North Carolina farm. She had been an avid bird-watcher, a passionately self-taught botanist who led the creation of a public garden of native Appalachian wildflowers and shrubs at nearby Lake Junaluska, North Carolina, and a spiritual seeker who discovered her affinity for Quakerism after a lifetime as a Methodist minister's wife.

I write these e-mails from North Carolina, where we have a small house in Waynesville, and from Minnesota, which is our home base. Because I was writing to friends of my parents, who knew them as Claude and Maxilla (Mackie), I refer to them both by their given names and as Mama and Daddy. Others who show up frequently in this story are my brothers (and their wives) Claude, Jr. (Jill), Bob (Lisa), and John; my husband, Chuck, and my children, Jae and Craig, the only grandchildren. Dogs, cousins, and a variety of friends also appear, and my mother calls me by my childhood nickname, Peachie.

DATE: Wednesday, October 25, 2006, 10:20 PM
SUBJECT: Claude and Maxilla—another transition
Dear Family and Friends,

This morning Mama and I met with a social worker and two nurses from Care Partners in Asheville in order to arrange for Daddy's admission to hospice care. They were wonderful, of course, and we were comforted to learn about all the additional services Daddy will receive as a result (a nurse to check in one or more times a week, a chaplain who will visit, volunteers to offer "compassionate presence," and a music therapist who will play her guitar and sing to him, Mama, and whoever else is around). This decision comes because there has been a rather dramatic decline in the past two months such that Daddy rarely walks on his own, cannot feed himself, and doesn't communicate much at all (though there is no doubt that he continues to know us). All of us now believe that it is time to let him go, to stop whatever medications he is on that have the purpose of prolonging life, and to pay attention to his comfort on every level—physical, emotional, and spiritual. There is no immediate emergency, but at the same time it does seem that he is gradually shutting down. We have no idea whether we are talking about weeks or months, but we are definitely in a new stage.

Mama is handling all of this incredibly well. Hospice considers her their primary contact person and will keep her apprised of developments and include her in things like music therapy. That is especially wonderful since I think too often she feels that she carries little authority with the powers that be [in the nursing home].

After Mama and I talked with the staff about hospice last week and set this process in motion, I found myself immersed in yet another wave of grief. Daddy has been fading away for many years, so there have been many points of palpable loss. As a friend whose father had Alzheimer's said, "You lose them a thousand times." This is, however, a new level of letting go. It is a relief to be able to do something positive to provide comfort, support, and solace as Daddy moves through this transition. Several years ago, when he had a small stroke and thought that he might be dying, I learned that he is absolutely not afraid of death. It is a comfort now to know that he has faced this passage already.

DATE: Thursday, November 16, 2006, 9:39 AM

SUBJECT: Claude and Maxilla—hanging in there

This is a quick update now that we have returned home to Minnesota. We left Maxilla in high spirits. Over the course of several weeks she was able to participate in picnics in the gazebo at Givens, drive to see the fall colors, and take an outing to the top of Eagle Nest mountain with her grand-daughter, Jae, grand-puppy, Guy Noir, and family friends from Durham who took the attached photo. This fall she has had good visits with all of her children, which led her to remark one day, "I am having a great old age!" The election galvanized her into action to defeat her congressman, who has done great damage to the environment and especially the national park system (just ask her and she will tell you about it, chapter and verse). She walked the halls of the nursing home to locate and help eleven people of like mind get registered and submit absentee ballots. When the election went her way, she was jubilant and ever so proud of her contribution. Mackie's arthritis is increasingly painful, but in every other respect she continues to be amazing. We are making arrangements to get her a motor-ized wheelchair so that she can visit Daddy even on days when her knees and hands hurt too much to make the walk. It will also preserve her inde-pendence in many other ways.

Claude has good days and days when he seems barely there, because (as we now understand) his brain just doesn't get enough oxygen due to arteriosclerosis. Mama called last night to tell me that she felt he was very responsive yesterday. He smiled, gave her a kiss, and talked a lot though she understood none of it. My last visit with him was Monday. I woke before dawn, saddened by the knowledge that he might not know me on my next visit and pondering the admonitions from hospice that it is important to let those who are dying know that it is OK to go. Actually, this is something Daddy has done for many others. As recently as 2003, he stood by the bed of our beloved aunt, Mackie's sister Sue, and told her that everything was OK, that death is part of life, and that she could go, surrounded by love.

Flooded with memories of his bass voice offering prayers in church services, at family gatherings, and by Sue's bedside, I composed a prayer that echoed his cadences. Later that morning I read it to him and then left it nearby. He was aware of my presence, but had lapsed back into what seemed to be sleep, so I told him that I was going to read this and he could hear it wherever he was. As I started, his face filled with emotion, as if he would cry. I read and wept, and he continued to respond to each phrase, eyes open, looking directly at me. I stayed awhile longer and he stayed present. He even gave me a sort of a hug and growled the affectionate grumble that has always been his hugging sound. It was very sweet. I'll be back briefly in early December and hope to have more times like that with him.

As always, thanks for surrounding our family with love and support. There are now 70 addresses on this list!

CLAUDE'S PRAYER

O God—in whom we live and move and have our being—be with
    Claude on his journey.
Surround him with love.
Remind him that his family—Mackie, Peachie, Claude, Robert, and
    John—are with him in spirit and sending loving thoughts even
    when they cannot be physically present.
Show your face in the people who care for him so that Claude can
    know that he is not alone, that You are always there.
Comfort him, lift him up, and when the time is right, welcome him
    home.
In the name of Jesus who taught us that God is love.
Amen

DATE: Monday, December 18, 2006, 3:33 PM
SUBJECT: Maxilla—another scan

Mackie had another scan last week with mixed results. The Rituxan cleared up several tumors, but others have appeared in her chest in the meantime, so the doctor no longer sees it as useful. At first she felt she was up against another hard decision when the doctor suggested a chemo drug (etoposide) as a possibility. Naturally we all googled it immediately and were concerned about the side effects, and there was talk of second opinions, etc. As of this morning, however, she has come to a new clarity that leaves her feeling greatly relieved. First of all, we all understand that any treatment at this point is to relieve symptoms. No one is talking about a cure. Put that way, she is clear that she wants to wait until there are symptoms (fatigue and short-ness of breath) before embarking on any treatment, since at the moment she has none. When that time comes, she will consider taking this drug, which apparently has much milder side effects than most chemo. It may be that the most important thing at this point is that she is still really in charge. That gives the rest of us a clearer role to play as well. Our job is to make sure she is getting good information and then to back her up. In the meantime she is enjoying her room full of books and flowers and some very good days with Daddy. He is thin and stiff, but has had a number of times lately when he is alert and present.

This is the darkest time of the year, a time of letting go. It fits my mood perfectly. I remind myself that last year this time was also very dark and that we have had the gift of many good months in 2006. Most of all, the firm, upbeat clarity in my mother's voice (and the political cartoons she clips and sends) call me back into the blessings and tasks of the present moment. She is still my teacher when it comes to living peacefully with uncertainty. If she can do it, we can too.

DATE: Saturday, January 20, 2007, 5:34 PM
SUBJECT: Maxilla and Claude—living peacefully with uncertainty
When I went to Asheville early this month, everybody was amazed at how alert Daddy had been for several days. Mama had told me on the phone about the time he saw her coming down the hall and smiled, saying clear as day, "I'm glad to see you," as she approached. The next day he said, "I love you." These have become moments to treasure. No one knows why Claude's decline seemed to level off and even slightly improve, but the fact is that however prolonged the journey, he is still appropriately served by hospice. This time he still knew me, but no longer called my name. We are all very grateful that he is not in pain or even discomfort most of the time and that the staff minister to him with warmth and affection. They all call him "Papa."

Mackie continues her lively interest in just about everything. She sent me to buy two more violets in specific colors, knowing the day that the store's shipment comes and the selection is best. We went out to eat several times, with Claude, Bob and Lisa, several cousins, and other friends. At the moment the only obvious sign of lymphoma is some increased breathlessness and the fact that she sleeps a bit more—and she even does that with a certain zest and relish. Her clear decision not to embark on additional chemotherapy (a decision her physicians fully support) means we all face unknowns as this disease progresses, but I do believe that she is surrounded by people ready to do whatever they can to make sure she feels as well as she possibly can under the circumstances. In the meantime she mostly doesn't think about the future but continues to read, think, and revel in the beauty of her flowers. This past week she weathered a respiratory infection. Her voice still sounds a little croaky, but the antibiotics have done their thing and she is getting better every day.

I'll be back in NC in mid-February and will send an update then or whenever there is news to report. We are all aware of your ongoing concern and love and want you to know it makes all the difference.

DATE: Friday, February 16, 2007, 3:08 PM
SUBJECT: Claude and Maxilla—together again

Last weekend I spent three wonderful days with Mackie and Claude and can report that they are doing as well as they possibly could. Daddy—who turned ninety on February 5—continues to have times when he is amazingly alert and other times when he is deep inside himself. It is hard to see him in the latter state, thin and slack-jawed, not really asleep but not responsive either. We do know, however, that even at those times, he is aware of things around and within him. The most amazing affirmation of that was Saturday morning. He woke up from a nap, alert and talkative. Some of his words were crystal clear while others tumbled around in his mouth, emerging as mumbles that—I am sure—frustrated him as much as they did me. I asked whether I could read his prayer. "Certainly," he said. And when I finished he thanked me. Then he volunteered, "I've had a rough couple of days," clarifying that by saying his troubles were "not physical" mainly. "Emotional?" I asked. "Yes," he responded. So the day before, when I felt that I could not get through to him, he was feeling depressed. Mama was so excited about his alertness that she reached for the phone and got through to brothers John and Bob. Daddy clearly knew who was on the phone and was very pleased to hear their voices. He could greet them and respond appropriately to some of their queries.

He tried to explain to Bob about the bad days. I stepped in to translate, telling Bob what he had told me earlier about having a couple of tough days, not so much physically as emotionally, and looking to Daddy for affirmation about whether I was correct. "That's right," he said clear as day. He also still has his sense of humor. More than once he chuckled over something that struck him as funny. Mama reports that early on Saturday, when a nurse who was getting him dressed in the morning asked whether he could roll over, he replied, "If you pay me enough."

There is no way to know what precipitates good days and bad days. The biggest change in his life is that last Tuesday he moved to the other bed in Mama's room. I wondered whether just the change—confusing as it has to be when one's comprehension is so murky—could be depressing. Mama thinks not. Several times I said something about how nice it is to have them back together, and on that very alert morning his response was, "at last."

Mackie was more energetic than I had expected. She had been laid low for several weeks with bronchitis. We know there are tumors in her lungs, and we know that one of these days she will be tired and not get better. She was afraid of that I think (and I know I was), but lo and behold, she is better. Three days we went out for lunch, shopped at the nursery for just the color of violet she needs, and visited with friends. And every night she stayed up late reading the book she bought for me on the intelligence of dogs so I could take it home. Her capacity for joy is undiminished. But all this activity does make her tired, and then she heads for bed. Daddy's move was her choice. He is her fifth roommate in one year. Two previous ones died. The last one was extremely stressful, and the quick way to deal with that was to make a switch with Daddy who has had no roommate at all for a couple of months. The nursing staff understands that they cannot expect Mama to care for him in any way, and I think he no longer expects that. It helps Mackie not to have to walk a long hall to visit with him or know how he is doing. We talked about the fact that much as we know what is coming, there is grief lurking close to the surface.

If you call, be aware that sometimes Mackie has a hard time hearing well on the phone. She will be glad you called, but may not want a long conversation. She is also happy to have visitors, even though she tires after awhile. So, stop by when you are in the neighborhood.

I am grateful for the nourishing time with good friends in Asheville and Waynesville when I am there. It is always hard to leave.

DATE: Monday, March 26, 2007, 1:37 PM

SUBJECT: Maxilla and Claude—still amazing

Claude and Maxilla have two grandchildren, my son, Craig (38), and daughter, Jae (25), each of whom was able to visit them for a few days while Chuck and I were in NC over spring break. Mama had been managing expectations for a couple of weeks, warning me that she tires more easily. Yet she seemed not to flag when we brought her to Waynesville at least four times and took her out to eat several more. Grandkids, trout lilies, a waterfall full from recent rains, a tiny orange tree she successfully pollinated with a soft paintbrush so that BB-to-marble-sized oranges have begun to grow, Bob and Lisa's new puppy, and Claude and Jill's weekend visit—everything fills her with delight. But I also had the feeling that she is trying to line things up in her life, find the loose threads and put them in place. We laid plans for a ninetieth birthday celebration in mid-April. Since I returned home, however, she has had second thoughts, worried that it would be "pushing the river" to try to spend an afternoon socializing with so many people at once. Stay tuned on that one. It is her call. Currently she is dealing with an intestinal virus that started on Tuesday and was just beginning to abate by the weekend. At times like this, living in a nursing home, even a good one, is difficult and lonely.

Daddy was amazingly present on several occasions during our week there. Each grandchild had an afternoon in which he knew him or her and was clearly glad they were there. Those days were a kind of blessing.

DATE: Friday, April 20, 2007, 10:57 AM

SUBJECT: Maxilla and Claude—declining gently

Last Saturday we celebrated Mackie's ninetieth birthday quietly and wonderfully. A bout of intestinal flu had left her so weak that she didn't think she could handle a full-fledged party, so she spent a cloudy, rainy day with us on Eagle Nest mountain while a few of the people who currently maintain the Native Garden stopped by at different times for banana pudding and strawberry shortcake. Her energy level surprised us, as if the presence of people she loves is a source of energy in and of itself. And then she crashes—which is OK too. Two weeks ago after a wonderful visit with Bob, Lisa, and their three-month-old puppy, Belle, she reported that the puppy's friendly antics had lifted her up, leaving her happily exhausted (I'm tempted to say "dog-tired"). Those of you who live nearby should not hesitate to pay Mackie a visit for an hour or so. Right now she is helping to make arrangements for a bog garden to be installed at Givens by her friend Darwin, who specializes in insectivorous bog plants. She would love to tell you all about it. My husband, who shares her passion for living things and the natural world, wrote a poem that captures Mackie's serenity and capacity for joy at this time in her life. None of us (including her) can read it without weeping. (Her sadness, she pointed out, is not about fear of dying but about leaving the people she loves.) She kept a copy of the poem to re-read and share with friends.

Claude is a bit of a miracle, though thinner than ever. The nurses report that he simply doesn't want to eat much and his physician confirmed that he is in decline and probably has only a few weeks left. He knew me, however, and he knew my brother Claude on Saturday. In fact, when I walked in on Friday afternoon, he reached out his arms and wept. Was he sad or just so filled with emotion that it spilled over? A month ago he had told me he wasn't sure he would be here on my return. This time I reminded him over and over that I would be back in three weeks, hoping he can hold on until then. One of the most touching things right now is the way that Mama looks after him. She can't do much—and is relieved that they take him to the other end of the hall near the nurses' station for substantial periods of time—but she gently wipes his eyes to keep matter from drying and irritating them, checks at night to be sure he is properly covered, tells the nurses when he needs a haircut, and on Sunday sent me off to buy him some comfortable pants with elastic waistbands and a couple of long-sleeved shirts to protect his fragile skin. I think his great loneliness is over.

DATE: Monday, June 4, 2007, 1:14 PM
SUBJECT: Claude and Maxilla—surprisingly stable

We have been here for about a month now and, as you might guess from my previous note, I would not have expected things to be as stable as they seem to be right now. Daddy, in particular, started eating again, so his decline is slower than anticipated though it definitely continues. The lovely thing is that he still knows us, mumbles "I love you," and even laughs occasionally. Sometimes he seems to have a private joke. Frankly I think he is amused by his situation. In the days when he was falling so much, the nurses would admonish him—"That's not funny!"—when they found him on the floor, laughing. He would reply, "Yes it is." A couple of weeks ago we spent an afternoon in the garden, watching our puppy romp with AJ, the black lab that lives there. Daddy was in his wheelchair, not very responsive until Mama told a funny story on herself whereupon he suddenly cracked up. [The story: Michael, a nurse we like a lot, complained jokingly to Mama about another nurse who had not followed his instructions. To his rhetorical question, "Why is it that women never listen to men?" Mama instantly replied, "Why should they?" At the time, Michael also cracked up and gave her a hug.] Hearing the story, Daddy laughed for almost a minute. What a treat to see the grin spread across his face.

Mackie is still astonishing. She always manages expectations, warning me that she gets tired easily, sleeps a lot, etc. And yet in the presence of friends and family she summons up that old vitality again and again. I know she is aware that the lymphoma is there, and growing, and when we first arrived she had a sense of urgency about several day trips she really wanted to take as soon as possible. So, we went to the Native Garden at Junaluska, and lo and behold she walked it from top to bottom. Of course it was very slow, and not just because of the logistics (walker before, oxygen tank behind, various ones of us positioned to assist). Every other step there was a story: when she planted this or that, where it came from, why she had to order some things from a nursery, things that refused to grow where she planted them. A week after that she paid a last visit to her old house, knowing that we are readying it to go on the market. She had imagined that she would find that good-bye hard, but with the house so empty and clean, she just walked through and then back out. The path was more important. She needed to walk the level path to the stream, pointing out plants and telling stories as before and loving every minute. The most amazing day, however, was one we spent first with Bob and Lisa followed by dinner with friends and a spectacular Memorial Day concert by the Asheville Choral Society and the Asheville Symphony. The final piece, based on a text by Walt Whitman imaging the United States as a ship carrying the world's hope for democracy, moved her to tears. She did take a long nap in the middle of the day, but for the rest of the time she not only didn't flag but seemed radiant with pleasure whether the source was puppies romping, friends talking, or powerful music. At this point I guess we're just trying to pile on the good days.

DATE: Tuesday, July 10, 2007, 8:33 PM
SUBJECT: Maxilla and Claude—slowly, slowly
I have not written in awhile because there really is nothing dramatic to report. We had a wonderful eight weeks in the mountains including lots of

quality time with my folks. Claude, to our total surprise, continues to be alert from time to time. By the time we left, I could sense further decline, though he still knew me and responded with momentary enthusiasm every time I showed up. Much of the time, however, we could not tell how aware he was of our presence, and when he did talk mostly it was muffled. The hospice nurse reports that this week she found him alert and able to respond clearly to questions like "How are you doing?" "Fine," he said. The honest truth is that this long good-bye may be harder on those who love him than on him. One of his losses, however, is that staff turnover in a nursing home means there are fewer and fewer people there who remember him when he arrived. Those are the people who talk to him, "love on him," and call him "Papa." The newer ones, in Mama's observation, are more businesslike, doing their job but unaware of the funny, gentle person the others had come to love.

Mackie is more conscious than anyone else of the decrease in her energy level and her increased need for oxygen. She has some days when chest pain is severe enough to call for morphine. But then it goes away. Even so, she still has several times the energy of just about anyone else in that facility. When I called to report that we were home safe and sound, she said she had "big news." She had planted seven tomato plants, which she lovingly tends by carrying fertilizer water balanced on the seat of her walker out to pour on them every couple of days. But several suddenly wilted and a bit of research revealed that they have a fungus (luckily some of the others are resistant varieties). That connection with the world of living things is an amazing source of sustenance for her. The visits of friends are also important, so don't hesitate if you are nearby.

DATE: Thursday, August 30, 2007, 9:24 PM
SUBJECT: Maxilla in the hospital; Claude's slow decline

Maxilla is in the hospital tonight with a heart attack that her doctors are hopeful they can get under control. It started in the early hours this morning. At Givens they gave her nitro and then several doses of morphine before the pain abated. After that really rough night, Mama proceeded to get up, go to lunch, and even walk outside to pluck a tomato to give to someone, but she was obviously weak from the ordeal. It was lucky timing that she already had an appointment scheduled at midday with her cardiologist. He called me to say that he thought she had had a heart attack and needed to be hospitalized for observation, allowing quicker intervention to control the pain. Mama later told me she felt very pressured by him, but we all really like this doctor and in conversation with me it was very clear that he understands the larger picture and will honor her wish to avoid any invasive procedures. So, she agreed to go. Tonight it is clear that was a good decision as the pain has returned and they are giving her nitroglycerin and morphine through an IV. The doctor on duty told me that Mama's blood pressure is good (wow, for once her high pressure is helpful) and they believe they can get her through this and manage the pain. Bob will drive up tomorrow and others of us are on standby.

Daddy continues to fade. I was in Asheville earlier this month in the aftermath of what was probably another small stroke. After several days of nonresponse, suddenly he was there and even mumbled, "I love you." When (brother) Claude visited last week he was never positive that Daddy recognized him, though there were some responses. The really hard part is that Daddy now has bedsores, which chips away at the comforting thought that he does not suffer. Inside that shrinking body and foggy mind is a powerful will to live. It is hard to know what to pray for.

I will send frequent updates as Mama's situation unfolds. The first 24–48 hours after a heart attack begins are the most delicate. She is in good care and we are hopeful that she will soon be stabilized and able to return home.

As always, we are lifted up by the incredible circles of people who care so much for Maxilla and Claude. Thanks for being there.

DATE: Friday, August 31, 2007, 6:31 PM
SUBJECT: Maxilla—holding her own

Last night was rough again, but thank goodness Maxilla was in the hospital. Bob was with her today and I talked with her several times—her voice getting stronger as the day went along. But there is still occasional pain and breathing is hard after even slight exertion. We have no idea how much that is a consequence of the heart attack and how much it is increased by the presence of tumors in her lungs and chest. She told me that yesterday she had decided the bad night was over and life was back to normal until the doctor became insistent about hospitalization. Even now she keeps thinking they will send her home soon, but I suspect she needs to be pain free for some amount of time before that can happen. It is hard for all of us to accept the reality that this was/is pretty big and "normal" may be different from now on. Bob and Lisa will be back and forth this weekend. I plan to go on Tuesday, assuming things stay stable.

Thanks for being there.

DATE: Wednesday, September 5, 2007, 9:00 PM

SUBJECT: Maxilla and Claude—turns in the path

Last night, when I arrived at the hospital Mackie was sleeping peacefully, and she looked wonderful. All the old sparkly self is there, though she is immensely tired. We met with her cardiologist in the morning who said she could leave the hospital and suggested that we be in contact with hospice because her pain (both heart attacks and congestive heart failure) will probably increase. Mama strongly wanted to return "home" to Givens, so I spent much of the day verifying that protocols to control pain will be in place. Though the cardiologist initiated the hospice connection, Mama—as always—spoke for herself, telling the hospice social worker, "I want to sign up with your organization." The first step will be to involve hospice in palliative care. They will review her records and make suggestions related to comfort. Later Mama can decide to move to full hospice care if she has no more need for physical therapy or other kinds of rehabilitative support. All of this is just another step on the path she has been on for some time, though I think for those of us who love her—and who see her intermittently—it comes as a bit of a jolt. That path is full of twists and turns, despite any efforts to make it linear and predictable.

Just as we were beginning the process of getting Mama discharged from the hospital today, word came that Daddy had taken a sharp turn for the worse. The hospice social worker—who had visited with us in the hospital—called in the early afternoon from Daddy's bedside to say that the staff had gathered around him, determined that "Papa" would not be alone. That was the scene we came into around three PM—hospice and Givens staff holding his hands, talking to him, hovering. His breathing was very labored and his face was ashen. Five hours and several doses of morphine later, he is resting easily and his color is good. When I asked the hospice nurse whether we were talking about days or hours, she thought hours and then quickly said that many people don't follow the pattern.

With Daddy's will to live, we should not be surprised by anything. When you hold his hand, he grasps firmly, and he gives tiny but meaningful responses to words of greeting and comfort, so I think he knows we are here. It is good that Mama and Daddy are together now, even though Mama is too tired to do more than wave across the room. My children maintain that Daddy hangs on because he is waiting for Mama. Perhaps her sudden disappearance for six days has something to do with the coma he seems to be in now. Hold him in your thoughts and prayers and I will send an update in the morning.

With all of this, I can't tell you how glad I am to be here. I'll be sleeping in their room tonight. Bob will join us late, and Claude (Jr.) is driving up tomorrow.

Thanks for being there, dear ones.

DATE: Friday, September 7, 2007, 11:13 AM
SUBJECT: Claude—free at last

Claude passed on very peacefully at 7:45 this morning. Claude (Jr.) was by his side when he opened his eyes and then breathed his last. We sat with him for awhile before the funeral home folks arrived and have spent the rest of the morning telling stories and beginning to make plans. I told the local chaplain, who has been immensely helpful, that she could expect an ongoing mix of laughter and tears from this crowd. Mackie is doing very well, having long anticipated this release.

DATE: Tuesday, September 18, 2007, 10:31 PM
SUBJECT: Celebrating Claude

Last week we celebrated Claude's life twice. On Tuesday the 11th I wrote the following but forgot to send it:

> The service at the nursing home yesterday was quite wonderful. A number of residents, several friends who live nearby, and an amazing number of staff attended to honor "Papa." My brother Claude and I expressed the family's gratitude for the way staff treated Daddy with love, understanding, and affectionate good humor. They gave Daddy this final persona—"Papa."
>
> Mackie is incredibly weak, though she got through the service yesterday just fine and was glad to see and talk to people. I learned from my cousin Martin, who visited her in the hospital, that she was really angry at the thought that they were "treating" her heart attack.

Fact is they were just treating pain and I think he was able to convince her of that finally. Given how things have unfolded, I think she is glad she survived this round.

This is a deeply bittersweet time.

Then on Friday, September 14, we celebrated Claude's life at the First United Methodist Church in Waynesville with a service organized around his prophetic roles on issues of social justice, his powerful presence in many familial roles (son, brother, husband "Sugarbunny," father, grandfather, and uncle—it was telling that every living niece and nephew came as did three from Maxilla's side of the family), and his final gentle, funny, and occasionally stubborn persona as "Papa" in the nursing home. Claude Jr. told stories in a voice and with a presence so like Daddy's that it was eerie. For many South Carolina Methodists—especially ministers—Claude Evans was a source of inspiration and support because he raised issues and spoke forcefully on topics that others were afraid to touch, starting with race but extending to gender, reproductive choice, and gay rights. Breaking silence and challenging taboos, he opened doors. Si Kahn wrapped it all together with a song. He had the entire congregation singing the chorus: "People like you help people like me go on, go on."

Mackie seems a bit stronger this week. She was awesome on Friday, staying almost an hour after the service to greet people from many, many parts of her life. Yesterday and today we moved her to a single room much closer to her beloved tomato plant. It is much brighter than the other one and looks out into a garden. She is learning to use a motorized chair and will be really good at it soon. In the meantime, watch out. The hardest part is the knowledge that her heart is damaged, and that the lymphoma, which we know is in her lungs and chest, is showing up again at the original site. Lymphoma doesn't hurt. It just makes you tired and can make skin itch. The damaged heart means that her body can never catch back up to the strength of her spirit and hurts fairly often. But we have good procedures in place to deal with pain, and I cannot emphasize enough how caring the staff is here.

As I said in my Tuesday note, this is a bittersweet time. We were deeply touched by the many cousins and friends from far away who came to tell stories, laugh, and cry with us and to offer Mackie so much, much love.

DATE: Friday, September 28, 2007, 7:36 PM

SUBJECT: Maxilla—learning from Mackie (again)

As we all begin to adjust to the new realities, Mackie is showing us the way. In her cozy new room, she has learned to be self-sufficient—getting around in the room on her own and riding her motorized chair (she calls it her "electric chair") to the dining room for lunch and dinner. She greets visitors with genuine enthusiasm, manages a pile of reading material by her bed, and keeps adding to the list of stuff we need to do (tie up tomato branches, water African violets, shop for more file folders, etc.). The bereavement counselor from hospice found her happy to talk about Daddy and tell stories. [Like how they met: he arrived for a summer intern position at a tiny local church, driving up to their farmhouse where he would be staying. She and her brother were riding bareback on a horse they had trained to follow touch commands with just a halter, no bridle. Mama said she and Daddy became very friendly so fast that the family packed Mama off to spend the rest of the summer with her older sister in Pittsburgh. But no one could stop their correspondence or future dating since Daddy was at Duke Divinity School and Mama was at UNC State in Raleigh.]

Since she came home from the hospital, Mama has been on palliative care in order for Medicare to pay for her training to use the motorized chair. Now that that is completed, she is shifting to full-fledged hospice, which changes the kind of Medicare coverage, so yesterday we met with the hospice intake nurse. We were relieved to realize that in case of extreme pain they could transport her to the hospice facility that—I am told—is absolutely the best place for pain control. Throughout the interview Mackie seemed both lively and slightly disconnected, telling the nurse that she is doing so well she really doesn't think she needs all their services. When the nurse asked why she was referred to hospice, I was the one who had to recount the conversation with Dr. Lim in the hospital and to point out that she has two conditions—heart disease and cancer—that are progressive and untreatable. Later, in the car, she allowed as how she doesn't think about the fragility of her condition but interviews like that are a reminder. The other reminder is anytime she tries to walk more than about fifteen feet. But she can enjoy picnics in the garden at Givens and rides in the car, so I think we will just try to get her outside as much as possible.

All of this leaves me feeling somewhat schizophrenic. I am never unaware of her fragility and the shortness of time. But I admire her ability to focus on present joy rather than living under that cloud and I aspire to do the same.

DATE: Thursday, October 18, 2007, 10:07 PM
SUBJECT: Maxilla

In recent weeks there has been little to report. I know, however, that many of you are concerned about Maxilla's frail and deteriorating condition, so I thought I would send a quick update.

Mackie can still get around in her motorized chair and carries out her daily life quite independently. She sleeps a lot, but still likes to read and pass along articles she thinks will be of interest. Last week, after several days of visitors, the staff recommended to her that she request visitors to stay around twenty minutes and not a lot more. The fact is that she is genuinely having a good time, but then her chest begins to hurt. I doubt that she can bring herself to enforce this suggestion, but I know that all those of you who visit would want to know how to pace yourselves. Our cousin Ann Evans, who herself is a physician, wrote the following to the gang of Evans cousins a week ago after a brief visit:

> Larry and I went to Asheville yesterday, and took our "puppy," Hercules, along for the ride. He was the hit of our visit with Aunt Mackie/Maxilla/Maxie . . . demanded a head rub of gargantuan proportions. Our visit was short, as Maxilla was having some chest pain, that nitroglycerin did not quite relieve, so she had to take some morphine and rest quietly for a while.
>
> She is an eternally amazing lady. Her mind is as sharp as it has ever been, perhaps even sharper, as her wits have been honed by her recent travails. She has us all pegged, and knows more about human nature than most folks. It is only her body that is frail at the present time. She is facing the end of her life with equanimity and grace, something I hope to aspire to, someday. She made the comment that one of her relatives visits for a need of their own, and I realized that is why I visit, *I need* to. She is a great example for us all.

This week her pain has eased off, probably because of the recommendation from hospice to give her a small dose of morphine in the early morning and again in the late afternoon. She can wake up without arthritis pain and some of the angina is averted before it begins. All in all, the quality of her life continues to be as good as it can be under these circumstances.

As any visitor can tell you, Mackie's sense of humor remains intact. A week ago I was there late, waiting to go to the airport to pick up Chuck. At the airport I realized I had left my cell phone in her room so we drove back to look for it. The night nurse let me in and I tiptoed into her room. Suddenly she sat up and pointed to the bedside table. "You missed one call," she snickered. "I called to tell you that you left your phone."

DATE: Saturday, November 10, 2007, 2:39 PM

SUBJECT: Maxilla—highs and lows

Maxilla's African violets are blooming again. When she was hospitalized at the end of August no one watered them for a week and the flowers quickly wilted. For awhile Mama assumed that she was going to get rid of them since she is unable to water, prune, and cover them at night as she had done before. But visitors and staff pitched in to keep them damp, and lo and behold last week suddenly every plant was covered with buds.

That burst of color came just in time, as things have gotten more difficult for Mama in the past week. She feels weaker, and her breathing has become very labored. The trip from her bed to the bathroom leaves her gasping. The doctor believes that her low red blood count explains the breathlessness—there simply aren't enough red blood cells to carry the oxygen she needs—and has prescribed a drug that stimulates the bones to produce more of those cells. That is not a quick fix, however, and so far it is not producing results. Luckily the morphine they provide when her chest hurts (which is fairly frequent) does ease her breathing a bit. Mentally she is still sharp enough to be totally delighted when someone brings her a New York Times that she can spend the week reading from cover to cover.

Last night my sister-in-law Lisa called to say she had "googled" Mama and turned up a humorous piece she wrote in 1996 about living with an African Grey parrot. I attach two recent photos of Mackie. In the first she sits beside her magnificent tomato plant that flourished until the frost a few days ago. She has taken immense pleasure in giving away dozens of tomatoes and hoarding a few for her bedtime snack. In the second, taken about two weeks ago, she is communing with a pitcher plant the day her friend Darwin Thomas installed a large bog garden at Givens. The garden was her idea, brought to fruition in a three-way partnership with Givens (preparing the land), Darwin who donated his own labor and the plants, and Mama who paid for Darwin's expenses in creating the bog. I was laid up with back pain that week, but Chuck put her on his cell phone to tell me about it. "Peachie, I'm in heaven," she exulted. We can only wish for more of those peak experiences.

DATE: Tuesday, November 20, 2007, 9:11 PM
SUBJECT: Maxilla—weaker but hanging in there

In the past week Maxilla has become noticeably weaker. Sunday a week ago, and again on Wednesday, we took her out to eat with friends, and each time she surprised herself by going, unsure until the last minute that she could do it. Then on Thursday she really felt sick, slept most of the day, and was confused and anxious when she was awake. The nurses took it in stride, as her vital signs remained stable, seeming to assume that this may be the way things are now. By Sunday, however, she had rallied quite a bit. While she sleeps a lot and breathes with difficulty (and the doctor now thinks this is due to lymphoma), she is still reading and thinking and ordering things from catalogues so her children will have something from her at Christmas. I've been re-reading the booklet from hospice and realize that at least some of the time she is experiencing the changes they describe in the last months: turning inward, less eager to engage in conversation, sleeping a lot. Short visits are still important, but don't expect the exuberance she has been able to mobilize in the past. Sometimes she just needs someone to water her flowers, fill her water glasses, and carry away a bag of newspaper and magazines to recycle. Other times it is good just to sit with her when talking takes too much energy. Presence matters.

I am writing you from Minnesota. Chuck and I drove home yesterday and today as planned, but late last week when Mama was feeling ill, it was difficult to imagine leaving. I spent time talking to nurses and other staff about Mama's condition and was comforted by their commitment to doing whatever can be done to make her comfortable. By Sunday, not only was she doing better, but also I think she was conscious of wanting to make it easy for me to go. We spent some time with cousins in the afternoon, and then we tried out a Yoga Nidra relaxation meditation CD. As she hugged me good-bye she asked me to reset the CD so that it would repeat the meditation track we had done. I left her listening. Chuck and I will return in about three weeks. In the meantime, brothers will be visiting and friends will be checking on her.

DATE: Wednesday, December 12, 2007, 11:15 AM
SUBJECT: Maxilla—hard times, slightly better

A cousin wrote recently that my silence seemed ominous. There was truth in that, though I was reluctant to write mainly because I haven't been here in three weeks. Shortly after we left in November, Maxilla took a turn for the worse. She was not in pain, but she really couldn't breathe and had no stamina—a scary, panicky place to be. Even in the middle of that, she kept going about her business. One night she called and her voice made me crouch over the phone with anxiety, "Peachie (gasp)?" "Yes, Mama?" "A group I don't know has asked for money (gasp) and they have an address in Minnesota (gasp). Do you know about the Center for Victims of Torture? (gasp)." "Oh yes," I responded, grinning at the friends around a restaurant table. "That's a wonderful organization linked to the University of Minnesota." "OK (gasp). I'll write a check (gasp). G'bye." Click.

Once again, to her own surprise, she is better thanks to morphine every two hours around the clock. She still rides her "electric chair" to lunch and dinner and gets herself to and from the bathroom. She was well enough to relish a week-long visit from her youngest son, John—sharing meals, watching the news, just being together. She can enjoy short visits, but can't do much of the talking. Friends seem to understand that easily. One friend regularly comes for twenty minutes, tells her some stories, and leaves. Another just sits with her or warms her cold feet. Several cousins keep showing up, just to be here. Yesterday was so unseasonably warm, we even took a picnic to the patio outdoors where we could look at the mountain view.

Chuck and I had planned a five-day visit, but I find it impossible to leave just now. Mama is acutely aware of the reality she is living. She wants to feel better, but she doesn't want a prolonged decline. It was strangely comforting to her when I pointed out that the medicines are doing their job, but they aren't stopping, or even slowing, the underlying progress of her condition. I think she knows that we are all in this grace-filled limbo with her.

DATE: Thursday, December 13, 2007, 9:09 PM
SUBJECT: Maxilla—still in charge

Today Maxilla made some key decisions about her own life. Claude (Jr.), I, and my daughter, Jae, were with her when "Dr. Liz" came by. In the midst of a meandering conversation about what could be done to make her comfortable, Mama pointed out that she didn't want them to do anything to prolong her life. Dr. Liz then noted that Mama was still on a number of medications to control her heart condition, and if they were discontinued it was likely that she would have a heart attack before the lymphoma completely blocked her lungs. I think we were all surprised to learn how much heart medication she still was taking. Mama's response was crystal clear. She decided to end them. This will not be an overnight process. Dr. Liz tells us that some of the meds will be discontinued slowly, with attention to maintaining the highest possible level of autonomy and comfort. But we really are now at the beginning of the end.

Yesterday, Mackie spent the day with Jae and Claude, looking at birding books she had ordered for Jae, who lives on the Texas coast. For many years, when Mackie lived in Dallas, she made pilgrimages to the Port Aransas Refuge to see migrating birds and to count the whooping cranes when they returned from their northern nesting sites. Today, she gave Jae a set of binoculars, so that she can stop at that refuge (which Jae drives by every day on the way to her work with the Coast Guard) and learn how to look for birds. It was a beautiful hand-off.

I will send updates whenever there is a change. It seems appropriate that we are coming to the darkest time of the year.

DATE: Thursday, December 20, 2007, 9:29 PM
SUBJECT: Maxilla—finding Solace

This afternoon Maxilla moved from Givens to Solace, the hospice inpatient facility in Asheville. As always, it was her decision once Dr. Liz suggested that this was the best way to control her symptoms, especially breathlessness. We were lucky that a bed was available, and within hours they made the move. When the word got around, staff started showing up in tears. These are people who do their work well by loving the people they care for and then letting them go. I couldn't find words to tell them how much that has meant.

For several days it has been clear that the morphine doses they could give at the nursing home were just not sufficient. Too many times I had to go ask them to give her more. Too often, at night, she would be so breathless after going to the bathroom that she had to sit for 10–15 minutes on the side of her bed waiting to be able to breathe well enough to lie down. She never complained about this, but I witnessed it last Sunday night when I slept in her room to avoid driving home in the snow. Anyone who has had asthma knows the terror when you just can't get enough breath. For Mama it would come out not only in a need for medicine but in a generalized anxiety that latched onto whatever presented itself (Was there enough oxygen in her tank? Would they run out of morphine? Did she have enough Wite-Out to deal with the mistakes she made writing notes and checks?).

Solace is a good name for the wonderful facility where Mackie is now. From the moment she arrived she was enfolded in a community of care-givers whose sole purpose is comfort on every level—physical, emotional, spiritual. An incredibly kind doctor interviewed her immediately. Nurses began administering morphine every 15 minutes. The nurse assistant turned out to be Sheila, who had cared for Daddy at Givens, where more than once she had draped an arm around me as I walked out in tears dur-ing Daddy's long decline. She greeted us like long-lost family. I watched Mama relax as she realized she doesn't have to struggle anymore. Her fierce insistence that she must do for herself had diminished in recent days, with an accompanying anxiety about how much help would be there when she needed it. For the last few days, it has been hard for me to leave in the evening, aware than she was steeling herself to get through the night. Late this afternoon, however, she told me it was time for me to go and assured me that she didn't need me to be there every minute. What a gift, for both of us.

We will know a lot more in the next few days. I feel sure that Mackie is in the right place now. You can visit her at Solace, just don't stay long as she can't talk much without using up too much breath.

Tomorrow is the darkest day of the year. For Mackie we can hope that the worst is over, that she will not suffer in these final days or weeks. She is not afraid.

DATE: Saturday, December 22, 2007, 4:15 PM
SUBJECT: Maxilla—peaceful, slipping away

I know many of you are feeling anxious about this next stage of Maxilla's journey. I've had a hard time getting my mind around the change. Thursday she was in charge: making decisions, getting to and from the bathroom, drinking thirstily but carefully (swallowing had become difficult), making herself eat at least some of her lunch, and on arrival at Solace expressing her wishes very clearly to the staff (make me comfortable, don't prolong, I'm ready to go). Friday morning she was taking in no food or water and her con-sciousness had retreated way deep inside herself. When I arrived, I was shocked to find her mostly unresponsive, calm though her breath was labored. She did open her eyes, look at me, and smile—a wonderful echo of that radiant smile you probably know, but fleeting this time. The fact is, she had worn herself out struggling to stay strong and independent and to breathe. Once she found herself at Solace, she let go. "It's wonderful," she had whispered to me soon after she arrived. Last night Claude joined me in the vigil, and Bob and Lisa were here most of today. Mama labored to breathe through the night. She was alert enough to recognize Claude briefly in the early morning, but the price of alertness was just too high. We made it plain that comfort is our only goal now, and this morning they seem to have figured it out: just the right position to let her lungs drain and a much higher dose of morphine. Since then Mackie has been sleeping peacefully—more relaxed than I have seen her in many months. Time is short now, but she has her wish. She may just rest for awhile, or she may let go entirely at any time. Once again it is up to her. I will let you know when she makes the passage.

DATE: Tuesday, December 25, 2007, 11:41 PM
SUBJECT: Maxilla—free at last

Maxilla breathed her last just after 10 PM today. Her final days were very peaceful, with the help of an immensely skilled and caring staff at the Solace Center. We should have known that she would be a tough cookie to the end, confounding everybody, and then when we had stopped having expectations, suddenly she let go.

Last night five of us (me & Chuck, Bob, Claude & Jill) and Mama's friend Betsy had a wonderful Christmas Eve dinner here in Mama's room. Bob created a feast from the deli at Earth Fare (a lot like Whole Foods). We ate and told Mackie stories and laughed. It really did feel like Christmas Eve.

We will celebrate Mackie's life soon—Saturday or Sunday—and I will send a note out tomorrow, as soon as there are plans. She was so vivid, so recently, that the void we feel now is huge, but we know she is also in us and with us and we need to celebrate that together.

Love, Sara

Epilogue

Following Maxilla's death on Christmas Day, we celebrated her life in a service that honored her spiritual journey and her connection to the earth.

Our central symbol was dirt. Each of four speakers placed in a beautiful pottery bowl dirt from a key place in her life: the farm where she grew up (FedExed by cousins), the garden at Lake Junaluska, the bird pens by her house, and the glen below her mountainside waterfall. The following day we spread her ashes and some of my father's above that waterfall on a misty winter morning. As we did so, a pair of pileated woodpeckers flew to a nearby tree and then took off.

ʃ

Whose Death Is It, Anyway?

CAROL K. OYSTER

The Beginning

It was a nasty, icy morning in January when I drove my father for his first biopsy. I knew he would need someone to drive him home after the procedure, but I was very surprised when he asked me to drive him there as well. My father was very invested in control in all aspects of his life and it seemed uncharacteristic of him to relinquish the driving to me. Although I had just turned forty, having grown up primarily in Southern California I had only in the previous year done any driving in snowy weather.

We left with plenty of extra time to reach the appointment and I drove with the advice of a friend—"drive as if you don't have any brakes"—ringing in my head. My focus on the road kept me from making any small talk, or talk of any other kind. My father was equally silent, perhaps contemplating the ramifications of the possible results of the morning's tests.

We were within a mile of the office when we reached a long, curving, downhill stretch of road. Despite my cautious driving, about halfway down I felt the rear of the car start to slide sideways. In the futile gesture familiar to those who grew up in a pre-seatbelt era, I threw my right arm across my father's body. "It's going to be okay," I murmured repeatedly. I don't know whether I was referring to the road or the biopsy. I was right about the car, wrong about the test. That morning we began our descent down the slippery slope to my father's death.

My father died on November 21, 1996. He was seventy-six years old. His death certificate lists cancer as the cause of death, and at least indirectly this is true. But his death might be considered a suicide by some because he chose the means and timing of his exit. As his daughter and a participant in the drama I was too involved to analyze what was happening to my father and to the family at the time. As a social psychologist, with the advantage of hindsight, I can now see a number of interrelated issues that affected our journey: the decisions involved; the process of my father's death; and, finally, the aftereffects of the experience on the surviving family members' decisions and choices about our own deaths as well as the societally related impacts of our experiences with a planned death.

The Medical Progress

The diagnosis was prostate cancer. While this wasn't good news, I remembered having heard that in older men the condition was often not treated since they would almost undoubtedly die of another medical problem before the cancer became a serious concern. What I didn't know is that the younger one is at the time of diagnosis (and my father was sixty-eight), the more likely it is that the cancer is of a virulent type which is, indeed, a matter for serious concern. And that was the type of cancer that was growing in my father.

The progress of the cancer was not extraordinary. The first attempt at treatment was surgery to remove his prostate. Despite the likelihood of side effects from the surgery, my father just wanted the cancer out—a sentiment I completely understood. After the surgery, he told me that the doctors had told him they had "gotten it all." I don't know whether that phrase came from my father or from his urologist, but I've heard it since from others after cancer surgery. If it is an attempt on the part of the medical community to placate patients and their families, it strikes me as a very cruel illusion to foster. As our family found repeatedly, it only takes one residual cell to restart the nightmare, and the doctors can never know for sure whether they do in fact "get it all."

After the initial surgery began the anxious bimonthly ritual of the PSA blood test (protein-specific antigen tests provide an indirect measure of whether the cancer is still present or active). The first few were close to zero, very good news indeed. In fact, for over a year we lived with the optimistic illusion that perhaps the suspense was over—that Dad really was cancer free. Then the numbers started to creep up, and it became clear that further intervention would be necessary. Because prostate cancer cells are fueled by the sex hormone testosterone, in order to quell the growth of my father's cancer he would need another surgery—an orchiectomy—a surgical removal of his testes, better known as castration.

At this point, I expected that my father would consult with an oncologist—an expert in cancer care. He refused because he said he could find anything on the Internet that a specialist might know about his treatment. I guess I should have expected that reaction. My father was a physicist by training and by disposition. He demanded to be in control of everything in his life. All of his adult life, for example, he kept a daily graph of his weight, which he measured on a physician's scale. I suspect he felt he could have more power over the urologist than over a specialist. Unfortunately, the aftermath of this surgery demonstrated how totally out of control he truly was at this point.

My father was an old-fashioned man who was very conscious of and proud of his masculinity. He was now living with what must have felt to him like one physically feminizing indignity after another: first incontinence and erectile dysfunction, and then the physical changes that accompany an almost total loss of hormones. His skin softened as did his shape. His previously muscular chest began to develop breasts. Perhaps worst of all, he began to experience the same hot flashes that menopausal women experience. He also, for the first time in his life, began to read romance novels. When teased about this, his reaction made it clear that he was worried that he was losing his masculinity.

After several more years of relative complacency, the PSA numbers crept up again. A scan indicated that the cancer had metastasized to his bones. We were at the endgame. It had taken six years. He was advised to contact hospice care—which meant the physicians felt he had six months or less to live. My father made it clear that he was not willing to go through the pain that accompanies death from bone cancer. Even before he knew for certain his condition was terminal, Dad joined the Hemlock Society and began researching ways to die. He had decided to take matters into his own hands.

What Was He Thinking?

My father was planning to actively end his life. During this period (and after his death) the philosophical question has been whether or not that plan was justified. Did my father—and by extension, does anyone—have the right to choose death? Always? Under what circumstances? I needed to find out.

The very definition of suicide is more nebulous than it might appear. There is really no consensus. Is the act of a hero who gives her life to save another a suicide? If not, why not? What about the person who smokes heavily, knowing the probable medical ramifications? Both acts result in a death over which the patient had some control.

Margaret Pabst Battin, who has written on the ethical issues in suicide, reports that a generally accepted definition of suicide used by coroners who must attribute a cause of death is "any death in which the proximate cause of death is deliberately (not accidentally) inflicted upon oneself, whatever its moral character."[1] Under this definition, both the examples above and my father's death would be considered suicide. There is another consideration in the identification of an act as suicidal, which is the motivation behind the act. This separates suicide from martyrdom and differentiates the hero from the smoker. The individual who gives their life for another or for a "higher cause" is generally not perceived as negatively as the suicide. The soldier who throws himself on a grenade to save his fellows is considered in a very different light than a rejected, love-struck teenager who ends his life with a firearm. The moral evaluation of suicide seems heavily dependent upon the values of the individual passing judgment.

From my reading, I identified three perspectives that have been debated in this regard: religious considerations, general moral evaluations (independent of religion), and social arguments. In the Christian tradition, while suicide is not explicitly forbidden in the Bible, it is considered a sin. This judgment is based on the idea that our lives are not our own, that they belong to God. Squandering this gift will result in eternal damnation. Even suicide to escape suffering is considered sinful because of the Christian belief that suffering is a valuable experience.

Even beyond religious concerns, the morality of using suicide as a means of escape has been perceived particularly negatively. The position that suicide is a cowardly act dates back as far as the philosopher Aristotle, who said, "to die to escape from poverty or love or anything painful is not the mark of a brave man, but rather a coward."[2] That this position continues to be held was brought home to me recently during an episode of the television series *CSI*. The crime scene crew was trying to determine whether an individual who died after a fall from a building was a suicide or a homicide. When it was discovered that the jumper had been wearing his glasses, Grissom (the *CSI* protagonist) pronounced it a homicide because, he explained, suicides always remove their glasses before they jump since they're too cowardly to watch what they are doing. Escape from pain is considered a morally deficient act in individualistic cultures because of general notions, both religious and secular, that physical or mental pain may be strengthening or character-building.[3]

Social arguments against suicide are based on the individual's implicit contract with and obligations to society and its agents, such as the family. This contractually based position argues that the consequences of the suicide for others must be considered in the evaluation of the act. Without such consideration, the act of suicide can be perceived as "the ultimate expression of selfishness."[4] The individual has obligations not just to herself, but also to the society at large, and to her survivors. Society is damaged in that it is deprived of the individual's contributions. Suicide is an injury to friends and family in that it causes grief and deprivation.

Viewed from a religious perspective, my father's death would be seen as a suicide and therefore wrong. My father was not a religious man; I cannot recall his ever attending church. He would have been unmoved by arguments against suicide based on the position of any church. Suicide is, in fact, more common in individuals who are not conventionally religious.

He was, however, a profoundly moral man. To his mind, a promise was a promise, and honesty was obligatory—even when unkind or unwelcome. I (and I believe he) would argue that his act does not rise to the arguments that would classify suicide as immoral. Because he was dying, grief and deprivation on the part of the survivors (our family) was inevitable, regardless of when his death occurred. I believe he perceived his suicide as moral in that hastening his death would lessen the length of time that the family would suffer. An earlier exit would, of course, also shorten the length of his own suffering, so perhaps there was an element of selfishness to the act.

A defender of suicide, Ernest van den Haag, draws a parallel between suicide and consensual homicide.[5] Homicide, he argues, is wrong because of the lack of consent of the victim, just as rape is similarly wrong. Consensual sex, however, is (at least under many conditions) legal and acceptable. Suicide, then, is homicide with consent, which should render the act morally acceptable. Since the actor and the victim are one and the same, any punishment that should be applied to the actor is an inherent part of the act. I believe Dad would have liked this reasoning.

As to whether his act was cowardly or morally deficient, I could not disagree more. Elisabeth Kübler-Ross, who has studied and written on the psychology of death, points out that "in our unconscious we are all immortal."[6] At some level, none of us really believes that we will die. Ever. To not only recognize the fact of impending death, but to hasten it is, to my mind, courageous, rather than cowardly. It seems to me that it takes even more courage to choose the path my father chose—self-starvation—because it does not involve screwing up the courage for a single act, but requires the decision be repeated multiple times to stay on the path and achieve the desired end.

So I would argue that my father's decision was not only brave, but rational. The concept of suicide as a rational act is appealing to some and appalling to others. The issue that appears to separate the positions is a question not of the rationality of the act so much as of the impetus and timing of the act—whether the suicide is an impulsive or a reasoned, deliberate act, and the circumstances under which the act occurs. A teenager who shoots himself would then be considered irrational while my father's act could be considered rational. As Charles McKhann frames the issue, "The seriously ill person who anticipates a bad death but wishes to avoid unnecessary suffering has a completely different problem, and consideration of an earlier death may be totally rational."[7] He identifies the rational suicide as a choice made independently, without any coercion or pressure, by a mentally competent adult, in the absence of a treatable clinical depression. Not everyone, however, accepts that there are any circumstances under which suicide can be perceived as a rational act.[8]

My father made his choice over a period of years and actually was pressured not to suicide. As to whether he was depressed, I honestly couldn't say. I think my father was a depressive personality throughout his life. But as his emotional state impacted on his decision, it seems to me that depression was a rational reaction to his impending death. As I will discuss later, depression is considered a normal stage in reaction to dying, and my father clearly passed beyond depression to acceptance before he died.

When he died, my father had come close to the end of his anticipated life span. Even without the cancer, he did not have a reasonable expectation of many more years. And with the cancer now metastasized, he had the expectation of approximately six months, months he anticipated would be filled with pain and suffering. Similar considerations appear to be among the reasons that the elderly have the highest suicide rates in our culture.[9] While the elderly represent approximately 12 percent of the population, they represent approximately 20 percent of the suicides. Between 60 and 85 percent of elderly suicides share with my father the fact of significant health problems. And in 80 percent of such suicides, poor health was at least a contributing factor. Under those conditions, isn't suicide a rational alternative?

As to permission, it strikes me as an act of overwhelming selfishness on the part of family members to demand that a loved one extend their suffering simply to give the family member more time. I also believe that an anticipated suicide might have positive effects in that it increases the potential for allowing the family time to adjust. It allows the dying person and family members time to take care of loose ends, to say the things that need to be said. A lot of preparatory grieving can take place before the actual death. Physician Sherwin Nuland states that "taking one's life is almost always the wrong thing to do. There are two circumstances, however, in which that may not be so. These two are the unendurable infirmities of a crippling old age and the final devastation of a terminal disease."[10]

Despite the commonly held notion that medicine can successfully deal with all physical unpleasantness, not all pain can be controlled. Opponent of suicide Ira Byock, a member of the Academy of Hospice Physicians, concedes that pain control is unsuccessful with some terminal patients.[11] His suggested response is to place these individuals under general anesthesia until they die. In 1990 the National Hospice Organization stated that this period of medical limbo can be beneficial for the families of the terminally ill in that it allows them time to prepare for the death and that this period of unconsciousness is "less of a burden to the family and the caregivers than having to *directly cause* death as the only way to relieve the patients' suffering" (emphasis mine).[12] I can only imagine the horror my father would have felt at the idea of being drugged out of consciousness until he died "naturally." I will discuss the other alternative, someone providing assistance (directly causing death, to paraphrase the hospice group), later. While suicide is no longer illegal, assisting anyone with their suicide is illegal in all fifty states (except the states of Oregon and, recently, Washington, where physician-assisted suicide is legal).

Our family found that even though, in the abstract, most of us agreed with the concept that people have the right to choose when to die, when it was real, when it was a member of *our* family, suddenly the issue became far more complex and troubling. We avoided confronting the idea head on by focusing on the details—what is referred to in the psychological literature as "trivializing." Instead of discussing the larger issue, we argued about the other aspects of the decision, such as the timing. Over time, every family member did come to accept that Dad had the right to end his life, though some far later than others.

We are not alone in considering suicide a right. Philosophers from Cicero to Seneca to Rousseau have acknowledged that, under certain circumstances, the individual has a right to commit suicide. As Cicero eloquently stated, "An actor need not remain on the stage until the very end of the play; if he wins applause in those acts in which he appears, he will have done well enough. In life, too, a man can perform his part wisely without staying on the stage until the play is finished."[13] In fact, there is even a conception of the right of suicide as requiring that others "at least where they can do so without serious risk to themselves and without violating other moral canons, are to assist in the exercise of that right."[14]

Decisions, Decisions, Decisions

Suicide entails more than a single decision. I should have known that. I was trained to deal with suicides on help lines and I knew the series of questions to ask to ascertain the seriousness of the caller's intent. But, in my father's case, I was still taken by surprise. The planning process took on a macabre likeness to the preparations for any other life-changing event, such as a marriage or the birth of a child. But those events signal the joyous start of a new life chapter. This would represent a beginning of sorts for the rest of the family although certainly not a joyous one, because Dad was arranging for his death.

The central decision, of course, was the actual decision to die. Dad was terminally ill, so in this case it was clearly an issue of when and not if, and we were still reeling from that fact. But there were major disagreements among us about whether he had the right to decide *when* he would die. The family was scattered across the country so there were long telephone conversations between pairs of us, and, for some of us, with Dad, about timing. What obligation did he have to the family in deciding the timing of his death? Almost all the remaining family members have birthdays between Halloween and

Christmas. Knowing that the date of this death would always be a grim anniversary, did he have an obligation to avoid dates that were important to the rest of us?

The decision to die changes the lives of all family members. Upon my father's death, everyone's role in the family would be altered. Of the survivors, my mother would experience the most profound changes. Her role would shift from that of a wife of fifty-four years who had been totally financially supported, to that of widow alone for the first time in her life. She had never lived on her own. The rest of the family lived various distances away, so she would have no one nearby to count on for help. Clearly this was a very frightening prospect for her. My siblings and I would lose our father, and our children would lose their grandfather—in the case of my daughter, her only grandfather. None of us wanted to face these changes any sooner than we had to.

The question of timing became a source of contention in the family. A lot of the disagreement was associated with the place each of us had reached in the process of accepting the inevitability of Dad's death. Although he had talked of the possibility beginning shortly after his first surgery, I don't believe my mother realized he would really choose to die until the day he stopped eating. My sister kept telling him it wasn't time yet. He did not appear to be in pain, and my brother's first child was due at the beginning of the next year. Why not wait? My brother and I both felt that only Dad would know when the time was right. It was, after all, his decision, his death.

The decisions just kept on coming. Beyond my father's decision to die and the decision as to when to die, there were decisions involved with the choice of the method of suicide. What materials would he need to acquire to accomplish his death? Would he need help either in acquiring these materials or in implementing his plan? Who would participate? How? What role (if any) do others have in the decisions involving implementation? How much input should the family have in the choices involved? Do family members have an obligation to facilitate a loved one's decision to die? What risks would family members be exposing themselves to if they did help?

The reality was, clearly, that my father was going to have to act alone. Why should he have had to end his life on his own, particularly if he has the inalienable right to commit suicide? Because in the United States, assisted suicide is a crime. No one, not family members or physicians (except in Oregon and Washington), can aid the suicide without fear of arrest. The actions of Dr. Jack Kevorkian, a Michigan pathologist who developed a suicide device and assisted over 130 people in ending their lives, resulted in his 1999 conviction on charges of second-degree murder and delivering controlled substances, and his subsequent incarceration.

As early as 1906, the Ohio legislature defeated a bill intended to legalize euthanasia (for those individuals who wished to die). The resistance to the concept of anyone assisting in a suicide, particularly physicians—those who would have the highest probability of facilitating a humane exit from life—is based on concern that such permission would be the beginning of another slippery slope, one leading to the killing of people who are deemed *by others* as needing to die (e.g., those individuals with disabilities). The concern is based on anxiety about coercion. Individuals with disabilities worry (perhaps with some justification) that their lives might be judged by others as having no value. The elderly might be particularly vulnerable to coercion from family members who want to avoid financial and emotional depletion waiting for the elderly relative to die. The Hippocratic oath, taken by physicians, states they should do no harm. As long as suicide is perceived solely as harm, and not an act of mercy, physicians may not help.

Physician Timothy Quill has set out a list of criteria that he feels should alleviate these concerns and allow physicians to assist someone to a welcome death. These criteria include a clear lack of coercion as evidenced by repeated, clear, independent requests by the patient; a demonstrated ability on the part of the patient to make rational judgments; the presence of a condition that is terminal and carries with it serious, constant, unbearable suffering; and validation of all the above.[15]

Why does Quill speak only of physicians? Because the average layperson lacks the resources and the knowledge necessary to make the death as comfortable, certain, and kind as possible. Due to the fact that physicians are not involved in assisting suicides, there are a large number of unsuccessful attempts that succeed only in injury and intensified suffering rather than a release. And certainly because loved ones cannot be involved, self-suicides are isolating and lonely.

My father's preferred method of suicide would have been something he could do alone. But as he investigated the options available, he was understandably concerned (as he told me the last time I saw him) that such an effort would not actually be lethal. Of the options he felt were still available to him, his first-choice method would have involved the participation of another. The Hemlock Society bible, *Final Exit* by Derek Humphry, recommended eating a pudding heavily laced with barbiturates.[16] In case that was not fatal, it suggested that a plastic bag be placed over the individual's head after he or she lapsed into unconsciousness (as was done by the Heaven's Gate cult). Dad asked my mother to help. She refused, which led to a heated exchange between them. At this early stage she was unwilling to consider that Dad would actually commit suicide. She certainly could not imagine being a part of the act.

Dad also considered a number of poisons and medications, but was unable to obtain what he needed. What he apparently didn't consider, however, was using the firearm in his dresser drawer, the method of choice of the "typical" elderly male suicide.

Finally, he decided he would simply stop eating and drinking. His research indicated this would be relatively quick (he estimated a week but lasted three) and painless (fortunately, this prediction proved to be absolutely true). This method would obviate the need to actively involve anyone else. It would also give him control of the process by making an ongoing series of decisions to continue on his course. I believe that for him the gun would simply have been too easy.

The Psychology of Dying

Physician Elizabeth Kübler-Ross described the psychological stages that individuals pass through as they approach death.[17] Not all patients complete the series, but the research shows that those who do are likely to experience a more peaceful death. The first stage involves the use of the psychological defense mechanism denial and also isolation. In this first stage patients refuse to accept that the diagnosis is correct, or that the prognosis associated with the diagnosis is correct. They may even insist that the physician has looked at the wrong chart. They could not possibly be dying. As Kübler-Ross states, "it is almost inconceivable for us to acknowledge that we too have to face death."[18] This is usually a temporary stage.

When denial is no longer a possibility, patients enter the second stage of the process. This phase involves anger, rage, envy, and resentment. And no one is spared the role of target. Patients rage against the medical establishment, family and friends, and even God. Patients are outraged that others will be going on with their lives when their own is drawing to a close. They are furious that God should take them when others, who clearly in the patient's mind are less deserving of life, should live. They are jealous and envious of those lives that will continue. This stage can render patients particularly unpleasant company. In fact, Kübler-Ross's initial interest in working with the dying was based on her observation that in hospitals the closer the patient is to death, the more infrequent the visits to the patient from anyone—including physicians and nurses. Her identification of this stage of the process makes that avoidance understandable. Who would want to visit a person who not only is going to excoriate them, but also might throw a bedpan?

I also believe that the dying patient in the anger phase evokes guilt in the observer. The patient blames the observer for living on—something for which she or he is not responsible. Also, the patient's anger may kindle reciprocal anger, which makes the nurse or family member feel guilty. How can one harbor angry feelings for a person who is in the process of dying? What kind of person feels that way? The answer, of course, is everyone.

The third stage involves an attempt to bargain one's way out of the dying process or to prolong life as long as possible. Kübler-Ross describes the case of a woman who desperately wanted to attend her son's wedding, although she was not expected to live long enough. With a lot of medical preparation she was able to attend the wedding. When she returned to the hospital, she reminded the staff that she had more than one son! Apparently she felt she could bargain with God, or fate, or the physicians, to again extend her life.

Depression is the next stage in the process of reaction to impending death. Patients are no longer able to maintain the fiction that this is somehow a mistake or that they can alter the course of the approach to death. There is also an element of preparatory grief. While loved ones are being forced to accept the loss of the patient, the patient must grieve the loss of everything and everyone. And there may be what Kübler-Ross refers to as "unrealistic guilt or shame."[19] Patients recognize that their death may be inflicting pain and hardship on those left behind. They may be leaving children with a single parent, one of the many emotional problems their death might create for those whom they love the most. And they may be concerned about the financial burden their end-of-life care may be inflicting on the family and the loss of income their death might cause the family.

The final stage involves acceptance. This is not an emotional stage. It is not a sad resignation, but rather is almost emotion free. During this stage the patient begins to detach from the physical and emotional world. It is often the family members of the patient who need the most support during this stage, as they often do not understand or cannot accept that the patient is pushing them away and slipping away emotionally before the actual death.

Psychologists now know that it is not only the dying individual who traverses these stages; family members (and friends) also make this journey. As a family, we lived through the stages at very different rates and our individual progress through the stages affected our relationships with each other and, inevitably, with Dad.

I believe that Dad moved past the stage of denial much more quickly than any of the rest of us. My mother managed to stay in this stage until several days after Dad stopped eating. Throughout the process she kept an attitude of unrealistic optimism about the ultimate outcome. While she appeared to understand that Dad had terminal cancer and had even requested she assist in his suicide, she never seemed to really get it. She felt that this was not really going to happen.

I quickly moved into the anger stage and stayed there for a very long time. I was angry at everyone, including Dad. In particular, I was angry because I felt he had not sought appropriate treatment. I am embarrassed to admit that a good part of our last weekend together consisted of me berating him for not doing everything he could to stay alive.

I believe my sister demonstrated the bargaining stage the most clearly when she tried to convince him to stay alive until after the birth of my brother's first child. She kept saying it was "too soon" to stop living. She tried to give him a goal, something to live for.

I cannot remember instances of the depression stage in any family members. Certainly we were sad when we weren't being naively optimistic or angry. But I cannot recall specific examples. Communication among family members was not optimal during the time my father was dying, partly because of the geographical space between us, partly because of the psychological distance. Perhaps we just kept our depression to ourselves.

Dad himself reached the acceptance stage first. One of the hallmarks of this stage is tying up loose ends. I knew he had reached this stage when he refused to talk to me on the phone in mid October. We had said our good-byes—any further contact would just reopen a closed book. After his death, we found that around this time Dad had created a stack of folders for Mom to examine after his death. They included, in the order they should be handled, all the information about his cremation, interment, insurance, and annuities—complete with contact names and phone numbers. He also purged all of his work-related files and his closet. He had come to terms with his death and done everything he could to make it easier for the family after he was gone. And perhaps these were some of his final opportunities to exert control.

Early in the summer of 1996, my father asked those of us living distances away to visit one final time. I didn't make too much of the date. All three of his children have lives that revolve around unique calendars—my sister's and mine around the academic calendar (my brother-in-law and I are college professors and my sister and I had children in school), and my brother's around the symphony season (he is a musician). I immediately made plans for my daughter to visit alone. I was still so angry at my father for what I felt was his mishandling of his treatment that I initially refused to visit. Almost as soon as I put my daughter on the plane I realized how foolish I had been. I was glad, however, that my daughter and I would spend time with my father separately. He was her only grandfather and they had quite a close relationship. At ten years of age, she didn't quite understand what was going on, although she was aware that her grandfather was ill. She didn't need to have my rage distracting from or interfering with their final time together.

When it came time for my visit, I felt like I got off the plane shouting. I screamed at my father for probably the entire first day I was at my parents' home. I attacked him for being so pompous that he would believe he knew better than physicians. I shouted at him about pretty much everything. And, much to my surprise, he took it. He didn't defend himself or respond angrily. He just sat there and took it. He had clearly advanced further than I had in accepting his death.

I finally ran out of steam. The next few days were a fine way to say goodbye. I baked him a pie—my own special recipe—which he pronounced the best apple pie he'd ever tasted. We baked chocolate chip cookies together. We had done that since I was a very small child. The ritual involved eating some of the dough before the chips were added, eating some dough with chips in it, and eating some chips. When I was a child we sometimes had only enough dough remaining for one or two cookies—so we ate that, too.

On the morning I was to leave, we left my mother at home, much to her chagrin, and went out to breakfast together. It was there that we finally spoke about the reason I was visiting. He told me he hadn't settled on a method, but was considering checking in to a hotel without telling my mother and ending his life. I told him I thought that was unfair for a number of reasons. First, he would involve innocent bystanders. Someone would find his body. Second, I felt it was unfair to Mom for him not to be honest with her.

I asked whether Mom really understood what he was considering. He said he didn't think she did. I told him he simply had to sit her down and make sure she realized that he was serious about ending his life. I told him that if he didn't, I would. (As it turned out, I was the person who ended up having that conversation with Mom.)

I asked what methods he was considering. He was still unsure because he had been unable to acquire a sufficient supply of any drug that would prove lethal—and he knew the inherent uncertainty associated with drug-induced death. I offered to bring him some poison. Dad was adamant in his refusal. He did not want to take the chance that the poison would be traced to me and I would be arrested for his murder.

Finally, we just reminisced about family matters. We talked about my daughter and their wonderful relationship. We stayed away from anything negative. I think we both knew that we were, in effect, saying good-bye. As my taxi pulled out of their driveway to take me to the airport, I knew, with a lump in my throat, that I would never see my father again. I was so grateful that I hadn't let my own issues prevent us from spending some last time together with all of our problems, if not totally resolved, at least no longer standing between us.

The Physical Process of Dying

Eventually Dad chose to stop eating, on November first. I think he chose that date to honor my request about the holidays. He didn't want to wait until after the first of the year and take the chance that he would be too far into the process of dying, either in too much pain or having advanced to the point where he could not carry out the act. He lived a lot longer than he expected to, lapsing into a coma on November 20, my sister's birthday. That he did not die until the next day was, I believe, an act of will on his part to honor my request.

Dad ate his last meal on Halloween, 1996. At that time hospice care was already in place, which presented a problem. Paradoxically, while the hospice movement and hospice care are intended to help the patient die, they sometimes don't or can't help in the way the patient needs. They provide physical and emotional care to the patient and support to the family. What they are often not prepared to do is help in the process of suicide. This is clear from the fact that the National Hospice Organization endorses placing the dying patient into a "peaceful pharmacologically-induced sleep" until the patient expires "naturally" rather than assist the process of dying in any way.[20] In fact, the discomfort with suicide goes even farther. "We are instructed that if a hospice patient has a firm plan for suicide, we absolutely must intervene," states a hospice nurse.[21] Unfortunately the hospice group working with my father shared these anti-suicide sentiments.

Once the hospice workers realized my father had a very firm plan, they began to try to undermine his intent. They told him that what he was doing would result in unnecessary suffering, that starvation and dehydration is a terrible way to die. They began trying to persuade him to drink "just a little water" or to eat a banana to prevent cramping from potassium depletion. As he remained adamant, they cut back on their visits, somehow forgetting that my father was not the only patient. My mother needed help she did not receive.

Were the hospice workers correct? Is starvation and dehydration a terrible way to die? My father's research had certainly indicated that was not true. And research published in medical journals supports this contention. A study my father might have read was published in the *Journal of the American Medical Association*.[22] It followed thirty-two terminally ill patients through the process of their self-selected death by starvation. They did receive palliative care (mostly medication for pain—as did my father). Sixty-three percent reported experiencing no hunger. Thirty-four percent reported no symptoms of thirst or dry mouth. And a remarkable 84 percent rated themselves as comfortable. In a study reported in 2003 in the *New England Journal of Medicine*, nurses rated patients in the process of self-starvation.[23] They reported that the patients suffered little pain, were peaceful, and experienced a high quality of death. That is certainly reassuring. Why should it be true?

Self-starvation, whether by abstaining from food and hydration or by the removal of a feeding tube (formally known as artificial nutrition and hydration—or ANH) results, within twenty-four hours, in a bodily process known as ketonemia. As the body is denied outside nourishment, it begins to break down body fat, which results in an increased production of ketones, which suppress hunger. If a patient is receiving appropriate medication to manage the pain of his or her disease and is not hungry, it seems reasonable to me that death might be peaceful and have a high overall quality.

My father's research had led him to believe that he would last slightly over a week after he stopped nutrition and hydration. He was wrong. He died three weeks later. However, he was only actively dying, from my perspective, the last two days. Before that time he was conscious, he was conversational with my mother, and, even as late as November 19, he still managed to get out of bed to add the final data points to his weight graph. Within twenty-four hours after that, he was unconscious.

My mother called me around 6 PM on the evening of November 21. She was alone with my father, and his breathing, she said, was "funny." She either didn't understand that this indicated imminent death, or her denial was making a reappearance. I asked her whether she wanted Dad to die in their bed or in a hospital. She was firm that she didn't want him to die in the bed where she would continue to sleep. If that was the case, I said, she should hang up the phone and call an ambulance immediately. She wanted to talk, perhaps believing in her denial that she could delay the inevitable. I got my then-husband on the line and explained to him what was going on. He also realized the end was very near. When he told her she needed to call an ambulance *now*, she hung up.

The next call came about 8 PM. My father had died in the ambulance on the way to the hospital. The long odyssey was over for him. My mother sounded dazed. Fortunately she had called a friend who would spend the night with her. Mom wondered aloud what would happen to her—she hadn't yet encountered Dad's final gift, which was on his desk, the stack of folders that would walk her step by step through the process of making his death official. But surely she meant more than logistical details. For the first time she would face life alone.

Aftershocks

As can be predicted, my father's death has had profound effects upon each family member. One of these has been our own decisions about personal end-of-life choices. My brother and sister and I have all made our own wishes known to the rest of the family. I have been clear that as soon as I am no longer "me"—when I can no longer think, interact with people, or eat without benefit of a tube—I want my body to die. While I do not know what my siblings have done, I have completed a living will and a medical power of attorney making my wishes formal and binding.

My mother surprised us all. Even after fighting my father's plans to die, when she began her final decline from Parkinson's disease, my brother, her executor, found a do-not-resuscitate order and an advance directive in place requesting that she not be subjected to artificial nutrition and hydration. I find it ironic that after fighting my father so hard, in the end she died the same way he did.

I found that the experience of my father's death strongly affected my reactions to events in the news. When the Terry Schiavo case was a topic of national debate, I found myself shouting at the television on more than one occasion. While the situation was not entirely parallel to my father's case (since it was her husband who was carrying out what he believed would be her decision to end her life), all of the debate, the frantic attempts to use the legal system to aid both sides, and the discussions about how cruel and painful her death by starvation and dehydration would be made me irrationally angry.[24]

My father's death was neither of those things. Yet the strength of my emotional reaction indicated that there was something not quite resolved. Clearly the case was evoking a state of cognitive dissonance in me. I had no sympathy whatever with what I perceived as her parents' attempted interference. I could not hear their claims about the agony she would suffer if food and nutrition were removed. If I believed that this type of death was agonizing, what kind of daughter would that make me to have allowed my father to die that way? I do not think I could have changed my father's mind if I had wanted to. But the important fact is that I didn't want to, any more than I would want anyone to interfere with my end-of-life wishes. And I think it frightened me to see a family try to keep someone alive for what I perceived as their own selfish reasons.

I also found that for a period after my father's death I was very selective about whom to tell how he died. I shared the fact that he had died. I mentioned he had cancer. But I did not tell many people that he had deliberately ended his life. I felt very protective of my father. I saw it as none of their business. I didn't want anyone's disapproval of his choice to diminish the loss I had experienced. And I certainly did not want to hear anyone call my father a coward.

I admire my father for his death as much as for anything he did in life. To me, he made a courageous, difficult choice. He took the time to make sure that the rest of us would be all right after his death. He faced down the inevitable fear of death for twenty straight days without flinching.

I always thought that I wanted to die quickly and unexpectedly, as in a car accident or by a fatal stroke while standing in front of a class. Perhaps that shows my selfishness since both involve other people, but in either case I wouldn't have to die alone. Since my father's death, however, I'm not so sure I want a dramatic, surprise exit. The time to tie up the loose ends, to say good-bye, and then the ability to put the period at the end of my life myself is very appealing. In the meantime, I have come to believe in the cliché that exhorts us to live every day as if it were our last.

A tiny part of me is still holding out for immortality. Since I realize that's neither likely nor even very desirable, I'll settle for savoring the time I have. But at the end, if faced with circumstances similar to those my father faced, I hope I have the courage to follow in his footsteps. After all, when everything is said and done, it was his death, as mine will be my own.

NOTES

1. Margaret Pabst Battin, *Ethical Issues in Suicide* (Englewood Cliffs, NJ: Prentice-Hall, 1982).

2. Quoted in ibid., 58.

3. Ibid.

4. Joni Eareckson Tada, *When Is It Right to Die? Suicide, Euthanasia, Suffering, Mercy* (Grand Rapids, MI: Zondervan; San Francisco, CA: HarperSanFrancisco, 1992).

5. Ernest van den Haag, "Why Does Suicide Have a Bad Reputation?" *Chronicles* 8 (1998): 20–22.

6. Elisabeth Kübler-Ross, *On Death and Dying* (New York: Simon & Schuster, 1969), 55.

7. Charles F. McKhann, "Suicide Can Be a Rational Act," in *Why Suicide? Answers to 200 of the Most Frequently Asked Questions About Suicide, Attempted Suicide, and Assisted Suicide*, ed. Eric Marcus (San Francisco: HarperCollins, 1996).

8. Adina Wrobleski considers the idea of suicide as a rational choice to be "a contradiction in terms—an oxymoron" (39). She argues that the survivors (family especially, but also friends) are blamed for the act. She continues that the survivors "certainly did not give permission for the devastation of their lives" (42). Finally she reveals that her experience with the matter was the unexpected suicide of her twenty-one-year-old daughter. Her words and ideas do sound like those of a wounded, grieving mother. She had no warning, no chance to try to intervene. She had every reason to expect that her daughter had many more years of life. Adina Wrobleski, "Suicide Is Never a Rational Act," in *Why Suicide?*, ed. Marcus.

9. Geo Stone, *Suicide and Attempted Suicide: Methods and Consequences* (New York: Carroll & Graf, 1999).

10. Sherwin Nuland, *How We Die* (New York: Knopf, 1994).

11. Ira Byock, cited in Stone, *Suicide and Attempted Suicide*, 98.

12. Stone, *Suicide and Attempted Suicide*, 99.

13. Quoted in Battin, *Ethical Issues in Suicide*, 177.

14. Ibid., 181.

15. Marcus, *Why Suicide?*

16. Derek Humphry, *Final Exit: The Practicalities of Self-Deliverance and Assisted Suicide for the Dying* (Eugene, OR: Hemlock Society, 1991).

17. Kübler-Ross, *On Death and Dying*.

18. Ibid., 55.

19. Ibid., 98.

20. Stone, *Suicide and Attempted Suicide*, 99.

21. Ibid., 98.

22. R. P. Mogielnicki, J. L. Bernat, and R. K. Gert, "Nutrition and Hydration for the Terminally Ill," *Journal of the American Medical Association* 273, no. 22 (June 1995): 1736–1737.

23. Sandra Jacobs, "Death by Voluntary Dehydration—What the Caregivers Say," *New England Journal of Medicine* 349, no. 4 (July 2003): 325–326.

24. Jon B. Eisenberg, *Using Terri* (San Francisco: HarperCollins, 2005).

The Family Tree

JEAN LEVITAN

I have often made the comment "when the time comes, I'm moving to Oregon." Oregon is that pioneer state far from my home where the citizenry and medical profession seem to support a person's right to die . . . to take control of the end of life. I suppose, if I were really honest, I should say that I hope "when the time comes, as Oregon goes, so goes the nation." But from where I sit now, the policies and politics in the United States make Oregon the exception, not the rule.[1]

I am the child of two World War II veterans. My mother was an army nurse. My father, much to my chagrin during the 1970s, had been a proud graduate of ROTC, leaving his senior year in college to head abroad and later distinguish himself as a captain in the army. Neither parent has ever gone to any great lengths to share war stories. The story we children grew up with was the romantic one: dad broke his leg in Austria skiing, and mom was his nurse. World War II brought them together, and their commitment to each other has extended over sixty years.

I know they each saw horrors. I know my mother cared for many injured soldiers in addition to my father. What I don't know is whether or not their wartime experiences shaped their pragmatic approach to aging and dying. My mother, in particular, and like her brother who was a physician, has always taken a very practical approach to life and death; she will discuss health-related articles in the newspapers, comment on the decisions of others, and sometimes give historical context for her opinions. On more than one occasion she has advised her children: "Put me in a nursing home when the time comes, if necessary." With the recent experiences our family has had with my father becoming seriously ill and being moved to a nursing home, my mother seems to have revised that advice. More than ever before she'll tell me how she hopes "to go in her sleep" or be hit by a bus.

Many years ago, as oldest child and executor of my parents' estate, I was given two separate advance directives, each notarized with instructions as to what each parent wanted if no longer able to voice his or her health-care preferences. I was told where their cemetery plot was located, the name of the lawyer to be contacted at the time of their deaths, and the basic parameters of their will. I put the documents away in a drawer and felt proud that my parents had been able to take such a practical approach to the end of their lives.

As my parents continued to age and confront more health problems, they met with their attorney and signed durable power of attorney forms. Those forms would enable me or my siblings legally to use our signatures in lieu of theirs, managing their finances and medical needs when and if necessary. Again, as demonstrated through so much of their lives, my parents were "taking care of things."

I pride myself on being able to think about life and death issues and talk openly about them. I've watched friends die from cancer and AIDS; I've attended many funerals of loved relatives and participated in both funerals and memorial services. As a college professor of public health, my teaching allows me to approach the subject of death and dying. I've tried in the classroom to pass along my mother's wisdom regarding "being prepared." I teach students about advance directives; they are encouraged to talk with their parents and other relatives about the end of life. I encourage them to sign organ donor cards, gently kidding them that they are prime specimens. We compare funeral rituals based on culture and background and their experiences to date with death and dying.

While I often share my own experiences with funerals, I have yet to tell the stories of my aunt and uncle—two people, from different sides of the family, who each ended their lives when they chose to. Perhaps it is more accurate to say: they ended their lives when they couldn't stand to live any longer with their illness and pain. From my perspective, my aunt and uncle accelerated the end of their lives, lives that were ending. Others may feel they committed suicide. The word *suicide* has so many negative connotations; it is so often framed as a desperate act committed by those who are profoundly depressed. From a traditional religious perspective, suicide is a sin. From a legal perspective, it's a crime.

Part of my hesitation in discussing the deaths of my aunt and uncle with my students has been that I don't view what they chose to do as wrong, and I've yet to figure out how to help my students understand that. I also find myself looking at such young faces and wondering if my students are ready or able to confront the complexities of dying when they're just starting to branch out and live as young adults. Now watching my own father suffer, I've come to realize how strongly I believe in the right of the individual to control the end of life. Working with the health-care establishment, I've also come to learn how inadequate all those end-of life documents, filled out in earlier moments of health, may be. The many questions that need to be thought through aren't there, and the personal struggles in finding the right answers can't be quantified on a piece of paper.

My Aunt

Anne Marie, always called Marika, was my uncle's wife. She was only six years older than I and, while I called her "aunt," it was often done somewhat teasingly due to the closeness of our ages. She was a complicated woman—beautiful, vain, opinionated, and someone who would not let anyone push her around. She sometimes made up her own rules if she thought the ones in place were ridiculous. I'll never forget the time the extended family was dining at a fancy restaurant where women were not allowed to wear pants. My aunt arrived in a lovely pantsuit, with a tunic top ending high on her thigh. When told she could not enter the restaurant wearing pants, she went to the ladies room, removed her pants, and returned just wearing the tunic top. It was the 1970s and mini skirts were in style, making her behavior slightly less outrageous.

Marika was a talented seamstress and gourmet cook, spoke seven languages, and yet never quite figured out exactly what kind of work she wanted to do. She had been an international flight attendant prior to her marriage, sold fur coats at Saks Fifth Avenue upon moving to New York City, and, while raising two children, briefly attempted to also manage a jazz musician. Throughout her marriage she also helped manage my uncle's office. She didn't have to provide financially for her family, yet she wanted to do more than be a "stay-at-home mother." Just prior to her diagnosis of ovarian cancer, she had finally discovered how useful her cooking and shopping talents could be at a local soup kitchen. At the soup kitchen she could excel by making her wonderful chicken soup and finding ways to cleverly stretch the budget to feed the hungry.

My aunt's diagnosis of ovarian cancer at age fifty-one caught everyone by surprise. What was worse was that, as is so often the case, her cancer, once diagnosed, was already advanced. This meant that she would need both surgery and chemotherapy. She accepted the medical advice and agreed to participate in the research efforts at Mount Sinai Hospital in New York City, a facility working specifically on ovarian cancer.

Marika was a fighter. She had lots of family support as she suffered through cycles of chemotherapy, including autologous stem cell treatments. That treatment involves the harvesting of the patient's own stem cells, the patient then being blasted with high doses of chemotherapy, and then the return of the stem cells to a weakened body. The goal is that, under close hospital supervision, high levels of chemotherapy can be administered, followed by a period of renewed strength once the stem cells are put back into the patient. During the process, the patient is especially vulnerable to infection, experiences intense nausea, loses body hair, and is also usually physically exhausted, just to name a few of the side effects. The patient must stay in isolation at the hospital, minimizing contact with outside germs until his or her level of immunity improves.

Marika somehow managed those weeks in isolation, becoming close to her nurses and hospital attendants. The treatment was incredibly challenging, both physically and mentally, yet she pushed through with courage and optimism. She seemed to dismiss the odds that "only one in four make it." She felt there was no reason why she couldn't be part of that survival percentage. Once the family could again visit, we were amazed at how gracefully Marika handled losing her hair. Here was a woman who valued her looks and for years had seemed to take great pleasure in being noticed. I'm sure she cried in private, as she witnessed so many physical changes. The public face Marika put to the treatment, however, was remarkable. She purchased two good wigs, alternating them with various scarves and cancer turbans. When her own hair grew back, she seemed to delight in the short curls, which grew in stark contrast to the longer hair she had worn for years.

The last time I saw her, my aunt was serving brunch as she had so many times over the years, and laughing that her family had better remember how to prepare an omelette. By this time Marika had received many different treatments both in the hospital and at home, including having fluid drained from her abdomen numerous times. The brunch had the extended family seated together around her dining room table, with Marika serving food as she had on so many other occasions. In contrast to the many months where she slowly sipped from her can of Ensure, that nutrient-dense beverage, or had her nutrition administered through a stomach tube, Marika was actually eating comfortably, for the first time in a long time. The moment had a very surreal aspect to it, for the food would go in her mouth to be tasted, down her esophagus, and then into a bag taped to her abdomen. It never actually was being digested. The irony was that, despite the seemingly festive occasion, she was ever closer to death.

When I got the phone call from my parents that Marika had died, I cried. When I got the phone call from my uncle, I screamed when he said, "You know, she threw herself off the roof." I kept sobbing and couldn't let go of the image. Seventeen floors down to a stranger's patio. She couldn't stand her life with such pain anymore. Somehow, despite her so very weakened condition, she had left her apartment, gone up in the elevator, through the door to the roof, onto the ledge, and jumped. I knew that roof. She had taken me there twenty years earlier to sunbathe, the place she, like other New Yorkers, lovingly referred to as "Tar Beach."

I knew Marika was dying but didn't know the extent of her pain until after her death. My uncle told me that the hospice care she had been getting was terrible, with mistakes and inattention frequent occurrences. The idea that there would be "death with dignity," as the hospice movement claims, had certainly not been her experience.

When Mount Sinai could no longer care for Marika—she had reached the stage at which there was no point to more treatment—she was released to the care of a hospice program associated with a hospital closer to her Greenwich Village home. She and my uncle were told that she would have regular visits from a hospice nurse, and because the program was "hospice," they assumed that death would come as peacefully as possible.

Instead, they ran into an incredible bureaucracy of paperwork, missed communication, incompetence, and cruelty. The transfer from one hospital to another resulted in over a week of crises and lack of hospice care. What was later explained as a "computer glitch" prevented hospice from giving care; care had to be paid for, and Marika was caught between being released from one hospital and into the system of another.

Once home care was begun, the provider assigned knew little of Marika's care plan and needs, nor was she familiar with proper pain management. My aunt was labeled "terminal" and that seemed to be all that mattered. Rather than truly getting the palliative care that is supposedly a staple of hospice, she was neglected, and both she and my uncle felt abandoned by a system that would only respond as long as all the paperwork was correct, ensuring proper payment once submitted. Responses to their requests for help seemed to be constantly framed within the need for medical personnel to first get the proper authorizations; attending to her pain was secondary to the need for the proper signatures and authorization for payment.

My aunt and uncle also felt silenced by the system. They had learned what worked best for her over the many months of treatment, yet their wisdom and experience did not matter. In particular, since my uncle lacked formal medical or nursing training, his knowledge about intravenous procedures, what pain medications and nutrients were best tolerated by my aunt, and so on, was not respected. My aunt's voice as to what she wanted for her care was also not heard. They were both frustrated in their attempts to get an answer as to who could provide the necessary authorization for action that would be in the true spirit of palliative care.

I learned the details of the last week of her life from a letter my uncle wrote to Mount Sinai Hospital. Marika's pain had increased, she was vomiting constantly, she couldn't eat or go to the bathroom, and the visiting nurse seemed to do little more than take her temperature and pulse. Where she found the focus and strength to end it all, I don't know. But on October 9, 1996, at 2:30 in the morning, she went to the roof of her building and jumped.

My Uncle

Uncle Harry was my mother's older brother by seven years. There had been another brother born between them, who had died from pneumonia at eighteen months of age. With my family settled in New York, and my uncle's in California, we seldom saw him and his family. I was sixteen when I first met my cousins; I don't remember many visits from my uncle prior to that, although a few did occur. My mother always seemed so proud that her older brother was a physician and often turned to him for medical advice. For me, Uncle Harry was this smart doctor on the West Coast, the uncle I really didn't know. Growing up, I would periodically look at the old, framed photograph on the wall of him and my mother as young children, but he didn't become real to me until I was in my teens and older.

On the occasions I got to visit with my uncle, I would search for traces of similarity to my mother. They didn't really look alike. They didn't talk alike. Despite the fact that he was supposed to be so smart, what struck me most was how quiet and soft-spoken he was. He wasn't fashion conscious, slowly drove an old Mercedes, and had a demeanor opposite to that of the more gregarious relatives on my father's side. I couldn't imagine him arguing with anyone or engaging in the loud discussions at meals more typical of the other side of the family. In all the years I knew him, and I didn't know him well, I never heard him raise his voice.

My uncle's obituary described a man who had served during World War II as a battalion surgeon and was awarded the Bronze Medal for valor during combat. After the war he and his wife settled in Pasadena, California. He and my mother corresponded by letter and shared in the long-distance care of their parents: for a period of time, my grandmother lived on the East Coast, while my grandfather lived on the West Coast. The two siblings each watched their parents age in pain and dementia, spending their last years in nursing homes. My grandfather suffered with Parkinson's disease, and my grandmother, while living into her early nineties, had dementia and didn't recognize her family for years. Neither, if I dare to judge, had a high quality life for a long period at the end of their lives.

My uncle, as an internist, had always followed good health practices. He ate properly, exercised religiously, didn't smoke, and left an unhappy marriage for a better one. The irony was that, for all his good habits, he entered his eighties battling hip replacements, diabetes, open-heart surgery, Parkinson's disease, and colon cancer.

My mother once shared with me that my uncle believed in the right to end his life when he wanted. He and his wife were going to stockpile pills and exit peacefully when they were ready. My uncle would write the prescription for the drugs needed, allowing them to feel in control. I'm not aware of the conversations between my mother and her brother, but I'd always heard her comment how she hoped for a quick and peaceful death as well. His plan undoubtedly made good sense to her; long years spent in nursing homes were not desired by either of them.

My uncle's life ended differently than he'd planned. Because he had stopped practicing medicine years before, he didn't have a stockpile of pills from which to draw when he wanted them. My aunt told my mother that all his physical ailments were increasingly interfering with his quality of life. Most recently, his colon cancer had returned, with all its accompanying problems. They didn't have the financial resources for private home health care, leaving my aunt filling most of her day taking care of him. Her own health was suffering, and she was facing possible surgery related to a recently diagnosed heart problem.

Uncle Harry apparently couldn't imagine not having his wife available to help with his care, nor could he be of any help to her with her needs. Between his many years of poor health, his wanting to let his younger wife attend to her own health, being eighty-seven years old, and being clear-minded enough to still implement a plan for dying, he had decided that it was time. There had been too many emergency calls to the police, too many ambulances, too many hospitalizations, too many surgeries, and too much dependency on a wife for even the most basic bodily care.

Knowing that my uncle was ill, but unaware of his imminent plan to end his life, my sister and I arranged to escort my parents to California for a visit. It was because of our announced visit, as I later learned from my mother, that my uncle postponed his death plan. According to his wife, Uncle Harry looked forward to seeing his sister once more. Just before our arrival, he fell and fractured his collarbone, necessitating a stint in a rehabilitation hospital. His wife seemed relieved to have some time off from constant caregiving and gladly escorted us to the facility. Our visits were pleasant, but the place certainly had the feel of a hospital. There were wheelchairs everywhere, hospital beds in rooms, institutional furniture, and, despite the friendly and attentive staff, you knew you were in a health-care facility.

Each day of that long weekend in California, we went to the rehabilitation hospital. My uncle greeted us with a smile, and we'd visit in the living room–type lounge on his floor. My uncle, the doctor, talked with pride about still methodically reading his medical journals. Despite being seated in a wheelchair, he seemed his same self. Good mind, quiet demeanor, and clearly pleased that his sister had visited.

In retrospect, I think about his dilemma—if you've decided you've had enough of life, you can't exercise your choice while a patient in a hospital. At least not easily. How frustrating it must have been to be close to so many medications and yet unable to get those you might want for a personal plan. Long retired, Uncle Harry could no longer write prescriptions. After the

California visit, I received an e-mail from my cousin, who had talked with her stepmother about my uncle's plans. Both my aunt and uncle preferred a drug overdose to other options. My cousin asked if either my mother or I had any access to pills for them. I didn't, and I didn't ask my mother.

A few months after his release from the rehabilitation hospital, I got the phone call from my mother: "Uncle Harry died." I suppose the weeks in the rehab hospital may have reminded him of how his own parents lingered for years and how he never wanted that experience for himself. He had had to implement plan number two; he starved himself. He knew that, as a diabetic, if he didn't eat he would go into a coma. And, if his wife respected his wishes, she wouldn't call 911 this time. She'd let him go. There had been other 911 calls in the past, and trips in and out of hospitals. This time no 911 call. He had left her with notarized paperwork so that no charges would be levied against her.

So much of what I learned about my uncle had always been through my mother, and his death was no different. She learned from his wife that it took two weeks for him to die, longer than they had expected for him to become comatose; at one point he had asked for water. I don't know all the details, nor did I need to at that time. He chose to be cremated; the same choice he had made for his parents, who had ended up under his care many decades before. I'm not sure his children approved of his choice, but he didn't leave them with any power to intervene. I do know that his failing body made life too difficult, despite the sharpness of his mind.

My Branch on the Tree

Like my aunt and uncle, and like my mother as well, I believe in the right to die. I don't want to suffer and have a prolonged death. I don't own *Final Exit* by Derek Humphry and The Hemlock Society, that best-selling advice book on how to engineer your death.[2] I still remember my mother's comments, though, at the time of its publication: "Who needs that book? You just take your pills with alcohol." I often think about what strategy I would attempt if I wanted and needed to end my life.

Over the years I still struggle to get that last image of my aunt from my brain. I know her building. I can envision her standing on the roof ledge, having unhooked all her tubes. It's the jump I could never do. My vertigo has always kept me away from ledges, and I can't imagine giving in to that fear of falling at the end of life. I know people jump to their deaths; I just don't think I could.

As for my uncle's approach, starving myself into a coma would be the ultimate irony after having lived a life in which food was my struggle and salvation. I've spent most of my life grappling with weight management issues, first enjoying foods and eating what I wanted, followed by dieting to reduce the weight gained by such patterns of eating. It seems unimaginable to give up food at the end of life, an effort that requires prolonged denial of what was once pleasurable. I vaguely remember reading about how applesauce can help one swallow the pills that could put you to sleep. I just don't know which pills or what dose. Give me a shot that puts me permanently to sleep. Let me and others go gently into that good night.

As I've watched my father struggle with becoming more and more mentally confused while he seems to still have the will to get physically stronger, the issues related to the end of life have come even more sharply into focus for me. My father was hospitalized for an infection and was so sick that I thought he might die. My siblings and I, along with my mother, were left to answer questions about his care that had never before been discussed. Ironically, even having durable power of attorney papers and a living will ended up being inadequate when we were forced to navigate the intricacies of care required. Should a feeding tube be inserted to help this frail man get stronger? Should physical strength be encouraged when his once sharp mind seemed to be alternating between hospital-induced delirium and already-diagnosed dementia? Does sitting up in a wheelchair for hours, only able to eat pureed food fed by an aide, qualify as a meaningful life to this once vibrant man who had filled his days, after retirement, with books, film, theatre, museums, and long walks? Those became only some of the many painful and challenging questions posed to my family.

We said no to the feeding tube and yes to improving his strength and quality of life. His meals went from pureed to chopped, and his trays started to include sandwiches and other recognizable food choices. My father could again enjoy desserts and has surprised the family by being able to chew the occasional hamburger. Weeks of physical therapy were required so that he could learn to walk again. He now walks, but instead of along city streets, he travels the hallway of his floor at the nursing home.

I've philosophically embraced the concept of death with dignity, yet it seems that for many, dignity is taken away. It's almost a cliché to comment that we start out in life relying on others to keep us clean and dry, and can end up with that same dependent situation at the end of life. I look around the nursing home and see people sleeping in their wheelchairs, watched from the nurse's station. The parallel image of babies sitting strapped in their seats napping is all too obvious. Both groups are in diapers, and both spend a good portion of the day asleep.

I cherish the moments of connectedness I can have with my father, yet afterward I go home and he stays. I struggle with guilt about making him adjust to his new home, and I struggle with guilt over my hope that he doesn't live there a long time. I don't ask him what he wants for the end; it seems those decisions will be made for him by his wife and children. We all agree that he must be kept comfortable and pain free. His signed living will just doesn't provide enough specific guidance to the family, and once in a nursing home his choices are limited by what is common medical practice and what is legal. I know my mother doesn't want her life to end the way his seems to be ending, yet to my knowledge, she has not made any plans like her brother's. To plan out one's end seems important, and to share how one feels with family essential. The words and plans, however, can ring hollow when you can't legally end your life nor secure the means to exit gracefully.

Since I realize that it may be difficult to control how I die, no matter how much I prepare, I've resigned myself to exploring the options for what will happen afterward. Recently, a piece on death by choice on television led me to the book *Exit Strategy: Thinking Outside the Box* by Michelle Cromer.[3] I saw the author briefly interviewed, responded to her upbeat humor about death, and quickly ordered the book. There were eighteen brief chapters, each outlining various options for one's cremains—aka ashes. Sprinkling your ashes over the ocean is only one of apparently many options offered today. Cromer explains how some have chosen to be sent into outer space, while others have chosen to become part of man-made reefs along the ocean floor. The back of the book provides a host of Web sites where interested parties can find the services they desire.

I found the book thought provoking, creative, practical, and above all, funny. At times I found myself laughing out loud. I wondered how best to tell my family that, of all the new exit strategies outlined, I think I'd like to become a diamond. According to Cromer, LifeGem is a company that extracts the carbon from your ashes to make a diamond. The cost ranges from $2,500 to $14,000; I suppose the range reflects the size of the diamond preferred. My mother always referred to her children as her "three jewels." I could take that to a literal level with a little help.

As I think about my students and what to include in my lesson on death and dying, I wonder what to share from my personal thoughts and experiences. Should I share the stories of my aunt and uncle? Do I burden my young students with descriptions of the pain of watching my own father's demise? Do I dare to use humor when talking about death and dying? At their younger ages, have they developed a dark sense of humor about life and death? Unfortunately, both the textbooks and classroom time allotted to the topic hardly match the depth of feeling and thought required to make good decisions around the practical aspects of funerals, determinations of death, organ donation, living wills/advance directives, funeral rituals, emotional states related to grief and dying, hospice care, and so on. Nonetheless, I emphasize the critical need for such family discussions.

On the home front for me, there are so many discussions still to be had. Recently, as my family visited the grave of my mother-in-law, I chose the occasion to mention that I'd prefer to be cremated, adding, "In fact, becoming a diamond might be a nice way to 'move on.'" One son shared that he too believed in cremation, but no one seemed to believe I could ever be reduced to a gem. We didn't pursue that option further. We've not had the more serious conversations about my views on the right to die and what kinds of choices there may be. For me it is easier to use humor and a twinkle of the eye to talk about ashes; it is so much more difficult to talk about the journey out and to verbalize what kinds of help I may want and need.

For now, I'll continue to focus on life and living. I always end my class on death and dying with a reminder to my students to live each day to the fullest, and not delay telling those you love that you love them. I've always been good doing that at home. Maybe this year in class I'll share the stories of my aunt and uncle as well. I know it's too hard to talk about my father without tearing up. But with a nod to the dark humor of it all, I may just tell my students about my wish to end up as a diamond.

NOTES

1. Editors' note: After this essay was submitted, Washington State passed a referendum (in November 2008) to allow physician-assisted suicide. This law closely resembles that adopted in Oregon.

2. Derek Humphry, *Final Exit: The Practicalities of Self-Deliverance and Assisted Suicide for the Dying*, 3rd ed. (New York: Dell, 2002).

3. Michelle Cromer, *Exit Strategy: Thinking Outside the Box* (New York: Jeremy P. Tarcher/Penguin, 2006).

Elegy for an Optimist

MIMI SCHWARTZ

"So Doc, when do we start?" my father-in-law said, hunched over from stomach cramps. My husband and I refrained from asking the oncologist, who had just prescribed a powerful, six-cycle dose of chemotherapy, a lot of what-if questions. How could we, after being warned that if we did nothing, "your father will starve to death, and that isn't a pretty sight!" Besides, this expert assured us that even at age eighty-four there were one-in-five odds for a cure. Charlie could be alive for his granddaughter's wedding in six months, we told each other as we left his room.

He was released from the hospital on day six, and everyone said he took the chemotherapy better than anyone they'd seen. No hair loss, no vomiting, the head nurse said, even though his blood pressure dropped on the morning of his checkout and his stomach cramps returned as soon as they fed him oatmeal. Constipation, they said. He'll be fine.

Three days later we half-carried him to the emergency room of our local hospital. He hadn't been able to eat, could barely drink, and had been up for three nights with pain. But eight hours after being hooked up to an IV (his first nourishment in days) and getting fresh blood from a transfusion, Charlie was talking about going home to his apartment the next week. He would hire a nurse's aide for a few hours a day, if he needed one.

My husband and I said, "Let's just see!" We kept saying it, even after they inserted a permanent catheter into Charlie's vein for easier transfusions and for a total liquid feeding that bypassed his stomach. We said it even after we asked the young resident how soon the first cycle of chemotherapy would shrink the tumor blocking his stomach. "Oh, that might take another five cycles," he said, very upbeat. "We have to build him up first before we can start again."

I have heard senior citizens complain about being written off by the medical profession, but not Charlie. With his gentle charm and solid insurance coverage from fifty years as a union man, he had everyone, from specialist to orderly, backing him 150 percent. His optimism was theirs as they took him daily for X-rays, CAT scans, MUGA scans, physical therapy, and endless tests. "You're doing great," they said as his blood pressure sank, his heartbeat became erratic, and he was moved to intensive care. We did mention a living will then, but Charlie didn't want to sign one. "One-in-five odds are good, remember?" He smiled.

"It's his choice," my husband kept saying, and I kept quiet, just as I had when my high school friend had brain cancer. Her family, desperate for a promising treatment, had asked me to ask my oncologist friend to suggest which of three experimental research trials to enter. After hearing the diagnosis, my oncologist, who practiced 1,000 miles away, said, "It doesn't matter what they try, she'll be dead in eight months." And she was—but not before having undergone eight months of experimental drugs given by doctor-researchers who kept saying she was doing great.

According to American Medical Association guidelines, doctors should elicit "informed consent," based on a patient's choice after discussion of "alternative treatments and consequences of treatment, including the consequence of no treatment." But is it choice when your doctor gives you one-in-five odds that contradict those, outside your personal medical loop, who say you haven't a chance? Is it choice when these odds are based on the whole population, and you are an eighty-four-year-old with a history of heart attacks? In a study of 917 cancer patients that I read in the *Journal of the American Medical Association,* most patients are overly optimistic and, like Charlie, choose aggressive, painful treatment that does not extend life, only discomfort. Their doctors, on the other hand, are highly accurate in prognosis; more often than not, they guess right about what to expect.

True, it is not easy to convey accuracy along with hope; and it is not easy to get patients to hear both parts of the message at once. But it is easy to avoid scare tactics like "starving to death is not a pretty sight." (We learned, subsequently, that people dying of starvation can be made as comfortable in hospice care as anyone else.) And, easy or not, it is essential to try for more informed realism so patients can make informed end-of-life choices.

Four weeks later I sat by Charlie's bed in a nursing home (where he had vowed never to be), hearing his chest rattle as it rose and fell. The cancer was everywhere, the morphine never enough, and the gentle man with his gracious optimism did not speak while I stroked his hand, except to whisper once: "If I had known I'd end in here, like this, I would have put a gun to my head."

But you should have known, I wanted to shout. We all should have known. Artificial feeding, chemotherapy, radiation treatment, blood transfusions. I kept remembering the nurse who monitored my father-in-law's blood on the morning after his first transfusion saying proudly, "We almost lost him yesterday!" As if dying in his sleep, at eighty-four, with cancer and a bad heart, meant failure.

Despite my vows to be more realistic, I can imagine an ending like his instead of at home on my third floor, looking over treetops, as planned. Even with my living will signed and waiting—No Extreme Measures. Do Not Resuscitate—what if, while at home, I run a high fever, or start choking for air, or stop eating? Will my husband be strong enough to hold my hand and not dial 911 to "save" me? Will my children not say to him, "Dad, how can you *not* call?"

I keep imagining someone saying these words to Charlie: "Mr. Schwartz, chemotherapy is a long shot, given your age and heart condition, but we could try if you want—and stop if it doesn't work out. Or you could buy a few good weeks or months with artificial feeding, but you'll have to go to a nursing home in order to do that. Or you could go home, and when things get too rough, we will provide hospice care to help you have an easy end."

But no one said them—not the doctors, not the social workers, not us. We were all seduced by high-tech tests and machines that keep urging you on, day by day, whatever the odds. But I say them now, to myself: rehearsing, rehearsing to remember them *if*—no, *when*—I need them.

Buddhist Reflections on Life and Death

A Personal Memoir

ALAN POPE

Death Becomes an Issue

When I was eight years old, my mother came home one day with fresh donuts. When I greeted her in the kitchen, my excitement over her offering yielded to the seriousness of her tone and the dampened nature of her energy. She told me that a neighborhood boy whom I knew had hanged himself following an illness. His mother found him in the closet with the belt from his robe tied around his neck. Stunned, I took one of the glazed donuts from the box held out before me, retreated into my mother's upholstered rocking chair in the den, and sat in stone silence. Staring into space, I was bombarded by a swirling mix of emotions for which I had no experience and no name. Biting into the donut, I tasted nothing.

I experienced on that day the magical transformation of a world that was safe and playful into one filled with ominous threat. The unfathomable image of my sometime playmate hanging by his neck in his closet defied all understanding. How could he have done that? How could he have been so unhappy? What was it like to have found him? Life now posed possibilities I hadn't known existed, possibilities whose proximity to people I knew made them frighteningly real. My innocence was robbed that day, and the comfortable sequence of events that moved through time in my ordinary all-American neighborhood suffered a disruption of which I could make no lasting sense. So I did all I could, and I forgot about it. I went about my life, my childhood, as though nothing had happened. But something had happened: a seed had been planted, one that would blossom into a fascination with death.

In high school, despite valuing mathematics and science above all else, I took a world literature class. It was fabulous. But as much as I loved reading writers such as Dante, Erasmus, and Molière, it was Leo Tolstoy's *The Death of Ivan Ilyich* that impacted me most deeply.[1] This slim volume, which inspired Martin Heidegger's massive existential treatise, *Being and Time*, revealed to me the inextricable link between how we live our lives and how we die.[2] I felt called to live my life with meaning and purpose, in such a way that I could die in peace, with a clean conscience. Putting that into practice, however, would prove difficult.

In Tolstoy's novel, the protagonist unexpectedly finds himself, in midlife, on his deathbed. In the course of dying, Ivan Ilyich initially denies not only the fact of his dying, but also the reality of how he has lived. Although the reader learns that Ilyich had abandoned his own moral virtue for the sake of professional ambition, and that he had married for status rather than love, on his deathbed Ilyich clings to the dogmatic assertion that he has lived his life as he ought to have—"pleasantly and properly." Nevertheless, such self-assurances are consistently interrupted by a sharp pain in his abdomen that abruptly brings him out of his head. Being grounded in here-and-now physical reality leads him to question the self-image he has developed and the choices he has made. Hearing the call of his own conscience, he realizes how miserable his adult life has been. Against all manner of psychological resistance, he eventually cannot deny the inevitable truth—that *he has lived his life all wrong*. This wrongness, as portrayed by Tolstoy, is in having lived a life of social conformity, a life of "shoulds" rather than "wants."

I was petrified by this possibility for myself! What if at the time of my dying I were to realize I had lived my life all wrong? How horrible! This concern amplified a brewing period of rebellion in my own life, and I came away from the story determined not to surrender my free will by blindly following the dictates of social convention. However, in so steadfastly adopting this stance, I resisted the conformity that *is* necessary for our healthy engagement with social life. The work of an adolescent includes adopting social personas from whose cloth our own unique person will be cut, and in attempting to avoid this process, I became bound in a web of confusion.

I also failed at that time in my life to appreciate the final scene of Tolstoy's novel. It is only when Ivan Ilyich's heart breaks open in compassion for others that he is able to die in peace. I understood the idea that redemption is always possible, but I didn't recognize the implication that the deepest meaning in life arises when we devote ourselves to the welfare of others. I wanted to be the unique person that I really am, without understanding that that person is inextricably bound to others and that the binding agent is love. Rather, I remained in a state of self-absorption that would only crack open later in life when I would struggle with chronic illness.

In the meantime, in my confusion I dropped out of college, felt tremendous guilt about it, and proceeded to make a series of decisions guided more by my head than my heart. Upon returning to school, I ignored my early connection to astrophysics, mathematics, and philosophy and majored in economics in an effort to please my father. By the time my father died, I found myself working in a corporation programming computers for business applications, rather than studying and researching the cosmos. My life lacked meaning and purpose. It was as though I had lapsed into the same system of conformity that had trapped Ivan Ilyich himself. My resistance had produced the very reality I had feared.

Chronic Illness and Spiritual Discovery

It wasn't until I developed chronic fatigue and immune dysfunction syndrome (CFIDS) that I realized how divorced my desire had been from my sense of what I should do with my life. I developed this condition in the spring of 1989 at the age of thirty. I was working on a doctorate in computer science, specializing in artificial intelligence. I had chosen this field more in order to validate years in industry programming computers than to satisfy an intrinsic interest. I saw my world in computational terms, which supported my tendency to live in my head as a defense against feeling my feelings. Perhaps I had found the perfect refuge from the possibility of death, for abstractions are not flesh and blood and therefore do not die. But in a manner eerily similar to Ivan Ilyich's relationship to his abdominal pains, the collapse of my physical health brought me back into my body, into that which is most immediately real.

I would suffer with this illness for four years—acutely for six months and substantially for two years. In the early stages, I was bound to my sickbed, and my eyes burned so badly that I couldn't read. One day my girlfriend drove me to a bookstore to select some novels on cassette with which I might amuse myself. I spotted the spiritual classic *Tao te Ching* and naively thought,

"Maybe this Chinese philosophy will do me some good." I had no idea how prescient that innocent thought would prove to be.[3]

Later, at home, I found that listening to a reading of a science fiction novel as I lay in bed taxed my energy and made me feel worse. When I replaced it with the *Tao te Ching*, I was instantly struck by the first words of the author, Lao-tze: "The Tao that can be told is not the eternal Tao."[4] I turned off the cassette player and lay there in wonder. "What was *that?*" I thought. I seemed to recognize that these words were at once profound and mysterious. Propelled forward, I listened to more, frequently turning off the cassette player to sit with what I had heard, as if absorbing a new way of seeing, a new way of hearing, a new way of understanding the nature of reality and of myself.

In listening to this work countless times, I realized that the eternal Tao is that realm of existence that is beyond concept, language, and time. So long as I tried to grasp this concept intellectually, it eluded me. But when I suspended intellect and entered into the immediacy of my lived experience, I gained a sense of Tao as the deep source of all phenomena, whether physical, mental, or emotional. Listening to the words of Lao-tze, I learned to view the world without the lens of abstract, computational models. The resistance that I had felt toward my physical pain and discomfort melted into an acceptance that allowed me to inhabit my body in a fuller way, discovering within it a reservoir of truth and wisdom.

As I gained strength, I read as much spiritual literature as possible, including works by Hindus, Sufis, and Buddhists. I learned how to meditate from a book, and for two years I diligently practiced breath counting, in both formal sessions and at odd times, such as when sitting in doctors' waiting rooms. Learning to concentrate my mind produced a welcome measure of calmness and serenity. I had tapped into a spiritual nature that all those years had lain dormant. My old priorities were shifting, and, like Ivan Ilyich, I recognized how dissatisfied I had been with my life.

Almost two years into my illness, after my level of functioning had increased, I saw an advertisement at the local food co-op for a Tibetan Buddhist meditation group in Delaware, where I lived. On a whim, I decided to attend one Sunday. The small practice community met under the auspices of two highly regarded Tibetan lamas (teachers) in New York. Although I at first found the practice strange and off-putting, I was intrigued by the knowledge and intelligence of some of its members. Chanting in

Tibetan, performing religious gestures, and visualizing deities were soon understood not as arbitrary religious acts, but rather as technologies for opening the heart and the mind. As I practiced more, asked questions, and read Buddhist philosophy, I sensed a peculiar familiarity in the understanding of the nature of mind and reality that this profound system articulated. It was familiar as ancient knowledge that has long since been buried, but, once exhumed, is obvious and true.

After meeting the lamas on retreat in New York that summer of 1991, I adopted Tibetan Buddhism as my spiritual path. Tolstoy's novel had shown me the importance of waking up before my time of dying, and Tibetan Buddhism offered me the tools with which to do that. This tradition has also taught me that the highest form of happiness comes from developing a compassionate heart and attending to the needs of others. The following year, I left the study of artificial intelligence to pursue my heart's calling—the study of *natural* intelligence. Withdrawing from one school (University of Delaware), I entered another (Duquesne University), where I eventually gained my doctorate in existential phenomenological psychology. Upon graduation, I spent five months on pilgrimage in India and Nepal before assuming my current post as a professor of psychology.

The Death of My Mother

As I was completing the coursework for my doctorate in psychology, my mother made the decision to discontinue the dialysis treatments she had begun two years previously. Whereas her kidneys had been the first casualty of the rare form of anemia from which she suffered, with the collapse of her lungs and heart in the offing, she in essence chose to end her life. My sister called me and I traveled to Virginia to be with them.[5]

When I arrived, my mother was excited to see me and asked to be helped to a chair by her bed. She had my sister bring out my birthday present, a marimba, or African tongue drum. I said that I could play this instrument, my sister could play the keyboards, and then I said, "What will you play, Mom?" Without hesitation, my mother said, "I'll be playing a harp." As the resulting laughter and tears subsided, she added, with a particularly reflective tone, "I always wanted to play a harp."

Although I initially had been perplexed by my mother's bold decision to end her life, I saw her open acceptance of dying as a great gift to me.

It suggested that she was facing death with awareness and with courage. But I was surprised by her next request. After we had positioned her back into bed and tucked her in for the evening, she asked that we keep the television set turned on to the old movies station. I immediately experienced a judgment about that, feeling that she should face her dying without distraction. However, in the face of wanting to comfort my dying mother, this thought didn't gain traction and we naturally honored her request. I also felt a passing judgment about a morphine patch on her chest, holding to a simplistic vision of what it means to confront one's own dying. But the sacredness of this occasion enabled me to let go of that concern as well.

My mother slipped into a coma that evening. When my sister came in the next morning and turned off the television set, Mom gave the death rattle and died. Gazing upon her freshly dead body was *awe-full* in the deepest sense, meaning that it was both inspiring and frightening. My own ideas about the rightness or wrongness of her decisions were made inconsequential by the power of this experience.

Now, years later, I reconsider my mother's decisions involving her death and dying and my judgments about them. In particular, I revisit my judgments regarding her act of passive suicide and her decision to die with a television on in the background, an act of distraction that ran counter to the values I had gained from reading Tolstoy's novel. In particular, I wonder about how in the face of her actual death those judgments no longer were compelling. For this understanding, I turn to the rich tradition of Tibetan Buddhism.

Buddhist Reflections on Life, Death, and Suicide

The Buddhist view of suicide is inseparable from its understanding of life and death.[6] Our present life is taken to be but one in an endless series into which we are born. To be born a human being, however, is considered extremely rare and precious. It is rare because the overwhelming majority of rebirths occur in realms of unspeakable torment, such as those of the hungry ghosts or hell beings; it is precious because the human realm offers the greatest opportunity for spiritual liberation.[7] Clinging to our ego-identity—a narrow sense of self that in reality has no inherent, substantial existence—pulls us into each round of rebirth until some future lifetime when we gain the wisdom and compassion to fully realize our true nature as the vast open ground of existence. Upon gaining such spiritual liberation, however, we take rebirth yet again, this time propelled not by lawful consequence, but by the compassionate aspiration to help liberate all suffering beings.

When we die, our consciousness enters a period of disembodied existence in which we must confront the projections of our own mind. If we can see them to be ephemeral and not solidly real, then we move closer to enlightenment, taking rebirth in a more favorable condition. However, if we go to our death in a chaotic state of mind, as when one commits suicide in desperation, our thick and heavy mental projections generate tremendous anxiety and perceptual distortion. When this occurs, we are apt to take rebirth in a situation of even greater terror and suffering than that which we are attempting to flee. In such cases, suicide offers no real solution for our suffering and can actually make it worse.

When we are in such desperate straits as to contemplate suicide, there are practices in the Buddhist tradition that can help. For example, we can aspire to take on the suffering of all similarly afflicted beings through our own misfortune. At one level, this exercise brings us into alignment with the reality of our mutual interconnectedness with all beings. It also reverses our habitual patterns of self-protection, thereby eroding attachment to ego and generating feelings of love and compassion for others. It provides a meaning for our pain and leverage for our awakening. Although Ivan Ilyich does not perform such a practice, Tolstoy portrays his constant pain as the factor that eventually awakens him from his deluded thinking. Ivan Ilyich comes to recognize the poverty of his life, and he makes amends through the experience of authentic remorse. As with the Buddhist vision, it is when Ilyich realizes that his family is suffering too that his heart opens in compassion and his pain no longer preoccupies him, allowing him to die in peace.

Owing to the rarity and preciousness of our human life, Buddhism naturally discourages suicide. However, it does not consider it to be a sin, for it posits no external agency, such as an all-powerful God, to cast judgment. Rather, Buddhism describes a natural, causal process, and its prohibition against suicide is in essence no more a judgment than would be a warning offered to a distracted canoeist approaching a precipitous drop. Therefore, if a person approaches suicide with positive intention and mental clarity, it need not necessarily be a problem. Similarly, despite the usual Buddhist injunction not to kill, it can be skillful to discontinue life support for a loved one in a vegetative state if performed with compassion toward the suffering person and with awareness that this incarnation has lost its usefulness for further advances on the spiritual path. In this sense, the Buddhist teachings are exceedingly pragmatic.

An exception to the prohibition against suicide is found in the highly realized practitioner who, having attained a profound nonattachment to his or her own body, commits suicide with the pure intention of liberating other beings. This situation is exemplified by the monks who immolated themselves to protest the war in Vietnam. These monks acted with tremendous poise and mindfulness, sitting in perfect meditation posture as their bodies burned. We can surmise that in having attained high levels of realization these monks had made the welfare of others their paramount concern. The Buddha said that his teachings are like a raft—when you get to the other shore, you leave the raft behind. Similarly, these monks had used their precious human lives for that which they were intended, and they were able to let go of them with pure, positive intent.

There are other kinds of extraordinary deaths within the Buddhist tradition. I once knew a Tibetan yogi who had fled Tibet in 1959 because of the hostile Communist Chinese takeover. Soon after arriving in India, his wife and daughters died from the arduous journey, whereupon he effectively went into permanent meditation retreat. He later was relocated to America, though he didn't speak a word of English. It is said that he performed 1,000 full-body prostrations every day, a feat requiring tremendous devotion and spiritual fortitude. Whenever I or anyone else saw him, he was chanting mantras, pausing only to flash a huge smile. When he developed cancer, well into his eighties, he faced it with complete equanimity and courage. One day, after he had grown quite ill, he asked for assistance in sitting up and putting on his ceremonial robes. He died immediately upon assuming perfect meditation posture. His body remained unchanged in that posture for three days. Students would come in and sit in meditation with him. When his body was finally removed for cremation, it was as soft and supple as a child's. Remarkable stories such as these are common in the spiritual literature.

Buddhist Reflections on Free Will

It appears as though this yogi knew that it was his time to die. On the other hand, consistent with some Buddhist versions of the deaths of advanced practitioners, it might be that he had deliberately ejected his consciousness through the crown of his head so as to end his present incarnation and advance toward the next one. We are left with the question of whether he sensed the time of his death or chose it. The Western philosophical tradition has long debated whether we have free will to choose our actions, or our actions are determined by outside forces, in spite of what we might otherwise think.

The Buddhist teachings on free will are complex and seemingly contradictory. Each position that is adopted, however, serves to build a progressively deeper level of understanding. The Buddha would offer one teaching or another depending on the capabilities and needs of the particular student. For example, if a student had a controlling nature, the Buddha would teach that our experience of free will is an illusion and that our actions are completely determined by our conditioning. What we take to be free will is nothing more than the allocation of greater cognitive resources to the process of choosing; what we experience as choice has nothing to do with free will because will doesn't exist. Rather, our choice arises causally from all of the factors associated with the patterns of our own minds in tandem with the situation in which we find ourselves.

In other instances, the Buddha said that while our conditioning determines much more of what we do than we might think, there actually *is* a sliver of free will. Because our minds are very chaotic, however, that sliver is obscured by an overlapping stream of thoughts, feelings, and impulses. If we could slow down the speed of our minds, we could find a level of detachment that would permit us to authentically choose how we respond to the situations in which we find ourselves. This view is actually quite similar to the existential position, which says that while we always are free to act, we tend to forfeit that freedom by following the dictates of convention. Buddhism's detailed understanding of this forfeiture of freedom can be succinctly cast as that of responding to life's situations along the well-worn grooves of our habitual patterns. If we could gain clarity in our minds, however, we could choose freely at all times. In this interpretation, we might suggest that the yogi, having thoroughly trained his mind, had consciously chosen when to end his life.

However, the Buddhist position on free will gets even more complex. These first two interpretations are regarded as not ultimately correct, even as contemplating them is necessary in order to arrive at complete understanding. Toward that end, consider the following example. Suppose you asked an innocent man, "Have you stopped beating your wife?" Either answer that he gives, yes or no, would be wrong because the question frames reality inaccurately. This is precisely the problem with asking the question, "Do we have free will?" This question is predicated upon the assumption that free will either exists or it does not, whereas in reality its existence is dependent on our point of view. It is like asking whether a flame passed from one candle to another is the same flame or a different one. We could say yes or no depending on how we look at it. But the absolute reality is beyond such dualistic ways of seeing.[8]

With this analysis we arrive at the idea that framing the yogi's actions regarding his death in terms of free will reduces the totality of the situation to a conceptualized idea. What we can suggest, however, is that because he had purified his mind stream so thoroughly his death was completely natural and spontaneous. The special powers that he had obtained were essentially those of the Zen master who eats when he is hungry and sleeps when he is sleepy. In abandoning all effort, the yogi simply died when it was time to die, but he did it with full awareness and spontaneity, in a manner transcendent of all concept and dualistic distinction.

The Death of My Mother Revisited

The judgments I made regarding my mother's means of dying unfairly pitted her actions against those typical of this yogi. For example, I questioned her decision to end her life on the grounds that she could use her suffering to arouse compassion for the suffering of others. In using a morphine patch and wanting the television set turned on, she was, I felt, distracting herself from the process of dying, possibly creating unfavorable circumstances for her next rebirth. It mattered neither that she was not a Buddhist nor that she had never read Tolstoy, for in my mind I had divined the general principles by which we should live (and die). Although I didn't wield these judgments against my mother in a harsh way, they lurked in the background of my consciousness as artifacts of my theoretical understanding.

However, as indicated earlier, when I gazed upon my mother's body in the moments following her death those judgments completely evaporated. I knew instinctually that everything was perfect just as it was, including the choices she had made. According to Tibetan Buddhism, we are all already enlightened and the entire world is suffused with enlightened energy. It is owing to our own emotional obscurations that we view reality through the distorting lens of our concepts and judgments. But the sacredness of my mother's freshly dead body momentarily lifted this veil of illusion and allowed me to see her in this open and raw way. In the same fashion that Lao-tse says "the Tao that can be told is not the eternal Tao," the mother that can be judged is not the actual mother. The death of my mother allowed me to see her as if for the first time, beyond the veil of concepts that had shaped my view of her.

In reality, this was not the first time I had seen my mother in this way, for in my infancy I had known her well before I even *could* form concepts and judgments. Although the sense of unmediated connection we experience with our mothers is perhaps deeper than that which we form with any other person, it necessarily gets obscured as we develop into thinking beings with our own sense of autonomy and self. As we come to understand the world conceptually, we form distorted ideas about ourselves and others. As we go through the adolescent stage of forming an integrated identity, we lose even greater contact with both our actual selves and our actual parents. By the time we form new lives as adults, our parents have become quite different people from those we had known previously, at least in the ways that we think about and interact with them. At that point, to see one's mother without distortion is quite an achievement.

Interestingly, in the year or two before my mother died, I had a moment in which I temporarily did see her without distortion. On a visit when she was feeling poorly, she was giving me advice that ordinarily would have annoyed me. For whatever reason, my consciousness spontaneously shifted in such a way that I saw her as being in a state of perfection, as if she were enlightened. It was as if my own filter had been lifted and I could see her as she really was. I disagreed with what she was saying to me, but I saw the love in it, and I saw my own disagreement as also being perfect, as if we were each playing our part in some cosmic play. It was a lucid moment I would not know with her again until I was standing beside her bed after she had died.

I am grateful to have had these experiences of genuine clarity with my mother, to have temporarily transcended the emotional conflicts that ordinarily colored our perceptions of one another. The decisions leading to my mother's death were indeed just what they needed to be, and my earlier judgments had been a product of my own habitual, narrowed state of consciousness. At the same time, these judgments reflected my own sincere efforts to seek the truth of how things are and to learn how best to live. Concepts and theories are helpful to that project, but can also interfere with it when we lose sight of the territory to which they point.

In a critical scene in Tolstoy's novel, Ivan Ilyich grapples with his memory of a syllogism he had learned in school.[9] If all men are mortal and Caius is a man, the syllogism suggests, then Caius is mortal. Ivan Ilyich realizes that as a child he hadn't connected the meaning of this syllogism to its implications for his own life. He starts to recognize that he had evaded the truth of his own mortality, and how that evasion had enabled him to marry for status and work for prestige, ignoring the call of his own conscience to live a meaningful life. Because disembodied abstractions cannot die, they provide a handy refuge from awareness of our own mortality, while rendering our experience opaque and removed from what really matters. We become concerned with our own welfare and with being right, even when doing so robs us of connection with others and alienates us from ourselves.

According to the Buddhist teachings, the way we use an ego-identity to function in society is similar to the way in which we use a body to move through the physical world. However, at the deepest level, we are neither our social identity nor our body. Rather, beneath the layers of conditioning and identification, the deepest nature of every person is love, compassion, and wisdom. And while negative judgments still arise in me, I am learning to see past them to my own deep nature so that I might love others more fully. Toward that end, I find the contemplation of my own inevitable death and the uncertainty of its timing to be an indispensable practice.

NOTES

1. Leo Tolstoy, *The Death of Ivan Ilyich* (New York: Bantam Classic, 1981).

2. Martin Heidegger, *Being and Time*, trans. J. Macquarrie (New York: Harper & Row, 1927/1962).

3. Stephen Mitchell, *Tao te Ching* (New York: HarperCollins, 1988).

4. Ibid., 1.

5. Part of this story appears in the preface to my book, *From Child to Elder: Personal Transformation in Becoming an Orphan at Midlife* (New York: Peter Lang, 2006).

6. The following discussion draws from multiple schools within Buddhist thought, but it does so from the perspective of Tibetan Buddhism, which incorporates all of them.

7. The six realms are, from highest to lowest: god, jealous god, human, animal, hungry ghost, hell. In the traditional literatures these are considered to be realms into

which one actually reincarnates, though contemporary Tibetan Buddhist teachers often portray them to Westerners as psychological states applicable to our experience in this lifetime.

8. The distinction between two truths, relative and absolute, to my mind resolves many of the problems of Western philosophy. A question such as the existence of free will only makes sense in relative reality, but not in absolute reality. As Albert Einstein suggested, we cannot solve a problem at the same level of consciousness at which it was created.

9. Tolstoy, *Ivan Ilyich*, 79.

Death as My Colleague

MARY JUMBELIC

I am a medical examiner, a term that is now familiar across the world. Television, film, and the written press have made this and words like *forensics* household terms. Courses are taught in college, high school, and even at the elementary level that emphasize solving crimes, evidence analysis, and legal medicine.

Of course, crime investigation and murder mysteries have fascinated people for centuries. This innate human inquisitiveness to solve puzzles explains the popularity of Arthur Conan Doyle's and Agatha Christie's works. Older board games such as *Clue* and TV serials such as *Quincy* sparked the human imagination and the satisfaction of solving crimes. Of late, though, my profession of forensic pathology has been glorified and glamorized. Newer shows such as *X-files*, *CSI*, and *Crossing Jordan* have intrigued a larger and even younger audience and introduced forensic pathologists as specialized, intelligent scientists working to provide answers to the questions surrounding the cause of death.

International news coverage of current murder investigations and trials details the work of law enforcement and the scientific professionals who diligently attempt to solve grisly crimes. This burgeoning interest emphasizes the resolution of the investigation and the capture of the perpetrator. The dead are objectified and dehumanized with explicit, gory photographs and video. Their bloody, open wounds are graphically depicted yet appear surreal and ghoulish, almost Halloween-like. This raw portrayal leaves the human being, so recently alive in the corpse, forgotten. Perhaps this anatomic objectification helps all of us to separate from the decedent and ironically to distance ourselves from death. The gorier, the more mangled, the more distorted the image of the dead person, the greater the gap that is created between the living self and death.

I see daily this physicality of death. For over twenty years, I have been performing autopsies, detailed internal and external examinations on dead people. I go to the scene of death and observe the body in its final repose. I interview the families, the police, and the witnesses to understand the circumstances that led to the dead one's final moment. My government office is responsible for investigating any sudden and unexpected deaths occurring in our county jurisdiction. This includes violent, traumatic, and suspicious deaths but also many natural deaths when there is no community doctor willing to sign a death certificate. I become the final doctor for those who avoid medical care either through extraordinary good health, or an unwillingness to succumb to the regimen of organized medicine, or an inability to afford health care. I am also there for the people whose physicians refuse to take responsibility either due to a patient's noncompliance with recommended care or the doctor's uncertainty over the exact anatomic cause of death.

I have seen infants who died unexpectedly, almost peacefully, in their cribs; the elderly wasted away and forgotten in a cluttered and filthy home; bodies torn by metal crunching against bones, producing unimaginable destruction due to a second of misjudgment on the highway; misplaced passion, with the very person who had been coveted lying in a pool of dried blood; and necks wrapped with frayed rope in the terminal desperation of teens.

Some experience painful, tragic endings of life while others die seemingly unaware in their sleep. Yet there is a simple, unifying picture of death that spans cultures, religions, ages, genders, economics, and politics: the last moment of life as we have come to experience it as human beings on this earth—a defined moment when the heart ceases to function and all bodily processes stop. Though this definition and experience of death is universal, it paradoxically remains unique and personal to each individual decedent, not just in the differences in the terminal physical manifestations but in the ramifications for those loved ones left behind in this world.

The majority of my professional life has been consumed with trying to explain death—the etiology of the injuries and diseases responsible for that physical moment when the heart stops beating. I live with death in the

background of my day, watching me as I try to replay in my mind the last few
moments of a person's life. For me, the truth I seek lies beyond the eviden-
tiary phase. It is not just a matter of recording organ weights, collecting body
fluids for drug testing, or retaining small pieces of tissue to look at under
the microscope. I am the deceased's advocate and final voice. Their damaged
organs, skin wounds, stomach contents, and drug tests all speak to me and
provide me salient details of their last few hours. I am the modern sleuth of
forensic medicine.

Yet I recognize death as a natural process, just as much a force of nature
as life. How else can one explain the mystery of one person surviving in a situation while another dies under the very same circumstances? Sometimes
death is a welcome victor to those who are suffering unbearably and sometimes a hated opponent who outwits and overpowers. The personification of
death is conveyed in epic tales as a dark, shadowy, robed stranger with scythe
in hand. To me it is the actual body of the person lying motionless on the
cold, steel gurney.

Individuals expend much energy trying to avoid personal and inevitable
mortality. A primitive and deep-rooted fear of death causes many of us to try
to control the very moment of contact with life's end. Within health care,
providers, especially doctors, use extraordinary means in an effort to
lengthen lives by an hour, a day, or a week. Modern medicine invades the
last private realm of the body with tubes thrust internally and mechanized
equipment performing necessary physiologic functions. Grim diagnostic
prognoses are ignored. False hope is doled out when the physician cannot
face his or her own fear of failure, of falling short of fulfilling the healing oath
so ingrained in the heart and mind.

The reliance on advanced diagnostic and therapeutic techniques,
improved pharmaceuticals, and other treatment modalities sometimes leads
both health-care providers and patients to pursue doomed therapies. These
treatments may be not only hopeless but also filled with complications and
pain. While they may be specifically mentioned in the consent form that the
patient signs, the therapies may be only superficially explained. Patients
ignore the possibility of a poor outcome related to the medical or surgical
therapy when their hopes are pinned on survival. The likelihood of therapeutic failure, no matter how real, pales in the face of the guaranteed alternative of death.

As patients travel down the road of treatment in the throes of a terminal disease, they are in an environment focused on the physical expression of that illness. Families and friends become marginalized and alienated from their loved one as health-care practitioners track the function but not the emotion of the patient's heart.

I review medical records daily from hospitals, nursing homes, and physicians' offices and learn about the physical signs and symptoms occurring before death: the established diagnoses, lists of disease processes, laboratory documentation, and medical assessments and plans. Absent from this analysis is the insight I gain from speaking with the next of kin of the decedent and hearing their versions of the medical course and illness in the days preceding the patient's death. In the chronically ill, a recurring story emerges of physical and emotional alienation at the time of the patient's final breath. This isolation is universally experienced by each of the patient's loved ones and, saddest of all, by the patient, especially when there are emergency medical lifesaving measures administered.

We humans have hubris about our own biology, an illusion of control over our own mortality. However, I have come to believe that death is a natural process, not one to be avoided and feared. If our own morbidity becomes so great as to bring death closer to us, perhaps choosing our way to meet death is an option. When we can approach the acceptance of disease with a realistic consideration of our alternatives, we may be able to choose our end in a way that is more dignified and peaceful than many of the deaths I have evaluated. Certainly having this freedom of choice and the availability of support might make a difference to an individual patient and his or her family.

To choose one's final moment might be empowering; to thwart death's stealth advantage—to pick the time and place. To have the support of those we love present at our last moment may help us live more fully in the hours or days preceding our chosen time of exiting this physical world.

For most people, this may not be an option due to religious beliefs, societal constraints, the absence of medical assistance, and/or the legal ramifications of choosing when and how to die. Families and even doctors have been investigated and prosecuted for homicides, even in the setting of terminal pain management with no intent to kill. This shortsightedness in most of the nation has stymied any open discussion of death and dying.

I have my own story, as each of us does. My interest in death began with what seemed at the time the premature passing of my father following lung surgery. Of course, at thirteen years of age, I did not understand how my daddy, under the best medical care available, could die in a hospital recovery room. This early inquiry into death's mystery profoundly shaped my personal life and ultimately my professional career. Nearly thirty-seven years later, I have had another personal encounter with death.

My mother was diagnosed with terminal metastatic pancreatic cancer two months prior to her death. We were in the examination room and the moment the internist palpated her liver edge during the abdominal exam on this wiry, youthful, yet recently fatigued seventy-nine-year-old woman, I knew the prognosis. Of course, since I am a physician as well as a daughter, we still went through the diagnostic processes, confirming the hopelessness of recovery. When I told my ever-optimistic mother the results of the CT-guided liver biopsy, she gave a primitive howl of horror like a wounded animal. She grieved then and never cried in sorrow again.

We made our decision in tandem: no chemotherapy, no radiation, no surgery, no further diagnostic testing. We went on a family cruise—my husband, our kids, mom, and I. We savored the time together; we rested, relaxed, and prepared emotionally for what lay ahead. Not that it was idyllic. My mother felt tired, couldn't eat, and had a reaction to antinausea medication that made her psychotic one evening. Even as physicians, my husband and I underestimated the importance of the liver and its function in helping to break down medication and the lack of function in one filled with cancer. Yet my mother accompanied us to the elegant dining hall, played cards, danced with her grandsons, and enjoyed silly trivia games poolside. We laughed and appreciated each minute as a gift. My husband and I cried, afraid that each moment might be the last to share with Mom.

We returned on a Saturday to the home we shared, having lived together since my first son was born. My mother had been the third parent in the upbringing of her grandsons, adding the experience of her Roman Catholic beliefs and participating in all of our rituals in our traditional Jewish home.

Mom and I drove to the grocery store to restock the family refrigerator. She pushed the cart and leaned on it for support as we strolled up and down each aisle in a ritual we had performed perhaps thousands of times before, each of us knowing this would be the last time.

At home, I tucked my tired mother into bed, where she slept peacefully. The next day, she awoke with a 104-degree fever. She was in and out of consciousness. I was the frightened daughter of the dying patient and perplexed about what to do. Should I call 911? Should I drive her to the hospital? I anxiously spoke to the oncologist and she explained (in that hopeful manner that only oncologists seem to be able to express) that this was a treatable episode and that a surgeon could drain the obstructed bile duct and treat my mother with intravenous antibiotics.

I hung up the phone and stared at the receiver. My mind seized up with the click of the disconnected telephone. I sat on the stair landing, my legs curled up to my chest in a classic fetal position of primordial comfort. As a physician, I feared my mother was septic, and I knew the bleak and painful consequences of her succumbing to its toxic effects. As a daughter, I knew she was actively dying. Shakily I went to her room, the portable phone still cradled in my hand.

"Mom," I whispered as I brushed the damp hair off her forehead. She opened her glassy eyes and a smile began at the corners of her dried lips.

"Sweetheart," she murmured.

I explained our choices with tears in my eyes, unable to make this weighty decision alone—the scared little girl, even then needing her to be my mommy, my guardian.

"I want to stay here. I don't want to die in the hospital with all those tubes and things," she said with great effort. I cried openly then and put my head on her chest. Her thin hand stroked my head. "I'll always be here," she whispered as she weakly squeezed my shoulder. "Right here."

That painful night passed, alleviating my feeling that my choice would kill her quickly. Yet the end of life was getting closer. Death's presence was hovering in the house, unobtrusive but waiting. My mother's body and spirit rallied—the fever broke. She began to call friends. After asking about their welfare, she would say unhesitatingly, "I'm dying and just wanted to talk to you one last time." Some were shocked; some offered condolences, mused about shared memories, said good-bye. Others were awkward and uncomfortable with this raw honesty, unable to acknowledge that she was dying. Close friends came to visit, said good-bye in person, and witnessed a human body in decay and a soul trying to leave this earth.

Every day she wanted a bath, so my husband and I would carry her to the tub filled with warm sudsy water and sponge her off. It wasn't difficult for us physically, as my mother weighed less than ninety pounds by then. Her skin hung from her bony frame, bright yellow from the cancer that had consumed her liver. Her abdomen was swollen and painful. But the water soothed as we poured it on her chest and back and she sighed with pleasure.

One day, she did not want to get out of bed for her daily wash.

"Not today," she mumbled.

I tried turning her to change the sweaty sheets and she groaned in agony.

"Okay, Mom, okay," I replied as I lay her slowly back on the bed. "I'm sorry."

Those two words carried so much more than an apology for the physical pain I was causing by moving her. I'm sorry you are dying. I'm sorry you won't get to see your grandsons become Bar Mitzvah or go to the Knights of Columbus dances you loved so much, or eat your nightly banana, or play pinochle with me. I'm sorry you won't be able to call me your "little princess" anymore. I'm sorry your life has to end like this. I'm sorry life has to end at all.

That night my husband woke me up as I fitfully slept. We took turns sleeping with my mother, never wanting her to be alone at the final breath.

"Mary, I think Mom is going to die tonight," he quietly said. "She has the death rattle."

I gathered our sons, aged nine, seven, and two years, and went to her room. I lay next to her, two boys on the other side of her, the third on a child's sofa on the floor, my husband next to him. Mom lay on her back, ashen colored even in her jaundiced luminescence, breathing erratically through cracked lips, encrusted secretions at the corners of her mouth and eyes, pain still visible in facial grimaces.

I hugged her gently and the boys did too. They easily fell asleep within the dreams of childhood innocence. Despite knowing this was the end, I drifted off as well. I awoke with a start. Something was wrong; I no longer heard her rattling breathing in my ear.

She was gone. Her skin was still warm to the touch as I felt for a pulse that I knew was not there. I put my ear to her chest, my face to her lips, feeling no air movement. Silence. I pronounced her dead.

I woke everyone, saying, "Mom just died." And then we all cried; even the toddler joined in because he sensed the tragedy surrounding him. We took turns having a final visitation with her, each of us placing a single red rose (her favorite) in her hands as we said our individual good-byes.

It was over. Seventy-nine years of life, two months of death. On the night of the fever, my family acknowledged death and invited him into our home. From that moment on, he sat politely in a corner, waiting patiently for the time and place. We sat with him, Mom and I; she with a conspiratorial look from time to time. They had a mutual agreement—she could take care of her last good-byes and prepare her only child for the hardest thing to face in life, and death would wait.

Death, which I have spent so much time interpreting, translating his physical descriptors for those that remain, gave me a gift. One I gratefully accepted.

We had chosen to avoid interventional therapy. It was Mom's wish—no hospitalization, no treatment, and no invasive tube to drain toxic fluid from a blocked system that would inevitably clog again. We watched as she refused to eat solid food and fed her like an infant with a small spoonful of strained squash or vanilla ice cream. Her intake was minimal; she did not have the stamina for more than a few mouthfuls. We watched as she stopped drinking, taking only sips of flavored water through a straw, and at the end allowed us only to wet her lips. These gestures of providing sustenance given by my older sons were tangibly comforting to them even though the physical aid they could provide was minimal.

Hardest of all, though, was watching her in worsening pain despite hospice providing pain medication. Even as I moved her body on her final day of life, my heart nearly broke when the slightest turn caused her excruciating pain.

Yet what if death had been unkind, slower and more cruel in its approach with my mother? Would we have done anything differently? As a loving daughter and a knowledgeable physician, I would hope to have had a frank conversation with her. I want to believe I would have honored her choice whatever it was and accepted her decision. Just as we were able to discuss the fever and the option of operation and hospitalization, I would have wanted to face any new options with the same raw honesty. But I am acutely aware of the reality that organized medicine would have been bereft of advice and not able to have assisted us in this decision. I know that legally an act of compassion could be prosecuted as a crime of violence. In the end, we would have been entirely, and utterly, alone.

In the past, I have been angry over senseless accidents to children or when a raging infection treatable by antibiotics overwhelms someone. Death has haunted me, leaving me unsettled with the scenes I envision of the last minutes of a decedent's life; that fine line between life and death is crossed in a millisecond when a singular action marks the difference between living and dying. Indeed, this vision of death does pit it as an adversary.

But, even in the unpredictable cases that I investigate, death is not simply a foe. For me, death has become a kind of colleague. The accumulated ghosts of those whose bodies I have examined help me to consider various alternatives in the new cases that I must face. This useful insight that death provides me in my daily work allows me to uncover the true source of the demise, and understand the malfunctioning of the human body on a deeper level.

I have seen the spectrum of death's role from antagonist to colleague in both the professional and personal worlds in which I live. Within the safety and security of my own home and family, in the confines of a predictable physical disease, death even became a friend.

My experiences have led me to believe that we should not limit our understanding and experience of death to the physical, as seen through the eyes of criminal death investigation, or the spiritual through the theories of religious beliefs. The choice does not have to be either/or. We must evolve from a primitive aversion to death to a closer, more realistic understanding of it.

Death is complex and no one choreographed response can work in every situation. In cases where the disease process is consuming our physical being, can we, should we choose the time and place of our death? Should we fight for whatever second of life is left to us or welcome the last moment in this world? Delay the process or expedite it? And, if not for ourselves, should we discuss this frankly with our terminally ill relatives? Should we at least recognize that we—and they—might have a choice?

If a person in pain can actually choose to have a peaceful exit, shouldn't we as a civilized society, as compassionate and sentient beings, support this? Should we pursue legal avenues for allowing access to this process? Should we legalize assisted suicide so that we can freely discuss our final options with medical personnel without fear of criminal investigation?

Life is a stronger, more evocative force that provides humans with purpose, hope, and a myriad of pleasurable feelings and experiences. Death is an opposing force of nature—a loss of living, an absence of sensate self, and sometimes a form of hopelessness or violence. However, taken in the context of the more predictable illness and disease that affects our bodies, death may possibly be viewed as a life-enhancing force—one to be encountered and understood from a new angle, on its own terms.

When our health fails and we look to our future and the finite possibilities of existence, death may be more of a comrade than we have considered him in the past.

PART TWO

Perspectives

In Part Two, writers from diverse backgrounds and representing sometimes conflicting points of view examine death and dying in essays less personal and more overtly political than those in Part One.

We open this section with two powerful essays that present sharply contrasting opinions on what constitutes "the good death" and whether it is achievable or not today, when most of us will face slow dying.

Award-winning journalist Stephen Kiernan details how and why the American way of death has changed. More of us will live longer, he writes: "by 2030, when the 1950s baby boomers reach old age, the number of people over eighty-five will have more than doubled, to 9 million." And more of us will need end-of-life care that we cannot get at home: "according to geriatric-care specialists, 56 percent of Americans alive today will wind up in a nursing home at some point." In light of this shift, Kiernan calls for a new approach to health care in America that moves from an overemphasis on acute and critical care to a focus on chronic care. He explains how treatment options—and resources—are dangerously misplaced: "In 1976 people struck by the major causes of death needed acute and critical care. They required aggressive interventions and techniques, responding to a sudden crisis and its immediate aftermath. That kind of treatment is precisely what an ICU is expert in delivering. And that expertise has been heroically successful. Today, though, when death is gradual, patients need a chronic-care model. They need more nonclinical services, greater consideration of their emotions, families, and finances. The ICU is as wrong a fit as using sports-medicine techniques to deliver a baby."

Kiernan advocates a more humane model for end-of-life care than he thinks hospitals and nursing homes typically provide. By treating pain aggressively through palliative care, while at the same time emphasizing the spiritual, emotional, financial, and psychological needs of the patient, as well as her physical needs, hospice cares for individuals, not cases, according to Kiernan. It thus represents a better option for the terminally ill.

While many of the writers in this collection share Kiernan's enthusiasm and optimism about hospice, Kathryn Temple disagrees.[1] She acknowledges that hospice has helped many, but she charges that it offers more than it can provide: "Entangled as it is with the other problems endemic to the American medical system, problems involving the institutional needs of hospitals, managed care, and insurance company mandates, hospice often comes up short in its efforts to provide what it calls 'a good death,' a death marked by dignity, choice, and strong family connections."

For example, while dying in a hospital might not be the best option for most people, for others it is. And dying at home may not be viable. Describing the final months of her husband's life, Temple makes her case: "He could not walk, use the toilet, or even manage the nurse's call button, which he seemed to confuse with the TV remote. Two or three times, he somehow managed to shift his body weight enough to fall, and on those occasions six to eight hospital staff would be mustered to raise him from the floor back to the bed. Once he was left on the cold hospital floor for hours while the staff tried to find enough people to help. Every few days he developed unexplained massive bleeding, bleeding that would be ejected all over the floor and, once, a complete wall of the hospital room. These late manifestations of imminent death would have occurred at home or in a hospice. Unpreventable, no matter what palliative care might have offered, they fly in the face of the hospice ideal of the 'good death.'"

Both Temple and Kiernan discuss the economics of the hospice movement. Temple writes that although hospice claims to be "'not a place, but an idea,'" nevertheless "it is an 'idea' supported by Medicare funds, covered by many health insurance plans, and relied upon by cancer centers, hospitals, and nursing homes to provide care for the dying." She claims that hospitals push hospice because it is cheaper than keeping patients hospitalized. Kiernan charges that, even if hospice is cheaper, the bulk of the nation's health-care dollars go not to hospice care but to "high-cost, low-quality end-of-life care" (like beds in the intensive care unit). While many have found hospice to be comforting and helpful, he sees hospice as underfunded and underused.

Temple's anger at the bad death her husband endured leads us to wonder just what a good death is. Certainly our religious beliefs, our culture, and other factors define a good death for each of us. For example, John Tsoi, director of Patient Advocacy at New York Downtown Hospital, says that for the Chinese a good death would include such factors as dying with a full stomach, knowing the children are married and self-sufficient, dying in old age after fulfilling one's moral duties, having immediate family members present and speaking last words to them.[2] A study described in the *Annals of Internal Medicine* identified six components of a good death: pain and symptom management, involvement in decision making, preparation for death, some process of completion, contributing to others, and affirmation of one's uniqueness.[3] Marilyn Webb, speaking out of her own experience in *The Good Death: The New American Search to Reshape the End of Life*, sums up the qualities of "good" and "bad" deaths that might transcend cultures: "those deaths that are good pull families together and leave a legacy of peace. Those that are bad leave a legacy of grief, anger, and pain that can continue across many generations."[4]

Other writers in this section bring their expertise to bear on key cases and laws that undergird the discussion of choices for end-of-life care. They discuss the Quinlan, Cruzan, and Schiavo cases mentioned in the Introduction—and others—as well as significant pieces of legislation in the United States and abroad, like the Oregon Death with Dignity Act, passed in 1994, which legalizes self-administered suicide in certain clearly defined cases and under specific conditions.

In complementary essays, Candace Cummins Gauthier and Natalie R. Hannon bring their considerable training and experiences to bear on how ethics should inform end-of-life care and decision making. A philosopher who has authored numerous publications in medical ethics and who teaches bioethics, Gauthier explains why the principles of beneficence, autonomy, and distributive justice should guide the decision-making process of health-care providers. Writing from the perspective of a hospital ethics committee member who also served as director of training and staff development, Hannon invokes beneficence, proportionality, respect for persons, justice, and the legal principles of self-determination and best interest as the principles guiding decisions in which her committee participated.

Both writers refer to specific, often complicated cases to indicate how such principles would be applied in practice. They deal with such issues as: withholding and withdrawing medical treatment, cases with and without advance directives, physician-assisted dying, and active voluntary euthanasia. And their essays demonstrate how principles, however clear in theory, become complicated in practice.

Besides discussing personal examples and those well-known cases referred to above, Cherylynn MacGregor includes a 2005 active euthanasia case that occurred after Hurricane Katrina in her essay, "Life or Death: Who Gets to Choose?" In this case, a doctor and two nurses were accused of murdering four older patients (between the ages of sixty-one and ninety-one), housed on the life-care floor of a New Orleans hospital, with lethal doses of morphine and Versed. While the New Orleans district attorney dropped charges against the nurses and a grand jury did not indict the doctor, this case sparked heated debate: "Many health-care professionals and attorneys have argued that the 'battleground conditions' after Katrina called for and justified 'battleground decisions' in the hierarchy of treatment and resources. However, others claimed that this case 'marks a major shift in American medical practice by expanding the frontier from killing consenting dying patients whose lives are deemed to be not worth living to killing non-consenting patients whose unhealthy lives are deemed to be not worth saving,'" MacGregor writes, quoting Charles Lugosi. Ironically, some of the challenges facing health-care providers in the Neonatal Intensive Care Unit are similar to those facing people working with the elderly and terminally ill, particularly the question of how to distribute often rare and/or costly resources, as Natalie Hannon explains in her essay.

In "Ageism and Late-Life Choices," Margaret Cruikshank brings a different perspective to the deaths of the four older patients after Hurricane Katrina, arguing that the "ageist implications of this tragedy have not been as prominent as the racial dimensions." She examines how ageism in our culture "compromises the quality of life for elders, inhibits their freedom to make choices, hastens or downplays the significance of their deaths, and may contribute either to suicide itself or to social attitudes that accept late-life suicide as natural, even desirable." Citing the former governor of Colorado Richard Lamm's approval of the rationing of health care to elders because old people have a "duty to die and get out of the way," Cruikshank declares that "neither profit nor convenience belongs at a deathbed."

In "Caregiving Beulah: A Relentless Challenge" (Part One), Susan Perlstein provides an example of the high cost of dying today. Once moved into assisted living, Perlstein's mother was spending her savings at a rapid rate, over $5,000 a month. As her daughter writes, "I was shocked at the exorbitant costs of her doctors, office visits, medications, and medical equipment as well as the residence— room, food, and aides." Then, after this experience, Perlstein writes about the complications of switching from Medicare to Medicaid. She would agree with Ira Byock's criticism of outrageous medical costs; he writes in his essay for this collection: "Adding insult to illness and injury, health insurance, Medicare, and Medicaid routinely pauperize people for being seriously ill and not dying quickly enough."

Later on, when the Perlsteins no longer had money for Beulah's home health-care worker, only the financial help of a cousin enabled them to continue providing their mother with quality care. It is "medical bills—not credit cards—[that] are the leading cause of bankruptcy in America," according to Kiernan, a statement echoed by others who have written on the health-care crisis in the United States.[5]

Thinking not only about the cost to her family, Perlstein wonders about the cost to society of end-of-life care: "I started thinking about health-care priorities and whether the government should set limits on costs for various procedures. . . . I wondered if these measures we were paying for were extraordinary and unjustified, given my mother's situation." Hannon and Gauthier also tackle the thorny issue of the distribution of health-care resources and fairness. "For example," Gauthier explains, "one theory says that a fair way to distribute health-care resources would be to give them only to people who can pay for them. Others provide criteria such as need, merit, contribution to society, and the best use of resources."[6] Whatever the solution, one thing seems clear, according to Ira Byock: "America's long-term care system is broken."

What isn't so clear is when and under what circumstances an individual should be able to choose death. In Part One, writing about the deaths of family members, Carol Oyster and Jean Levitan explored the social, religious, and moral arguments against suicide. For them, the term is inappropriate and too judgmental for what they witnessed. "The word *suicide* has so many negative connotations," says Levitan; "it is so often framed as a desperate act committed by those who are profoundly depressed. From a traditional religious perspective, suicide is a sin. From a legal perspective, it's a crime." Looking at the statistics for suicide among the elderly, Oyster raises the possibility of suicide as a reasonable option: "While the elderly represent approximately 12 percent of the population, they represent approximately 20 percent of the suicides. Between 60 and 85 percent of elderly suicides share with my father the fact of significant health problems. And in 80 percent of such suicides, poor health was at least a contributing factor. Under those conditions, isn't suicide a rational alternative?"[7]

In Part Two, Kathryn L. Tucker, a lawyer and advocate for the terminally ill, enters the debate, not only criticizing the term *suicide*, but also rejecting the commonly used terms *assisted suicide* and *physician-assisted suicide*. Tucker cites medical organizations and legal experts who recognize that the terms *suicide* and *assisted suicide* are inappropriate when discussing the choice of a rational, terminally ill person to seek medications to bring about a peaceful and dignified death. Tucker endorses the American Medical Women's Association position statement: Whereas "the terms 'assisted suicide' and/or 'physician-assisted suicide' have been used in the past, . . . to refer to the choice of a mentally competent, terminally ill patient to self-administer medication for the purpose of controlling time and manner of death, in cases where the patient finds the dying process intolerable, the term 'suicide' is increasingly recognized as inaccurate and inappropriate in this context." Instead, these less emotionally charged, more value-neutral and accurate terms are now being used: *aid in dying* or *physician-assisted dying*. Active in challenging right-to-die laws in the United States, Tucker provides an instructive review of the legal history in her essay.

"Dying Down Under: From Law Reform to the Peaceful Pill" by Philip Nitschke and Fiona Stewart provides a personal and historical account of the right-to-die movement in Australia. As a physician disgusted by what he saw as the medical profession's "insufferable paternalism" toward seriously ill and dying patients, Nitschke has dedicated his energies to ensuring that "the issue of when and how we want to die becomes another of a growing list of human rights in the industrialized West," like those for women, indigenous people, and gays, for example.

After "the heady days of the world's first voluntary euthanasia law," the Rights of the Terminally Ill (ROTI) Act, passed in the Northern Territory of Australia in 1996 (but overturned a year later), Nitschke developed what he calls the "Deliverance Machine." Consisting of a laptop computer attached to a syringe driver, the device "allowed patients to self-administer lethal drugs," and Nitschke provided it to Bob Dent, the first man to use the ROTI Act to end his own life. Nitschke was the presiding medical practitioner at the deaths of three other people who used the machine.

The authors describe the founding of Nitschke's and Stewart's nonprofit organization, Exit International, and the group's development of a homemade "Peaceful Pill" ten years later.[8] After telling the choosing-to-die stories of Bill and of Lissette, Nitschke and Stewart explain how they and others came to conceive of the pill as being accessible to all, "devoid of any qualifying criteria—other than old age," which put them "at odds with legislative reform in the area of end-of-life choices all around the globe."

A 2007 study of end-of-life practices in six European countries indicates that "the Dutch and Belgian parliaments voted in favour of euthanasia in 2001 and 2002. In Switzerland, assisted suicide has been implicitly authorized for many years and in the Netherlands it was legalized by an Act of 2001 which came into force in 2002. In France, an Act passed in April 2005 and brought into force in February 2006 authorizes doctors to withhold unnecessary medical treatment or to intensify pain relief, even if this unintentionally hastens death."[9] Physician-assisted death is not frequent in these countries, representing 0.1 percent of deaths in Italy, 1.8 percent in Belgium, and 3.4 percent in the Netherlands. In most cases medical decisions liable to hasten the deaths of very old people involve the alleviation of pain and symptoms. Rarer in Italy but more frequent elsewhere is the withholding or withdrawal of treatment.

While Nitschke and Stewart see some European countries at least addressing the question of the right to die, from their point of view individuals should have

that right without any strings attached. They explain what they see as the limitations of existing laws. In Oregon, and now we can add Washington, the person
must be "terminally or hopelessly ill": "In the Netherlands, for example, to qualify
to use the law a person must be experiencing extreme unrelievable suffering. . . .
In Switzerland–the only place in the world that allows foreigners to receive an
assisted suicide–the organization Dignitas only accepts people who are 'terminally
ill' or who have 'an incurable disease' or who are in a 'medically hopeless state.' In
none of these places can well, older people legally ask for assistance to end their
own lives at a time or place of their choosing. While suicide is legal, obtaining
the means to a peaceful, dignified passing–particularly if it is barbiturates
that are being sought–is illegal and can incur significant legal penalties in most
jurisdictions."[10]

Many of us worry that, at a certain age or at some point, we will lose our ability to make decisions or take action regarding the end of life. Given this situation,
who should speak for us when we can no longer express our own wishes?

If we have prepared advance directives, our wishes might seem obvious; but
Gauthier writes that some people argue that they should not be honored because
"the person who filled out these documents is not the same person as the one
presently suffering from advanced dementia, a devastating stoke, or persistent
vegetative state. [These same critics] also argue that when we are not yet suffering
from these kinds of conditions we cannot make an informed decision about what
we would want if we had them." Gauthier strongly disagrees: "If we are not qualified to make these decisions for our own future selves, then who would be? Even
if we do, in some sense, become a different person as an Alzheimer's patient or in
a persistent vegetative state, the earlier capable self is still the closest anyone could
be to the later incapable self. Furthermore, the earlier and later selves still share the
same body that will suffer and die one way or another, whatever we want to say
about the person before and after the onset of the relevant medical condition. . . .
I maintain that we are each in the best position, of all possible candidates, to make
these decisions for our own future medical treatment when we are conscious and
capable of doing so. We each know our own tolerance for pain. We know whether
or not we value length of life or quality of life more." However, Cruikshank adds a
note of caution about advance directives: "Although advance directives are praised

for encouraging autonomy for elderly persons, they may not always have this effect." They could be used to coerce older people into forgoing full care.

Both cultural norms and religious beliefs affect end-of-life decision making. For example, Hannon notes that in patriarchal cultures (such as in Latino and West African countries) medical decisions are given not to the patient but the husband or eldest adult son. She cites a conflict for the hospital's ethics committee when a Korean woman wanted to be told her full and truthful diagnosis, but her son, authorized by his mother to make decisions for her, told the staff not to tell her that she had terminal cancer. In his country, such a diagnosis would lead her to become depressed and not want to live out her remaining days, the son felt.

This idea that no news is hopeful news is prevalent in many other cultures; for example, a study in Ireland found that while 83 percent of patients wanted to be told the truth, only 55 percent of their relatives wanted them to be informed of the diagnosis and prognosis.[11] In a talk on "End of Life Issues and the Chinese Patient," John Tsoi explained why Chinese patients he has worked with are reluctant to discuss advance directives: *Death* is a forbidden word in Chinese culture and talking about death will make it happen.[12]

According to news articles in 2007, studies show that minorities are more likely to want aggressive care, and as a result "they are more likely to experience more medicalized deaths, dying more frequently in the hospital, in pain, on ventilators and with feeding tubes—often after being resuscitated or getting extra rounds of chemotherapy, dialysis or other care."[13] Minorities are also underrepresented in hospice and palliative care: 7.5 percent of hospice patients are black and 4.8 percent are Hispanic, less than half their representation in the general population. The California HealthCare Foundation report found that "some minorities and immigrants view hospice care as a way for doctors to deny them the medical care they've been fighting for."[14] While the focus is on race in many of these studies, a significant part of the explanation of differences is socioeconomic. Not surprisingly, "one study found that people with higher income and more access to treatment are about twice as likely to feel comfortable with withdrawing care as those of more modest means."[15] If you don't speak English, and if you are black, Hispanic, poor, elderly, or a woman, argues Ira Byock, there is a greater chance of dying in pain.[16]

The perception of doctors has changed over time. Natalie Hannon writes that, up until the sixties, patients trusted physicians to do what was in their best interests; back then, we did not question medical authority. But this is no longer the rule. Hannon claims that the feminist movement was one of the key factors in this loss of trust and new questioning of doctors' recommendations, since it "criticized the paternalism of male physicians and the medical establishment in general." Unethical and racist research was another factor, Hannon cites the most well known example, the Tuskegee Study of Untreated Syphilis in the Negro Male, "which was conducted from the early 1930s to the 1970s. Poor, southern African American men who had syphilis were denied treatment, so that the course of syphilis could be studied, despite the fact that the course of syphilis was known. . . . Besides Tuskegee, there was exposé after exposé of other unethical medical studies. For example, patients at Willowbrook, a home for retarded children in Staten Island, New York, were infected with the hepatitis virus to study the infection; in Texas, Mexican American women participated in a double-blind experiment to see the effects of birth control pills, without the women's consent or knowledge. (All the women believed they were receiving birth control.)"[17]

They may no longer be seen as absolute authorities, but doctors still play a central role in the process of death and dying. So it is heartening that, in recent years, a number of medical practitioners—and others—have called for changes in the way medical schools train them. As many have pointed out, medical students are taught to win the fight over death, to cure their patients, not to oversee and support a comfortable journey out. Usually, they are not trained in end-of-life-care. As Stephen Kiernan wryly notes, medical educators spend "more time teaching students how to deliver a baby than how to deliver an adult into eternity." Atul Gawande admits that "most of us in medicine . . . don't know how to think about decline."[18]

There have been some changes. Surgeon Pauline W. Chen finds hope in new specialized medical school curricula in end-of-life care and an increase in membership in the American Academy of Hospice and Palliative Care to more than 2,000 members in 2005 from 250 in 1988. Nevertheless, she maintains that most doctors still "remain unwilling to talk with patients about death."[19] Physician Jerome Groopman teaches a course to first-year students at Harvard College called "Insights from Narratives of Illness." He uses literature—from Tolstoy to

Philip Roth—because "no insight into its more existential aspects is found in clinical textbooks, properly devoted to physiology, pharmacology, and pathology.
Rather it is literature that most vividly grapples with such mysteries, and with the
character of physician and patient."[20] Unfortunately, until this is a required course
for doctors, it will have little effect on doctor/patient relations.

In this collection, Cherylynn MacGregor mentions factors besides their training that affect how doctors treat or do not treat patients in severe pain at the end
of their life. Government sanctions for physicians prescribing pain medication
(which can lead to reprimands, fines, or imprisonment) and insurance regulations
that monitor doses and services keep doctors from providing optimum care.

Long-time palliative-care physician and advocate for improved end-of-life
care Ira Byock addresses the problem with medical schools today in our last essay:
"In medical schools across the country, students are required to take classes and
rotations in obstetrics amounting to 150 hours or more of training, much as they
were in the 1950s. Yet today few doctors in the United States deliver babies in
their practices and every physician who does has completed post-graduate residency training in obstetrics or family medicine. In contrast, the large majority of
physicians participate in the care of people who are chronically or acutely ill, yet
required medical school curricula remain scant in topics such as communication,
pain assessment and management, ethics of decision making, and guidance for
people facing life's end."

In the debate for and against physician-assisted dying, Byock claims that both
sides are wrong and gives reasons that he has come to this conclusion, having
been "a former partisan (for the con side)." The issue, for Byock, is larger than a
debate over whether physicians should be allowed to assist their patients to die,
although that debate did call attention to the plight of dying Americans in the
1980s. Instead, he recognizes that end-of-life care itself must change: "In the context of the contemporary crisis that surrounds dying, a complete life-affirming
moral position would include a call to individuals and communities of faith to act
on their fundamental responsibilities to care for people who are dying and support
their families during caregiving and in grief."

What would such change look like? Byock calls on "faith leaders, congregations, faith-based medical centers and social services organizations" to become

involved in fixing our broken health-care system. Admitting that "substantial, possibly unprecedented commitments of time and money would need to be invested in large-scale initiatives in health care, independent and assisted living, long-term care, and community-based social support," he contrasts this spending with what has already been spent on political battles to advance one side or the other.

Citing solutions ranging from paying a living wage to nurses and aides, to organizing volunteer groups to visit nursing homes, to promoting legislation to mandate that state insurance policies include adequate hospice and palliative-care coverage, Byock calls on us as individuals and citizens to respond to the crisis. As he concludes his essay, "In the current and future crisis that surrounds the way we die, solutions . . . can be reached by taking the social and cultural high road of building common ground above and beyond the fray. By our words and, far more importantly, by our actions we can demonstrate how a civilized society cares well for its members through the end of life."

We end this section—and the collection—with a poem by the feminist writer and cat lover Marge Piercy.[21] In "End of days," Piercy writes that she wants to die like a beloved cat who senses that death is near, quickly and painlessly, in the arms of someone who cares.

She thus sums up the hopes and fears of many writers in this collection—and many of us—when she writes that, if she reaches a point where she can no longer choose,

> I want someone who loves me
> there, not a doctor with forty patients
> and his morality to keep me sort
> of, kind of alive or sort of undead.
> Why are we more rational and kinder
> to our pets than with ourselves or our
> parents? Death is not the worst
> thing; denying it can be.

NOTES

1. Differing experiences of hospice care are also described in Part One. For instance, Sara Evans's parents shared a room in a nursing home. Both participated in hospice care with Maxilla (her mother) moving to a hospice inpatient facility named Solace, where "[f]rom the moment she arrived she was enfolded in a community of caregivers whose sole

purpose is comfort on every level–physical, emotional, spiritual." June Bingham also praises hospice. In contrast, the experience of Jean Levitan's aunt with hospice was negative. Because she was entering hospice, "they assumed that death would come as peacefully as possible." Instead, she ran into a bureaucracy of paperwork, caught between hospital and hospice, not getting care. Susan Perlstein's mother, in her nineties, wanted to be independent, but finally agreed to assisted living and home hospice. While she did not always follow the hospice team's advice, she loved her hospice doctor.

2. John Tsoi, talk and PowerPoint presentation, at the Closing Plenary, Twelfth Annual Jarvie Colloquium, "Preparing for and Coping with the 'Last Chapter of Life': The Older Person, Families, Friends, and Workers," New York, June 8, 2007.

3. Karen E. Steinhauser, Elizabeth C. Clipp, Maya McNeilly, Nicholas A. Christakis, Lauren M. McIntyre, and James A. Tulsky, "In Search of a Good Death: Observations of Patients, Families, and Providers," *Annals of Internal Medicine* 132, no. 10 (May 2000): 825–32. Discussed in Jane Brody, "World Enough and Time for 'a Good Death,'" *New York Times*, October 31, 2006.

4. Marilyn Webb, *The Good Death: The New American Search to Reshape the End of Life* (New York: Bantam Books, 1997).

5. See "The Health Care Crisis and What to Do About It" by Paul Krugman and Robin Wells, *New York Review of Books*, March 23, 2006, where they review three books: *Can We Say No? The Challenge of Rationing Health Care*, by Henry J. Aaron and William B. Schwartz, with Melissa Cox, Brookings Institution; *The Health Care Mess: How We Got into It and What It Will Take to Get Out*, by Julius Richmond and Rashi Fein, Harvard University Press; *Healthy, Wealthy, and Wise: Five Steps to a Better Health Care System*, by John F. Cogan, R. Glenn Hubbard, and Daniel P. Kessler, American Enterprise Institute/Hoover Institution.

6. The intensity and cost of care provided to Medicare patients with chronic illnesses vary widely among top-ranking hospital in various regions. See Robert Pear, "Researchers Find Huge Variations in End-of-Life Treatment," *New York Times*, April 7, 2008.

7. An early article on the subject is Lisa Belkin's "There's No Simple Suicide," *New York Times*, November 14, 1993. The suicide rate among midlife Americans (forty-five-to-fifty-year-olds) increased nearly 20 percent from 1999 to 2004. For women in that age range, the rate leapt 31 percent. Patricia Cohen, "Midlife Suicide Rates, Puzzling Researchers," *New York Times*, February 19, 2008.

   On suicide research, see "When a University Kills Suicide Research," *Inside Higher Ed*, July 7, 2008.

8. In "In Tijuana, a Market for Death in a Bottle," *New York Times*, July 21, 2008, Marc Lacey quotes Philip Nitschke on the availability of Mexican pentobarbital.

9. Johan Bilsen, Joachim Cohen, and Luc Deliens, "End of Life in Europe: An Overview of Medical Practices," *Population and Society*, no. 430 (January 2007): 1. See also Mark Landler, "Assisted Suicide of Healthy 79-Year-Old Renews German Debate on Right to Die," *New York Times*, July 3, 2008.

10. Jane Brody's article "Terminal Options for the Irreversibly Ill," *New York Times*, March 18, 2008, names some organizations that provide help for people nearing the end of life, like Compassion and Choice and the Final Exit Network. She refers to the book *To Die Well* by Sidney Wander and Joseph Glenmullen. See also *Jane Brody's Guide to the Great*

Beyond: A Practical Primer to Help You and Your Loved Ones Prepare Medically, Legally, and Emotionally for the End of Life (New York: Random House, 2009) for information as to options and choices.

11. Jane Brody, "Tough Question to Answer, Tough Answer to Hear," *New York Times*, March 6, 2007.

12. Tsoi, "Preparing for and Coping with the 'Last Chapter of Life.'"

13. Rob Stein, "At the End of Life, a Racial Divide: Minorities Are More Likely to Want Aggressive Care, Studies Show," *Washington Post*, March 12, 2007. Research has shown differences in life span based on socioeconomic grouping and racial and ethnic background. Robert Pear, "Gap in Life Expectancy Widens for the Nation," *New York Times*, March 23, 2008.

14. "Few Minorities Use End-of-Life Hospice Care," Associated Press, July 15, 2007.

15. Stein, "At the End of Life, a Racial Divide."

16. Ira Byock, *Dying Well: The Prospect of Growth at the End of Life* (New York: Riverhead Books, 1997), 242. The subculture of terminally ill people has been compared to a "minority group that lacks social, cultural, or economic power." See *A Few Months to Live: Different Paths to Life's End* by Jane Staton, Roger Shuy, and Ira Byock (Washington, DC: Georgetown University Press, 2001).

17. Hannon cites Robert Veatch, "Experimental Pregnancy," *The Hastings Center Report* (June 1971): 2–3.

18. Atul Gawande, "The Way We Age Now," *The New Yorker*, April 30, 2007, 55.

19. Pauline W. Chen, "The Most Avoided Conversation in Medicine," *New York Times*, December 26, 2006. See also her book, *Final Exam: A Surgeon's Reflections on Mortality* (New York: Knopf, 2007).

20. "Prescribed Reading," *New York Times Sunday Book Review*, May 13, 2007. The article "The Do-Not-Resuscitate Order [DNR]: Associations with Advance Directives, Physician Specialty, and Documentation of Discussion 15 Years after the Patient Self-Determination Act [PSDA]," by E. D. Morrell, B. P. Brown, R.Q.K. Drabiak, and P. R. Helft in *Journal of Medical Ethics* 34 (2008): 642–647, observes that still in 2008 DNR orders are written very late in a patient's hospital course. The researchers attribute doctors' reluctance to write DNR orders earlier "to diverse considerations, including the unpredictable nature of critical illness and the emotional and time-intensive character of this type of conversation. Many initiatives over the past decade have been aimed at improving care for the dying with regard to DNR orders: ethics committees, palliative care consultation services, medical school competency-based curricula for students and residents designed to teach and evaluate skills such as effective communication and ethical awareness, and the hospice care movement. Despite all of these interventions, our data suggest that patterns of DNR ordering have changed very little since the passage of the PSDA."

21. Piercy writes at length about the joys of living with cats in *Sleeping with Cats: A Memoir* (New York: HarperPerennial, 2002).

The Transformation of Death in America

STEPHEN P. KIERNAN

The nation's leading cause of death for much of the past century has been heart disease, and its most common manifestation in 1976 was the heart attack. Back then Americans suffered more than 750,000 heart attacks annually. Stroke—the bursting of a blood vessel in the brain—was another major cause of death. Accidents rounded out the top tier of the list.

A generation ago life ended swiftly. Death fell upon most people with nearly the speed and severity of a guillotine blade.

It is no longer so. Over the past thirty years the rapid causes of death have declined, while gradual causes have grown exponentially. Most people today do not die suddenly; they die incrementally.

Not only is the manner of death changing, but also the change is accelerating. A few numbers describe the transformation succinctly.

First the big one: Deaths from heart attack now occur at a rate 61 percent below that of thirty years ago.

Stroke fatalities have plummeted, too, by 71 percent in the past thirty years.

The rate of fatalities from accidents has plunged 36 percent.

The way we die has been utterly altered.[1]

Today people's dying occurs gradually, from sicknesses that take their lives by degrees. In a recent fifteen-year span, deaths from chronic respiratory disease increased 77 percent. Fatalities from Alzheimer's disease have doubled since 1980. Some 24.3 million people have that illness today, living an average of eight years, and the number is expected to reach 42.3 million in 2020.[2]

The list of gradual killers is long and growing. People now succumb to congestive heart failure, lung disease, diabetes that leads to kidney failure, ALS (or Lou Gehrig's disease), Parkinson's, osteoporosis that results in falls, confusion, and immobility. Today people face a whole battalion of incremental illnesses. AIDS is the brutal newcomer—unheard-of in 1976, the leading killer of twenty-five-to-forty-four-year-olds in 1995, and still among the top causes for that age group.[3] But the granddaddy of them all is cancer.

Despite decades of research, yielding near-heroic advances in detection, diagnosis, and treatment, cancer fatalities in the past thirty years have increased 22 percent. Smoking offers a tempting target for blame. Cancers from tobacco take about 180,000 people's lives each year. But cigarettes are only part of the problem. The panoply of various carcinomas, myelomas, and melanomas now accounts for almost 550,000 deaths in America yearly.

The situation will undoubtedly worsen. More than 16 million people were diagnosed with cancer between 1990 and 1997. The American Cancer Society estimates that the odds of Americans having cancer sometime in their life are one in two for men and one in three for women. If current trends continue, by 2010 cancer may replace heart disease as the nation's leading killer.[4]

The change, for a growing number of people every day, is this: dying today is gradual. For the first time in human history, we can anticipate our mortality. We can watch its slow approach. We can look it in the eye.

Quite apart from the statistics cited, people know that dying is different today simply from their own experience. They mourn the friend who found a lump in her breast and lymph nodes, then underwent chemo, radiation, and surgery, and eighteen months later was dead. They recall the neighbor who began acting erratically, later could not finish a sentence and, after a cruelly long decline with his body sound but his mind absent, died unable to recognize his own family. People know the smoker with congestive heart failure who took years to slip from pale skin and cold fingers to a life tethered to an oxygen tank to dying in his nursing-home bed. They remember the diabetic who ignored symptoms until it was too late, surviving after kidney failure thanks only to the mixed blessing of dialysis every few days and spending years on the transplant list only to die before a matching donor could be found. They know the unfortunate soul whose advanced Parkinson's lasted ten years, or whose Lou Gehrig's disease took away one function and one piece of dignity at a time. They watched a person far too young waste away from AIDS.

Yes, gradual death has its own savagery. Its result is no less final than a sudden passing. But death by degrees does mean that *dying* is different. It takes months, not minutes. For a rapidly growing number of people, dying has become a process. There are options and opportunities; there are choices. To understand the enormous potential that now exists in the dying process, and to learn how to maximize that opportunity, it is instructive first to contemplate how the change in death occurred.

Medical advances offer some explanation. Beta-blocker drugs that prevent heart attacks, for example, are post-1976 medicines. Prescription drugs have helped treat incremental illnesses, too, from tamoxifen thwarting breast cancer to AZT's success in slowing the onslaught of HIV. Medical researchers predict gains against all manner of diseases once they grasp a fuller understanding of DNA—a day they herald as fast approaching because the mapping of the human genome finished three years ahead of schedule.

But medical discoveries are only part of the story. A more complete answer is that Americans have sought—nay, demanded—better delivery of the medical capacity that already exists, and better access to it regardless of cost, because they believe this improvement will give them longer and healthier lives.

They are not always right. Replacing an aging ambulance with a medivac helicopter is no substitute for sensible eating and regular exercise. But when it comes to sudden death, the demand for improved delivery of care—an insistence on better service—has made a demonstrable difference. The change has come at many levels of society, from government programs to hospital facilities to communication tools to skills that Americans have learned for themselves, all to thwart sudden death.

Think of this achievement. About 6.4 million people now survive angina chest pain *each year*, while an additional 700,000 people survive a heart attack *each year*.[5]

Even though many people do not receive ideal care quickly enough, medical intervention in heart disease saves literally millions of lives. In 2002 alone there were 2,057 heart transplants, 93,000 heart-valve replacements, and 515,000 cardiac-bypass procedures. The success of these procedures is astonishing: right now there are 13 million victims of heart disease alive in the United States.

Treatment of strokes, the second-leading cause of death in 1976, remains complex. It's not as simple as giving aspirin, and stroke remains a major cause of permanent disability. Still, there have been gains. About 700,000 Americans still suffer a stroke each year. Some 530,000 of them survive. Consequently, about 5.4 million stroke survivors are alive in America today.[6]

The point is that progress in the fight against sudden death is not solely a result of medical advances. It is a result of spending huge sums to battle the causes: The American Heart Association estimates the cost of heart disease and stroke at $393.5 billion annually. Another factor that must not be under-estimated, even in light of such a massive expenditure, is the consumer-driven improvement in delivery of existing medical tools.

The decline in accidental deaths follows this pattern. Although recent years have brought many lifesaving improvements in emergency medicine, the factors in reducing accidental fatalities are as varied as bike helmets and flotation vests, occupational-hazard protections in factories, car-safety recalls, and utilities' more vigilant pruning of trees along power lines.

The evidence of a national mobilization against sudden death is consid-erable. At about the same time as Lyndon Johnson's order that led to EMTs, the Red Cross began offering lifeguarding courses to reduce drownings. Starting with the National Traffic and Motor Vehicle Safety Act, Congress began a series of mandated safety standards, from compelling auto manufac-turers to include seat belts to requiring children in the 1990s to ride in car seats.[7] The Federal Aviation Administration began investigating air crashes in painstaking reconstructive detail; today no other form of mass transporta-tion is safer. The food supply had to meet higher standards under the Wholesale Meat Act and the Wholesale Poultry Products Act.

In fact, Washington repeatedly bolstered the push for a safer America. Pollution that caused illness or death diminished under the Clean Water Act and the Safe Drinking Water Act. When Congress created the Consumer Products Safety commission, establishing government standards in areas as varied as medicine bottle caps and children's pajamas, the rate of death and injury from accidents fell 20 percent in a decade.[8]

Courtrooms have been a factor, too. It's easy to argue that American society has become too litigious. Yet one welcome side effect of consumer and employee lawsuits has been improved product and workplace safety. From 2002 to 2003 alone, the rate of deaths due to injury on the job fell 13 percent.[9]

Quantifying the actual number of lives saved is harder than with heart attacks or strokes. Statisticians can't measure a death that didn't occur. But the impact on American lives can certainly be counted in the tens of thousands each year.

How did accidents decline? People demanded it. And they took personal responsibility, buying safer cars and suing unsafe manufacturers while developing skills for their own benefit. How did heart attacks and strokes decline? The same way, from consumer demand coupled with changed public behavior.

So it is that life expectancy in America continues to grow. Social advocacy, governmental policy, and personal action combine—and succeed. In 1900 the average American lived to be forty-seven. His counterpart in 2000 lived to be seventy-five, a single-century jump of twenty-eight years. Yet the latest data, from late 2005, indicates an even better average expectancy of 77.6 years. Note, too, that the extension of life is accelerating. Almost two-thirds of the gain—nearly two decades of life—has been accomplished since 1960 as a result of the mobilization against sudden death. That is what such a comprehensive societal response can bring: eighteen years.

Some demographers argue that using average life expectancy may actually understate the gains. Another statistic may be more telling: In 2000 there were 4.2 million Americans aged eighty-five or older; by 2030, when the 1950s baby boomers reach old age, the number of people over eighty-five will have more than doubled, to 9 million.[10]

It is a signal accomplishment of the postwar generation that despite the public's many complaints about the cost and complexity of medical care, and despite the well-documented decline in exercise rates and increase in obesity, people today simply live longer.

Here are the realities of where and how Americans die.

Depending on the region of the country, between 50 and 60 percent of people's lives end in hospitals. They go to these institutions for advanced care like surgery or because of an emergency or for medical equipment such as ventilators and feeding tubes. If they are near death, these patients typically land in intensive care. However, many terminally ill patients come to wish that their desire for late-stage heroic interventions had gone ungranted. There is nothing wrong with hospitals, of course, nor with people who work in ICUs. On the contrary, intensive care saves thousands of lives each year. Countless trauma patients would never recover without the powerful tools and specialized expertise of intensive care.

Yet there may be a great deal wrong with using intensive medicine on a person whose death is certain and near. To begin with, for the patient, everyone in the ICU is a stranger. For the family, the head clinician comes into the patient's room, introduces himself, and promises to have the unit's other doctors stop by during their shift. Those visits may actually happen over the next few days, if the unit is not too crowded. Even if family members can keep these people straight, though, not one of the doctors knows the slightest nonmedical thing about the patient. There is negligible opportunity to personalize the care, much less help the sick person pass time in a fulfilling way. Visitation hours are limited, and there is little flexibility for making the room more comfortable or comforting. If the patient is conscious as he dies, breath by dwindling breath, he is also monumentally bored.

It is not crass to consider as well the cost of dying this way. An ICU bed costs about two thousand dollars a day, not counting lab tests and special equipment fees. That burden falls in part on health insurers (and thus whoever pays the premiums) and in part on taxpayers (when Medicare pays ICU bills). But the fundamental strain is heaviest on patients' loved ones. Medical bills—not credit cards—are the leading cause of bankruptcy in America. A 1995 study found that 31 percent of the families of dying people spent "all or most of their savings" on the patients' hospital care.[11]

This extravagance would be worthwhile if it resulted in a better experience for the person who is dying. But definitive research has found the opposite to be the case. Half of American patients who died in hospitals, one authoritative study found, experienced "moderate or severe pain at least half the time" during their final days.[12] Those last hours were not filled with quiet dignity and compassion, either. The same study found that 38 percent of patients who died in hospital spent ten or more days in intensive care or on a ventilator.[13] Researchers have revealed how unwelcome that level of intervention was to patients and families: 44.9 percent of ICU deaths came after life support was withdrawn or withheld.[14] In essence, people in that situation were almost eager to die.

Sometimes patients try to take control of the situation. They draw up legal documents that either permit another person to speak for them when they cannot or dictate what treatments they want and which they consider excessive. However, only a fraction of people have these instructions in place. Moreover, ICUs routinely act contrary to these directives, because staffers either are unaware that the documents exist or are too busy to read them.[15] One study found that 70 percent of physicians failed to determine whether dying patients wanted to be resuscitated in an emergency.[16]

The situation is no better in the second most common location where death occurs: nursing homes. About eighteen thousand of them are spread across America, housing almost 2 million people. Today more than 20 percent of Americans' lives end in these facilities, a number almost certain to rise.

There's nothing inherently wrong with nursing homes. They allow for a modicum of personal care, and families generally can visit whenever they wish. But the national nursing shortage, plus cost constraints that lead to fewer staffers being medically trained, have compromised the quality of nursing-home care.

That is not conjecture. The federal agencies that fund and oversee nursing homes make quality information public about individual facilities. Researchers at the University of California in San Francisco collated all that data to provide a national overview.[17] The truth is ugly.

- Residents were strapped down: 11.2 percent of nursing homes used physical restraints "for purposes of discipline or convenience" not related to the patient's medical symptoms.
- Residents were hungry: 9.3 percent of homes provided inadequate food, 7.7 had food that was nutritionally inadequate, 5.3 percent served "infrequent meals," and a stunning 36.2 percent failed to prepare and serve food in a manner sufficiently sanitary to prevent illness.
- Residents were dirty: 19.9 percent of nursing homes had poor housekeeping, while 13.8 percent failed to help people with daily living tasks such as grooming and oral hygiene.
- Residents grew sicker for avoidable reasons: 17.5 percent of nursing homes failed to "ensure that residents without pressure sores did not develop them." Another 11.8 percent failed to treat people with bladder incontinence well enough to prevent lost function and restore what had been lost. Some 18.4 percent of the homes failed to provide a comprehensive plan for residents' care, and 9.3 percent were cited for improper infection control. The general quality of care was deficient in 30.5 percent of the facilities.

- Residents were at risk: 22.4 percent of nursing homes provided insuffi-
  cient measures to prevent accidents, and 25.5 percent had environmental hazards. Another 24.6 percent had poor professional standards for
  staff, 13.6 percent hired "unemployable individuals," and 8.6 percent
  failed to follow proper pharmacy procedures.
- Residents were humiliated: 17.5 percent of nursing homes failed to maintain the dignity of their residents. Another 10.7 percent were deficient in
  protecting residents' privacy and confidentiality.

Strapped down, hungry, dirty, humiliated—that is the experience of
American elders. Each of these scores, not incidentally, reflected a decline in
care quality since 1997. The number of problems per facility leapt 40 percent
in six years. Living in a high-end home provided no guarantees, either. The
number of facilities with no deficiencies at all was 9.5 percent in 2003, less
than half the number in 1997.

Regardless of whether consumers know these grim details, they have
strong opinions about nursing homes anyway. In a 2001 survey of 3,262
seriously ill patients, only 7 percent said they were "very willing" to live
in a nursing home. In fact, 26 percent said they were "very unwilling" to do
so. A striking 30 percent said they would "rather die" than live in a nursing
home.[18]

Here's the really bad news: According to geriatric-care specialists, 56
percent of Americans alive today will wind up in a nursing home at some
point. Of those who stay longer than two weeks, 76 percent will die in that
facility. Twenty percent will spend more than five years in a nursing home.[19]

People would rather die than face a fate that, in growing likelihood, certainly awaits them.

Because neither the public nor policymakers have known that dying has
become gradual, they continue to treat the final stages of slow dying mistakenly, as if it were a sudden trauma. Consider two trends. First, the number of
hospitals across the country fell from 5,803 in 1980 to 4,895 in 2003, a drop
of 16 percent. Second, during that same period the number of intensive-care
beds jumped from 54,633 to 60,826—a leap of 11 percent.[20] That happened
while Americans were living longer and while more of them were succumbing to incremental illnesses. In other words, the manner of dying and the
manner of its treatment have been moving in opposite directions.

So, today there are machines to breathe for the patient, medicines to sustain blood pressure, tubes to provide nutrition, equipment to perform the tasks of the heart, lungs, kidneys, and bladder. Of course, using these devices is imperative if a patient might recover. The question is their usefulness for a person who will never be cured. The technology is so complete, neither a beating heart not a functioning brain is required to enable a body to persist on this side of what was once considered death. The machines can even keep a body's parts viable after the person has certifiably died; hospitals routinely do this while arranging organ transplants.

When high-tech medicine is most successful in preventing an all-but-certain death, however, it is also most dehumanizing—in the cases when medicine saved a life but not the person. There are now roughly thirty-five thousand people in the United States living in a persistent vegetative state.[21] That's thirty-five thousand people with no consciousness and no chance of recovery, the body's organs kept alive by ventilators and feeding tubes. Imagine the agony for their families. Imagine the expense. And to what gain?

Perhaps these thirty-five thousand lives may yet serve a societal purpose, if their plight awakens people to the change in dying from sudden to gradual and compels society to act upon that knowledge. Aware that death is likely to come slowly, patients could prepare for their passing with deliberation and calm. Families could offer and receive care while helping their loved ones close out their life with peace and unrivaled richness. Friends could provide the best that friendship is, the shared experience and common values. Medical professionals could deliver the kind of care that first led them to choose that line of work, the empathy and intimacy, the respectful treatment of a patient's ultimate trust.

But this is not how it happens. That is not what America has done with gradual death. The profound opportunity is almost always missed.

Until recent years the only people who knew for certain that death was approaching were criminals facing execution. Indeed, anticipating his life's end, at a fixed time and place and by a predetermined means, was a key component of the condemned man's punishment. America's attitude toward gradual dying remains locked in that thinking. People unfamiliar with death in any form are unequipped to capitalize on the unique potential of its present manifestation. The result? At a minimum, dying people experience preventable suffering. At the maximum, patients, families, and caregivers miss some of the most precious, compassionate moments life has to offer. We turn to medical technology that invades instead of curing, prolongs instead of healing, at a time when we, across the whole of society, could all be expanding our hearts.

Considering this opportunity, some of the obstacles are painfully practical. One example is physicians' worries over getting sued. Doctors routinely perform extra and perhaps unneeded medical actions out of fear that they could face a malpractice suit if they fail to use every treatment option. They likewise do not use the full power of pain medications, out of concern that they could trigger a criminal investigation of their prescribing practices.

Doctors' caution is entirely understandable. Yet surveys confirm that more than 90 percent of Americans want limits on their medical care at the end of life, no long-term feeding tubes or ventilator, for example, if they are never going to regain consciousness. Even more people want their pain managed aggressively. Thus, at the end of life, doctors and patients have directly conflicting purposes.

A further contributor to the problem may be misuse of medical powers. The word *misuse* ordinarily implies questionable motives, but in this instance it means a lack of awareness of how death has changed, and thus a mismatch between what patients need and what they receive.

Health care is typically delivered using one of three clinical models: critical care, for people with traumatic injuries such as those from a car crash; acute care, for people in a physical crisis such as a heart attack; and chronic care, for people who have an ongoing illness that is not in crisis but requires sustained treatment and attention. In 1976, people struck by the major causes of death needed acute and critical care. They required aggressive interventions and techniques, responding to a sudden crisis and its immediate aftermath. That kind of treatment is precisely what an ICU is expert at delivering. And that expertise has been heroically successful. Today, though, when death is gradual, patients need a chronic-care model. They need more nonclinical services, greater consideration of their emotions, families, and finances. The ICU is as wrong a fit as using sports-medicine techniques to deliver a baby.

There is another way. Poll after poll has found that Americans do not want to die in hospitals or in nursing homes. Consistently more than 90 percent say they want to die at home, among friends and family, with their pain treated aggressively.

There are organizations in every state that provide exactly this kind of care, through the hospice movement. The guiding premise of hospice is that people's needs at the end of their lives are much more than medical. They are spiritual, financial, emotional, psychological. Hospice strives to deliver the dying experience people say they want, attending to details many patients don't consider until someone asks: Which friends will you allow to visit, and whom do you want kept away? What foods do you want to eat until your appetite wanes? What faith, if any, do you wish to celebrate or observe? What old conflicts do you want to reconcile, and which would you rather leave unresolved? How do you want to balance receiving pain medication with remaining alert for visitors? In the final hours, what music do you want playing at your bedside?

Many people mistakenly believe that hospice is a kind of facility, akin to a nursing home. Hospice is actually a set of beliefs, a philosophy of health care that relies on medical facilities only some of the time.

The first hospice did resemble a nursing home, though it was considerably nicer. Founded by Cicely Saunders on the outskirts of London, St. Christopher's Hospice boasts gardens, a room for taking tea, a chapel. As a nursing student during World War II, Saunders received a thorough instruction in suffering. After the war she obtained a degree in social work, then went to medical school and became an M.D. She opened St. Christopher's in 1967.

The hospice philosophy places the patient at the center of care. That means managing pain is paramount, because pain-free people are far better able to attend to other important business. Medical concerns are only a subset of treatment and do not automatically take precedence over a patient's emotional or spiritual needs. As a result, a team of people is involved in the patient's care—doctors, nurses, social workers, clergy, and often volunteers who meet essential nonmedical needs such as driving people to appointments. The philosophy is not geared solely toward the patient, either. Hospice also attends to the sick person's family, their fears and challenges and grief.

The principles of hospice may seem like common sense, but they actually represented a radical departure from conventional medicine. Ordinary health care is organized around certain settings—the doctor's office, the lab, the hospital. Hospice care is designed in accordance with the patient's wishes, which may be to receive care in one of those places or in a nursing home or, most often, at home. Ordinary health care is about treating disease. Hospice is about caring for individuals. Everyday medicine treats only the person who is afflicted. Hospice treats family members as part of the plan of care.

Unfortunately, too often conventional health care believes that when there is no possibility of recovery, nothing more can be done. People in these systems often find themselves abandoned just when they most need attention and care. Hospice believes that as long as a person continues to live, a great deal can be done. The patient is only as alone as he chooses to be.

Finally, regular health care places people within systems, with schedules for medication and tests, fixed hours for meals, and no time or personnel to provide individualized care. Hospice is all about spoiling the patient, personalizing care down to details as specific as the art on the walls, the content and timing of meals, the music in the air. This approach can turn slow dying into something incredibly loving, calm, and even funny.

Hospice may provide cancer patients, for example, with a wide array of services. They may receive pain-control drugs. They may receive radiation to ease their suffering without aiming for a cure. They may obtain counseling or help from clergy. They may formalize in writing what steps they want taken to prolong their lives in its final days, and which measures they do not want. They may get help managing their household. Their families may receive respite care, as an aide or volunteer visits the home so loved ones can have a few hours' reprieve from caregiving—to shop for groceries, attend to other responsibilities, or just take a break.

When a person's condition worsens, hospice does not embark on futile adventures to prolong the suffering or delay the inevitable. Instead, the focus remains on keeping the patient as comfortable as possible and supporting her family as much as possible. If there is no one available to provide care at home, or family members are too old or too ill or otherwise unable to do the job themselves, hospice becomes an inpatient service, a kind of hospital that specializes in caring for people who are dying. Regardless of where they receive services—and here is perhaps the most dramatic break from conventional health care—when people in hospice care enter their lives' final stages, they are not abandoned. They continue to receive care up to and beyond their last breath. When a patient dies, his or her body is treated with respect. The family receives bereavement services if they wish. The people who cared for the patient, too, are given time and means to mourn.

While defining what hospice is, it is important to make two points about what hospice isn't.

First, hospice isn't alternative medicine or an alternative to medicine. Hospice care is directed by a physician and provided primarily by nurses who specialize in end-of-life care. It employs traditional medical tools for treating pain and other symptoms. Hospice is virtually as much its own form of medicine as cardiology or pediatrics.

Moreover, hospice respects the gains against illness that medical advances have wrought. One seasoned hospice worker notes that of the top twenty childhood diseases she encountered while providing terminal care to children in the 1970s, sixteen have since been eradicated. Medical science is a mainstay of hospice care.

Second, hospice is not about surrender or passivity or hurrying death along. Rather it is a vigorous, active effort to make the quality of a person's life as optimal as possible for as long as possible. The hospice ethos is that death occurs in an instant, and until that instant the patient is fully alive and fully deserving of respectful care. Often the quest may involve matters that are completely nonmedical. For example, a person with advanced terminal illness may wish for reconciliation with an estranged loved one. This issue may be paramount in the patient's mind. Regular health care shows little if any interest in such concerns. Hospice care, by contrast, would involve social workers, intermediaries, whatever means the patient approved, in the effort to achieve reconciliation.

In America, however, hospice is barely a sapling. Fewer than 20 percent of dying people use hospice resources to control and personalize their care. With the potential demand for dignified end-of-life care that exists today, just imagine the flood that will come in 2011 when the first baby boomers reach sixty-five years of age and are able to use hospice resources.

The trends are not encouraging. The number of sites providing hospice care has been increasing at about 3.5 percent a year, and the number of hospice patients has also grown.[22] But the number of intensive care beds also increased, the revenues they generate expanding at a rate averaging $17 billion a year. That means a larger share of the nation's health-care dollars winds up in high-cost, low-quality end-of-life care.

Hospice usage rates vary widely around the country. Rural areas score low, either because there are too few nurse providers or because the widely dispersed financial resources cannot meet the funding needs. Large cities fare poorly, too, perhaps because their academic medical centers accept hospice's role only with reluctance. In New York City in 2002, for example, 12.8 percent of terminally ill patients were found suitable for hospice; one hospice director in the city said it should be closer to 60 percent.

Many people who do enroll in hospice receive only a fraction of its potential benefit. The portion of hospice patients who die within one week of admission has increased 67 percent since 1992. Even hospice's strongest advocates admit that one week is far too brief a time to get pain under control, learn the patient's particular needs, and establish support systems for the family.[23]

These trends raise a central question about living well while dying slowly: If hospice is so effective, so compassionate, and so relatively inexpensive, why don't more people receive this treatment? Since the hospice model aligns so closely with how Americans say they want to be cared for at the end of their lives, why do so few people benefit from it? After all, everyone who goes to the emergency room with a broken leg receives an X-ray. Is end-of-life care so different?

Yes, it is. End-of-life care is different to medical educators, who spend more time teaching students how to deliver a baby than how to deliver an adult into eternity. It is different to health insurers, especially government programs, which will pay for extravagant medical interventions but not the tender loving care people want and deserve in their last days. It is different to hospital administrators, who generate huge revenues from inpatient intensive care units but don't make a nickel if a person dies quietly at home. And because people experience a loved one's death privately, one family at a time, end-of-life care is especially different for health consumers, who often do not even know that the hospice option is available to them.

The result is that hospice is sorely underused. The need is growing: financial pressures from the status quo are mounting. That ought to foster a booming increase in hospice care rather than a modest decline. Why is this happening?

- Until the 1980s Medicare—the nation's largest health-insurance program—did not pay hospice organizations for providing care. Even now, much of the cost of care is not reimbursed.
- Only a fraction of U.S. hospitals have staff trained to identify patients who are candidates for hospice and to help families tap that resource.

- Hospices struggle to provide care to people who live in nursing homes, because of turf and funding issues.
- Medicare's eligibility rules discourage doctors from considering hospice as an option for their dying patients. For people with kidney failure to qualify for hospice, for example, they must cease dialysis—even though that ensures their death from blood poisoning in weeks if not days.

The same is true of all curative treatment: for Medicare to pay a person's hospice bills, the patient must effectively stop seeking a cure. In other words, the patient must choose between living as long as possible or as well as possible. Government policy does not allow someone to pursue both. Here's a grim example of eligibility rulers that chill hospice use: The physician must provide a signed certification that the patient will be dead within six months. In addition to heartlessness, the problems with that policy are many. First, studies have found that doctors are notoriously bad at predicting when patients will die. Second, if a doctor's patients outlive the prediction, the physician may be prosecuted for Medicare fraud. No wonder doctors resist directing patients to hospice. No wonder a growing number of hospice patients enter its home-care program only days before dying. But the worst aspect of this eligibility rule is the effect it has on patients and their families. Because of the six-month certification requirement, patients equate entering hospice with surrendering the fight to stay alive. Families consider the suggestion of hospice a sign that the doctor has given up.

Add these forces together and the result is clear: While seven-eighths of the population want to die at home, without needless suffering, less than one-fifth actually does so. All the positive attributes of hospice are not enough to make it popular.

Not surprisingly, there is a growing effort to bring some hospice principles into hospitals, by providing what is now as "palliative care." In general, to palliate means to reduce the violence of something, to mitigate or soften its negatives. In gradual dying there inevitably comes a point when patients are not ever going to get better. But the fact that they cannot be cured does not mean that the tools and techniques of medicine cannot make their remaining life much better, that the negatives cannot be softened.

Consider a palliative approach to a woman with advanced lung cancer. After months or years of her battling the disease, it has finally spread throughout her body. She is not going to recover. She may have months before the cancer takes her life, but one morning she has difficulty breathing. She experiences panic and desperate coughing. Her oncologist finds a tumor in her esophagus. He promptly orders radiation therapy on that tumor. This treatment will not stop the disease, but it will prevent future episodes of compromised breathing. The patient will still die of lung cancer, but she will not gasp and choke in her remaining months, nor suffer prematurely because of a preventable blockage. Her treatment has been palliative, providing not a cure but comfort.

Palliative care is important for many reasons. First, there will always be patients who feel more secure within a health-care institution, people for whom the size and resources of a hospital are reassuring. A preference so central to their emotional well-being merits respect. Second, physicians observing the shift toward gradual dying may find it easier to advocate for better care within existing facilities than to create new programs. Third, palliative care's attention to comfort is applicable to many patients beyond those whose death is imminent.

"We're working way upstream of hospice,' says Diane Meier, who runs the palliative-care program at Mount Sinai Hospital in New York City. "From the moment you are diagnosed you receive both life-prolonging therapy and palliative care, until the very end when the patient is no longer able to benefit from the life-prolonging work, at which point care should focus one hundred percent on palliative care."

Like many hospice advocates, Meier partly defines her work by what it is not. "Palliative care is not about convincing people that it's okay to die. Palliative care is about helping people achieve the best quality of life they possibly can, for as long as they possibly can."

Finding demand for palliative care is not an issue, Meier says. When Mount Sinai started its program in 1997, "we expected fifty patients that year. We had two hundred and fifty. Last year we had nine hundred new patient consults, and we've had roughly five thousand patient visits since '97."

Doctors who direct patients to palliative care often become allies, because it lessens their workload. "You take a doctor, an oncologist, say, and he's got forty patients in his waiting room. He cannot spend an hour in a family meeting, discussing issues and options. We can. We do."

In addition to her medical duties, Meier is an advocate. She directs the Center to Advance Palliative Care, which works to spread palliative care around the country. "We provide technical assistance to local leaders on how to make the business case," Meier says, "how to project the need and the value of palliative care, how to measure your work to ensure quality, how to bill, how to launch a program that actually delivers on what it promises."

From a technical standpoint, palliative care is not difficult to provide, Meier says, yet most doctors don't know how. Persuading cash-strapped hospital administrators to undergo the expense of teaching them—and then to adopt palliative care principles permanently—is a real challenge. "Doctors don't know how to do this stuff, it's so arcane. There is plenty of content available on how to manage pain, but it is not enough to get the care to the bedside. You have to justify your existence."

Yet hospitals have many reasons to provide palliative care, Meier says. "There is both conclusive data and widespread public awareness that patients are suffering. And the business argument for change is also powerful. Hospitals with a growing population of increasingly frail patients are not going to make it without a palliative-care approach."

Meier is quick to boast that the number of hospitals moving into palliative care is fast growing, nearing 20 percent. Those inroads have resulted in part from the success of palliative care in hospitals that have embraced it, and in fair measure because of $23 million in Robert Wood Johnson Foundation funding for the advocacy center Meier runs. Despite all that spending and the clear need for improved care, however, 80 percent of U.S. hospitals have not embraced a commitment to ensuring patients' comfort at the end of their lives. Like hospice, palliative care has a long way to go.

It is fair to ask, too, why a matter as important as patients' comfort should be shuttled off to a distinct service within a hospital. Why should regular medicine shrug off these responsibilities? The job of compassionate patient care needs to be done everywhere, just as every doctor and nurse needs to know how to take vital signs. If something affects 100 percent of patients, shouldn't at least its rudiments be known by 100 percent of practitioners, with expertise available in 100 percent of institutions? The lessons of empathy and understanding, of responding to patient needs, are valuable not only in terminal care. Virtually every aspect of contemporary medicine could benefit from greater humanism and heart.

Shifting health care to accommodate today's manner of dying may sound like a daunting task. But there is a role model: the dramatic improvement in emergency care over the last generation. Institutional medicine has played a modest role. Far larger has been the influence of health consumers, who insisted on emergency services that reflected their genuine needs and who learned how to participate in their care and that of people they love.

The needs for end-of-life care are analogous: Just as 911 phone service activates emergency medicine, America needs to establish a responsive system for summoning excellent end-of-life care. In the same way that a half-day CPR course prepares ordinary people to help others avoid sudden death, America needs a class that teaches people how to seize the opportunity presented by slow dying.

Given this analogy, there are two encouraging factors in end-of-life care. First, unlike emergency medicine, decent treatment for dying people is relatively inexpensive. Rather than revolving around doctors, it relies on nurses, volunteers, and families to provide care. Instead of powerful drugs that restart hearts and open clogged arteries, it requires common pain medicines. Compassionate end-of-life care minimizes recourse to costly surgeries or heroic technologies. And it uses patients' own homes rather than hospitals' expensive trauma-care beds. Second, emergency medicine is complex, requiring advanced diagnostic tools and personnel with special training. Proper end-of-life care is often simple, from a medical standpoint, and the paramount job qualification is empathy.

When it comes to dying, American society today is like a subterranean explorer trying to find his way out of a cave. First we must light the inner cavern, so we know where we are. Then we need to illuminate the winding paths ahead, to find our way to daylight and fresh air.

NOTES

Editors' Note: This essay is excerpted from *Last Rights: Rescuing the End of Life from the Medical System* (St. Martin's Press, 2006), in which the author examines how death and dying in America have changed in the thirty years from 1976 to 2006.

1. Data drawn from the *National Vital Statistics Report*, a publication of the Centers for Disease Control and Prevention, and from the Web site of the National Center for Health Statistics (www.cdc.gov/nchs/hus.htm). Several years' publications provided material, generally in the charts on death rates for selected causes. The data concerned 1972–1992. For the subsequent ten years, the information was supplemented by data for selected causes of death provided by the American Heart Association and the American Stroke Association. This source was confirmed and supported by "Preliminary Data for 2003," 53 *National Vital Statistics Report* 15

(February 28, 2005). The incidence of heart disease and stroke remain high because the nation's population has grown, but the trends in rates of death from those causes have been consistently downward. For example, the number of deaths from heart disease dropped 9.9 percent from 1992 to 2002, but the rate of deaths from heart disease in that period fell 26.5 percent.

2. "Preliminary Data for 2003," 53. The period of increase in chronic respiratory disease mentioned here was from 1979 to 1994; data on Alzheimer's disease was supplemented by information on the current number of people with the illness provided by the American Alzheimer's Association. The estimate of future cases came from Ed Edelson's December 15, 2005, report in *HealthDay*.

3. AIDS data from the HIV/AIDS Prevention Division at the Centers for Disease Control. The period under study was 1987–2000.

4. Data from the National Cancer Institute and the American Cancer Society. The 2005 statistical compilation of the American Heart Association also provided information.

5. "Heart Disease and Stroke Statistics—2005 Update" and "Open Heart Surgery Statistics," American Heart Association Web site (www.americanheart.org).

6. Ibid., and Andrew Murr, "To Save the Stricken Brain," *Newsweek*, December 8, 2003.

7. Norman Finkelstein, *The Way Things Never Were* (New York: Atheneum, 1999).

8. National Center for Health Statistics Web site and "Preliminary Data for 2003."

9. Ibid.

10. "Life Expectancy Hits Record High," *National Vital Statistics Report*, February 28, 2005. The report, based on data from 2003, found life expectancies for white males at 75.4 years, black males at 69.2 years, white females at 80.5 years, and black females at 76.1 years. Each is a record high. Supplemental material about life expectancy came from the Rand Institute Study *Living Well at the End of Life*, by Joanne Lynn and David Adamson.

11. The $28 million "Study to Understand Prognoses and Preferences for Outcomes and Risks of Treatment" (hereinafter "SUPPPORT project study") is considered definitive because it surveyed 9,105 seriously ill patients in detail, including following about half of the group until death. Numerous subsequent studies stemmed from SUPPORT's findings. Data about people spending their savings on dying patients' hospital care, about hospital patients' pain experiences, and about spending time on ventilators also come from the SUPPORT project.

12. Data about hospital patients' pain experiences come from the SUPPORT project study.

13. Data about people spending time on ventilators come from the SUPPORT project study.

14. Nicholas Smedira, "Withholding and Withdrawal of Life Support from the Critically Ill," *New England Journal of Medicine* (February 1990).

15. Information on disregard for advance directives is from SUPPORT project study.

16. The study on physicians failing to find out whether dying patients wanted to be resuscitated was conducted by the National Institute of Mental Health through the Robert Wood Johnson Foundation.

17. Research by several scholars at the John A. Hartford Center of Geriatric Nursing Excellence at the University of California at San Francisco, which in turn relied upon individual facility data made public by the federal Centers for Medicare and Medicaid Services. The percentages reflect the situation in 2003. The primary source for that information and for comparisons with past findings was Charlene Harrington, Helen Carillo, and Cassandra Crawford, *Nursing Facilities—Staffing, Residence and Facility Deficiencies* 1997–2003.

18. Thomas Mattimore, "Surrogate and Physician Understanding of Patients' Preferences for Living Permanently in a Nursing Home," *Journal of the American Geriatrics Society* (July 2001): 45:7.

19. Information on percentage of Americans dying in nursing homes from geriatrician Allen Ramsey.

20. Information on number of intensive care beds from interviews with officials at the American Hospital Association, as well as several editions of the book *Hospital Statistics*, published by Health Forum, an affiliate of the AHA.

21. Up to 25,000 adults and 10,000 children are in a persistent vegetative state, "Medical Aspects of the Persistent Vegetative State," by the Multi-Society Task Force on PVS, *The New England Journal of Medicine* (May 1994).

22. According to Stephen Connor, vice president for research and international development at the National Hospice and Palliative Care Organization, in 1996 the United States had 2,722 licensed provider sites for hospice care, serving approximately 450,000 patients. In 2000 there were 3,100 sites, which served 700,000 patients.

23. Barry Yeoman, "Going Home," *AARP Magazine* (January/February 2005).

Unintended Consequences

Hospice, Hospitals, and the Not-So-Good Death

KATHRYN TEMPLE

Some families find hospice a dependable, even indispensable resource, a way to avoid hospital care and instead provide a warm environment for the terminally ill family member. More than a mere alternative to hospital care at the end of life, hospice can offer a terminal patient and his or her family dignity and security during difficult times. Unfortunately, my family found that neither hospital nor hospice had much to offer. Instead, we encountered an inhospitable, even hostile hospital environment, made worse by what may be the inevitable inadequacies of the hospice system—its inability to meet the expectations that its very existence creates. While this essay is informed by my experience and that of my family, as well as by my research and reading, I recognize that our difficulties with hospice are not universal. Regions differ, hospice organizations differ, families differ. But, as I suggest here, hospice tends to promise more than it can offer. Entangled as it is with other problems endemic to the American medical system, problems involving the institutional needs of hospitals, managed care, and insurance company mandates, hospice often comes up short in its efforts to provide what it calls "a good death," a death marked by dignity, choice, and strong family connections.

Like most families confronted with the imminent, untimely death of a family member, my family had only the vaguest idea of what hospice provided. When I checked our insurance policy the week my husband was diagnosed with what proved to be an incurable, aggressive cancer, I was reassured by the very general claim that hospice was "covered." I assumed we were covered by what I thought of as a benign, palliative-care system that would provide resources for both our family and my husband, a system that would understand what we were going through and help us with the physical, emotional, and financial issues that accompany death from terminal cancer. That understanding of hospice—though encouraged by my reading of the hospice publicity I'd run across over the years as well as by a discussion with a hospice representative during the early weeks of my husband's diagnosis—turned out to be unreasonable, ill informed, and naive.

Our story (for it is my husband's and my daughter's story as well, and, to a lesser extent, the story of all of those who loved my husband—his family, his colleagues, and his friends) is one of hospice's best intentions thwarted, in part by the underpublicized problems that plague the medical system as a whole. Our experience calls into question some of the very ideals that the hospice movement holds dear—"choice," "care," and "the good death"— ideals at the core of its identity. While hospice has helped many, gained many devotees, assisted many "on that final journey," it has also escaped scrutiny through relying on the repetition of these generalized ideals that, until placed under pressure, seem almost immune to critique. In particular, my understanding of what choice might mean in this context, my belief that hospice would offer care as promised, and ultimately my faith in what seems to serve as a sort of mantra for the hospice system, "the good death," would be shattered before we were done. *Choice* became a relative term; *care* did not include the care we needed. And while some deaths are better than others, no one can guarantee what hospice calls a "good death."

"Hospice is not a place, but an idea," asserts our local hospice Web site.[1] If so, it is an "idea" supported by Medicare funds, covered by many health insurance plans, and relied upon by cancer centers, hospitals, and nursing homes to provide care for the dying. In other words, it is a highly funded, institutionalized, and concretized "idea," one that operates not only on the levels of idea and ideal, but also on the level of the real world where real people become ill and their families struggle to help them. For hospice does not exist alone but at the nexus of life and death, of hospital care, home care, and no care, of patient, caregiver, and survivors. Hospice operates in these interstitial spaces: here is where good intentions meet unintended consequences, where ideals meet real patients and real caregivers.

The modern hospice movement arose, of course, from good intentions. Hospice, brought into being in England in the 1960s primarily by Dame Cicely Saunders, evolved out of her perception that dying patients had little choice in their own care and that the care they were offered was less than adequate. In response, Saunders established St. Christopher's Hospice in London, an institution that became the modern model for hospice facilities all over the world.[2] While other facilities had offered palliative care for the dying, St. Christopher's combined such care with research and program development to suggest a model for the medical system at large, a model based in compassionate care that allows the dying to choose how they wish to end their lives. Funded by charitable giving and the government, St. Christopher's offers services to local residents at no cost while also helping to organize and promote hospice services throughout Great Britain and internationally. In the United States, the movement was slow to take hold until Medicare added a hospice benefit in 1982.[3]

At its core then, hospice was seen as a response to the very limited options of the dying, not as the substitution of one set of constraints for another. Shouldn't the dying and their families be permitted to choose the location and circumstances under which death occurs? Why should they be forced to remain in hospitals, regulated by institutional rules, their visiting schedules controlled by hospital schedules, pain and other symptom relief predicated on the needs of those who would live, rather than of those who were going to die? When understood in this context, hospice can be seen to have offered a necessary, even crucially important, challenge to the dominance of institutional control of the dying. Indeed, in its heady early days, hospice may have seemed akin to other cries for liberation common in the late 1960s and early 1970s. In essence, the hospice mission was to free the dying, to give them choices in how their deaths were to occur.

Familiarity with these origins helps us understand how the uncritical and unexamined use of what is often called the rhetoric of choice has come to dominate hospice advertising and promotion. If one googles the words *hospice* and *choice* together, over four hundred thousand hits appear. "Your hospice choice . . ." says one hospice Web site. "Everyone has choices," claims another. "Of course, it's the patient's decision . . ." claims a third. Somewhat more darkly, one site suggests that choices may seem "few or unpleasant," but most of the hospice literature claims "choice" as a primary characteristic of the hospice system. Given hospice rhetoric, one imagines competent, well-advised, calm patients and caregivers, sitting in a sunny kitchen, reading the literature and talking over their "options," then "self-selecting" into the hospice system.

But what is the meaning of *choice* in this context? Our family discovered that both the psychology of illness and the institutional needs of hospitals worked against the patient's right to choose. The Princeton law professor Beth Kiyoko Jamieson outlines what she calls the "agency principle—that individuals have the right to make their own decisions about how to live their lives, that individuals must be assumed to be capable of making ethical decisions, and that social reprobation . . . must not inhibit the decision-making process" as one that should be incorporated into theories of liberty.[4] But as Jay Katz has pointed out in the legal context and Joan Williams in the feminist legal theory context, choice is never free but instead is constructed by social, legal, and cultural constraints. Law professor Williams is especially adept at deconstructing the rhetoric of choice when she points out that all choices (even choices made by the professional, highly advantaged women she studies) are constrained and that often the "constrainer" of such circumstances is the very social entity that most loudly advertises choice as a primary value. As Williams argues, choice is only choice in the sense of something freely chosen, but every choice is made under constraints of some kind.[5] Like everyone else, potential hospice patients do not choose hospice in an ideal world of infinite choices or in a social vacuum. The choice of hospice, perhaps more than most choices, is peculiarly shaped by the gradual narrowing of options faced by the terminally ill.

If choice is not free under the best of circumstances, can even a remnant of its free-wheeling nature remain at the end of life? What goes unreported in the hospice literature is the imposition of the idea of rational choice on the lives of the dying, an imposition that overrides what outside observers sometimes see as the irrational belief in the possibility of a cure or the likelihood of continued life in the face of an obvious terminal illness.

Take, for instance, our situation, which was shaped from the beginning by my husband's powerful embrace of, first, denial, and, later, a determined refusal to act, as coping mechanisms. From the day of diagnosis with a rare and fatal cancer, known for its zero five-year survival rate, he rejected his six-to-twenty-four-month prognosis. He fired doctors who insisted on discussing it, replacing them with those more willing to speak positively about "treatment" and "options." In the face of chemo's two-year assault on his body, frequent hospitalizations, increasing debility, a failed heart, and eventually rejection by every heart transplant facility in our region, my husband insisted that he would recover and even convinced some of our friends and colleagues that he would "beat this thing." Those few friends who raised the issue of prognosis were politely cut off and redirected to more general topics. His attitudes were reflected in his advance directive—the one document most strongly associated with the patient's right to choose—executed before his first major surgery. There, he demanded every possible form of care that would keep him alive, including aggressive interventions such as feeding tubes and respirators. If in an irreversible coma, his preference was to live indefinitely. No measures were to be rejected in the pursuit of life.

My husband was not singular in his denial, nor in his insistence that every possible measure be taken. Denial is a common, well-recognized coping mechanism among the dying. As Sherwin Nuland argues in *How We Die*, "Denial is one of two factors that immeasurably complicate our best intentions when, as physicians or the beloved of a dying person, we seek to enlist him as a full participant in choices that must be made in the days remaining."[6] Typical is a caregiver who reported that her friend continued to talk of coming home until the day of her death, despite having spent her last months in a well-regarded inpatient hospice facility, one with a full array of counseling services. Another patient insisted on continued treatment in the face of a stage four gastric cancer. The family coped by offering her placebo treatments, yet placed her in a hospice program and cared for her at home. She was never told she was "in hospice" since, as a nurse, she would have recognized and protested this form of "giving up." Grief counselors recognize denial as a positive coping mechanism; at least one such counselor told me to "celebrate his denial," to build it up, as otherwise he would be miserable. And why should someone be miserable at the end of life if he need not be? Some of the hospital staff understood and helped. As one of the physical therapists told me two weeks before my husband died, "I know the physical therapy doesn't mean anything, but if he thinks it will help him go home, I'll give it to him as long as he can do it."

Though sometimes shocking to the uninitiated, denial represents a phenomenon so widespread as to become a frequent topic of conversation in online chatrooms and e-mail listservs. What is the spouse to do when the terminally ill partner refuses to accept that death is an option? Depending on how experienced any individual caregiver might be, responses tend towards a desire to "make him face the truth," rather than acceptance of the patient's point of view. Caregivers often take on all of the financial and practical concerns of the household, sometimes unexpectedly, and, as a result, feel particularly alone, even abandoned by a spouse, when the spouse is unable to discuss the ramifications of a diagnosis or to plan for a future in which the caregiver may have to face life alone. Few caregivers find it easy to tiptoe across the tightrope that denial creates, to plan for the worst while hoping for the best.

My own response shifted over time: in the beginning I felt strongly that my husband needed to understand his prognosis, that understanding would allow him to make choices about his treatment and his legacy, bring him closer to his family and friends, and, in short, help him face his future in the full knowledge of what his life had meant and would mean. Later, as I learned more about the function of denial, I began to believe that he should be respected for the choice he was making, that he was choosing to believe in a future that made him feel whole. It was not my right to impose my own negative, "realistic" view on that choice.

The commonplace use of denial as a coping device has led to a wide literature addressing the contradictory and flawed nature of advance directives. Advance directives are usually written by healthy people or by newly ill patients, often by those who have never experienced severe pain, never taken care of a sick person, never seen anyone die. Thus, it's not surprising that most find it easier to imagine survival than their own demise. Familiar only with autonomy and self-direction, such a patient cannot imagine a future in which such concerns become irrelevant, indeed, a future in which his only desire would be to avoid more pain or to end his suffering or worse, one in which he could not experience or express desire, but was instead so drenched in pain and so mentally incapacitated that his experience was beyond articulation. Lack of knowledge about the dying process governs many advance directives.

Conflicts between autonomy and dependence are embedded in the concept of the advance directive itself. As Robert Olick, a Georgetown professor, suggests, the advance directive is an autonomy-shifting device: "The point of an advance directive is to guide others in promoting our interests for us more strongly, to charge others with this responsibility."[7] Perhaps advance directives attempt too much. They seem as often violated as followed, so often violated in fact that there is an entire literature around their violation. Turning to Olick, we find him describing (but not endorsing) a "current interests" approach. Under this scenario, when the patient becomes unable to decide, the advance directive (designed with exactly this situation in mind) becomes unenforceable and the patient's prior interests are replaced by what health-care providers or family members imagine to be her "current interests." Any prospectively imagined autonomy fails to survive competency, because with incompetency, all of the aspects of the self that the patient was trying to protect have ended. The incompetent patient has no dignity or "self" left to protect under this theory: "incompetence extinguishes a person's autonomy-based critical interests."[8]

As the research predicts, our family found that the advance directive became less useful as my husband became sicker. Although copies were placed in his hospital file and his desires were restated every time he faced a new procedure or hospitalization, little was made of all this on a practical level. For instance, despite his advance directive, I was told that the hospital planned to stop transfusing him with their limited blood supplies. Transfusions saved his life five or six times in the months leading up to his death, but, according to the doctors, there were limits on how much blood could be used. While these limits were never explained in detail (if he had needed one unit to live, would that have been provided?), I was told several times that he had almost reached his "limit," implicitly a threat to deny the care that he had demanded in his advance directive.

The hospital was not alone in this push to ignore the advance directive. As my husband neared death, his siblings joined me in serving as what Olick refers to as "rebel proxies."[9] While we did not wish him harm, when asked, for instance, to approve a painful and traumatic procedure that might have slowed brain tumor growth (but would not have offered a better quality of life or longer lifespan), we found ourselves unable to move forward. His sister and brother, who loved him dearly, were horrified at what the doctors were suggesting while I, having watched him endure two years of aggressive chemo and two useless major surgeries, had lost faith in his doctor's advice. At this late stage, we were more able to move toward accepting his death than trying to prevent it. As his condition worsened, the advance directive seemed less and less relevant. The medical personnel, his doctors, nurses, and the hospital social worker never mentioned it, while various hospital and hospice representatives continued to pressure all of us to "choose" hospice. The pressure increased after he was declared incompetent. At the very moment he was in the mental condition that should have triggered the advance directive, it became the one thing that everyone wanted to ignore.

Denial often takes the form of refusal, "the refusal of many patients to exercise their right to independent thought and self-determination."[10] My husband adopted this tactic, consistently refusing to discuss his "choices" until his final descent into unconsciousness made any such discussion impossible. During one of the brief periods when he seemed out of pain and yet alert, I decided to bring up hospice. Still clinging to the notion that he should have a right to choose and, indeed, to the belief that hospice would require him to make a knowing choice to discontinue treatment, I found myself forcing a discussion that he did not want to have. Under considerable pressure from the hospital social worker and other administrators to move him into a hospice program, I began with: "We need to talk about what we're going to do. Remember the people who came to talk to you about hospice?" Enlisting more strength and purpose than he had in weeks, he suddenly remembered how to use the TV remote well enough to crank the volume to high. "Why did you do that?" I asked. "Because I don't want to talk about it," he shouted over the noise of the set. Yet, was this Nuland's refusal to "exercise independent thought"? In a setting where his choices were largely meaningless, one in which hospital staff, not to mention wife and family, saw only one choice, he had decided to exercise the choice still remaining to him: the choice not to choose.

Even if one were fortunate enough, rational enough, competent enough, to imagine a freely chosen, autonomous decision under conditions defined by one's upcoming death, one would also have to contend with hospice's own internal deconstruction of choice. For hospice claims to treat not just the patient, but the family. And the family, at least in the literature, is also granted a choice. As Fiona Randall points out in her work on the philosophy of palliative care, hospice often presents its goal as one that gives both family and patient the same rights. As she says, the goal is "the best possible quality of life for the patient and family."[11] Constance Putnam, author of *Hospice or Hemlock*, emphasizes this as well. Hospice has multiple purposes: "the terminally ill person's own preferences and lifestyle must be taken into account . . . and . . . family members and other caregivers also have legitimate needs and interests that must be taken into consideration."[12] One does not have to review Randall's lengthy argument to understand the conflicts inherent in the spreading of "choice" across parties with different goals and concerns. Even my limited time on the cancer ward (two months) exposed me to several conflicted situations: families often wanted the patient to "keep fighting" while the patient, exhausted and beginning to turn inwards towards death, wanted to be left alone. Meanwhile, other patients, like my husband, vowed to live on, despite family, clergy, and hospice workers who wanted him to "face facts," "find closure," or (in the case of hospital administrators) simply agree to stop treatment.

While "choice" is obviously an important component of the hospice ideology, "care" may be even more important to hospice's identity. As Putnam suggests in her work comparing hospice to assisted suicide, hospice "emphasizes comfort care. The basic idea is that palliative care [is] offered on a continuing basis, and aggressively, to all dying patients. Such care is viewed as especially important at the point when 'cure' is no longer possible."[13] Google *hospice, care*, and *caring* and your hits will soar, to about 1 million. The online description of our local hospice program uses the words *care* or *caring* six times in one short paragraph. Hospice provides "care" and is a "care" program. It is a "special form" of "care" offering "caring" professionals and a "program of care." Or put more broadly, "For patient, family, and loved ones, hospice is a special form of multidimensional care designed to treat the full human being, not the disease. Hospice assists people who are dying and their loved ones with a full range of medical, emotional, spiritual, and social needs." *Care* substitutes for *cure* in the hospice lexicon.

But what does care actually consist of in the hospice context? Let's return to the modern hospice mantra: "Hospice is not a place, but an idea." This has not always been the case. For millennia, hospice was a place, not an idea at all. The Latin word *hospes* means both "host" and "guest," thus linking the role of carer and cared-for. Over time, the word evolved into *hospitium* (from which we get *hospitable*) as well as other words related to the French and English *hospital*. More important, *hospice* originally meant a place where weary travelers could rest and where the sick could recover.[14] How did such a humane understanding of the meaning of hospice evolve into today's system, one in which patients are often sent home to family members ill-equipped to care for them or offered inpatient hospice only when critically ill or when death is "imminent"?

For in truth, the hospice system assumes that care will be provided by family members and at home, not by a "caring team of professionals" as so many hospice Web sites suggest or in a hospice facility. Inpatient hospice facilities are few; only the wealthiest patients can afford access to anything more than crisis care. Indeed, most inpatient hospice facilities accept only those patients in crisis, those who can be stabilized after a few days and returned home. Long-term hospice care may be provided in nursing home or rehabilitation settings, but while direct hospice services are often covered by insurance, unskilled care is not. Unable to lift or bathe my husband, unable to care for both him and my elementary-school-age daughter, I found one nursing home that would accept him. They asked for $9,000 a month and needed a guarantee up front that I could pay. Under these circumstances, the routine daily care of the debilitated, incontinent, dying patient becomes the caregiver's or loved one's responsibility; the location of that care, often the living room or den. Choice is, of course, related to the hospice conception of care, for while a patient may "choose" hospice, his family may not be able to carry out his wishes. What to do given that hospice is ill-equipped to help when patients do not have a wide and deep support basis? For hospice is, as the literature says, "not a place, but an idea" and it is an idea that assumes that someone else (not hospice itself) will actually care for dying patients.

One could be forgiven for failing to understand this. Few family members do: As one hapless caregiver told Renee Royak-Schaler, an oncology researcher, "I think there is an assumption that everybody knows what hospice is. It's not true . . . the physician did not give a realistic picture as to what hospice was going to be like."[15] Even the most astute caregiver might have difficulty getting past the hospice promotional literature to discover just what the limits of the promised "care" might be. Some clues appear in the hospice promotional material on the Web: there one can find a list of actual services, one of which is "specially trained volunteers who can provide a few hours' respite care." Another is "help in securing all the medical equipment, medications, and information needed to care for a loved one at home." An alert reader might wonder why, given all this promised "care," respite care is necessary. If "care" is provided, then why "respite"? But perhaps the answer appears in that last item, in the words "to care for a loved one at home." Or buried even deeper in the Web site, where one finds the advice that one must learn to accept help from others, "especially from family, friends, and the community."

Turning from hospice promotional literature to journalistic accounts, one finds an even less helpful description of the care hospice provides. Reed Abelson, writing for the *New York Times*, inadvertently suggests the confusion that plagues talk about hospice: "Typically, the patient is cared for at home, supported by a team that might include a doctor, nurse, social worker, home health aide, a clergy member and various counselors and therapists."[16] Note the passive voice here, not common in news reporting. If the patient "is cared for at home" who is doing the caring? If there is "support" provided by a "team," who is the support supporting? Presumably not the patient, since she is already being "cared for." Not until one digs deep into its Web page does our local hospice reveal that "caregivers" are the ones actually providing whatever care the patient receives. As their Web site asserts, "the hospice team supports the caregivers," and "Almost all . . . patients spend more than 95 percent of their hospice experience in routine home care." Where do these caregivers come from? Again, the hospice promotional copy is vague on this concept, but a careful reader will discover that the family is expected to provide not only care, but twenty-four-hour uninterrupted care (except in those rare cases when "volunteers" may provide respite care). Indeed, most hospice programs require that the family guarantee twenty-four-hour coverage for liability reasons.

This system works wonderfully for those wealthy enough to afford quality inpatient services. Art Buchwald did a well-publicized stint in a swank Washington, D.C., hospice, until he decided he wasn't going to die anytime soon and discharged himself. Even in-home hospice care works for some in more traditional communities where families have remained close, the social network is strong, and expectations of help from the medical community are low. But for mobile urban families, for families dependent on the well spouse's employment not only for income but also for insurance, or for patients without family support, in-home hospice fails miserably. As Joanne Lynn notes in her essay against living wills, "societal support for hospice . . . serves mostly relatively well-off cancer patients with homes, in contrast with the societal denial of adequate support for long-term care for those who are severely disabled and alone."[17] But one need not be alone for hospice care to fail: one need only belong to contemporary society, where most people work, few remain at home full time, and extended families are almost nonexistent.

Sadly, as I discovered from my participation on caregivers' listservs, cancer listservs, and on a listserv for those anticipating the death of a loved one, in the area of care, hospice often fails to meet the expectations and the hopes of hordes of families and patients. Again and again, caregivers (meaning family members, untrained and ill-prepared to offer care to the dying) report that they needed help, not counseling, not twenty-four-hour phone lines, not medical supplies or hospital beds. One wife reported, "For the most part, my house was full of people 'checking' on us for the last thirty days of my husband's life. I felt trapped in the house with people who had no medical training and were just stopping by 'to see how we were doing.' One day my medical provider sent a guitar player! No nurses, but a guitar player and various 'managers' who were not coming to provide care, only 'checking' to see how we were doing."[18] Another wife complained that she "can't seem to shake the visions of our horrible experiences with home hospice. Thankfully, my daughter is an RN and she came every day to help. The nurses I was promised never came." And a third noted, "The myth of hospice is that they will dash around and do the patient care while the family hangs out with the patient. In my experience, hospice did nothing. I did patient care; a friend of mine was generous enough to run all of our errands, food shop, and do laundry; and there was really very little time to spend, except for the very end." Ironically, in one case, the very hospice provider who could not provide "care" managed to find someone to supervise the disposal of drugs after the patient's death. "Priorities, priorities!" as the wife put it.

Even hospice's much-vaunted emphasis on pain control, perhaps the most important kind of care from the patient's and caregiver's point of view, is not always realized. One wife reported that after her husband died, hospice sent a nurse and a minister to talk to her. She mentioned that the narcotics didn't seem to provide her husband with pain relief and was told that "this happens sometimes." As the wife said, "The only reason I involved hospice was because I wanted his pain controlled. IT WAS NOT CONTROLLED." A close friend's mother recently died after an uninspiring bout with in-home hospice. Fortunately, my friend had two sisters to spell her; the family was on shifts for six weeks and their mother was never alone. But at the end, hospice care failed. On her last day, in excruciating pain, their mother sobbed and, finally, screamed uncontrollably. When the family decided to call for an ambulance, the hospice nurse announced that there was nothing she could do and left them with their agonized mother. Only in the hospital was her pain brought "under control." She died a few hours later, in the hospital, blessedly free from pain, but leaving the family traumatized.

Perhaps the most difficult issue our family faced involved the continual pressure to care for my husband at home. Why is home care the hospice "gold standard"? Why are patients told repeatedly that it would be "better to die at home," that they would be "more comfortable at home," that "no one wants to be in the hospital"? Anyone who gives the reality of dying a moment's thought can see the problems: family members may or may not be capable, emotionally, physically, or otherwise to care for a dying family member. Emergency services are not readily available at home. The living room, den, or other accessible place, often the only spaces in the home large enough to accommodate a hospital bed and equipment, do not necessarily offer the dignity and privacy that many dying patients prefer. Children may be in the home and not every child is equipped to cope with the visible, imminent death of a loved one. Hospice advocates themselves agree that home care is not always appropriate. As David J. Casarett, a hospice researcher, points out, "A discussion of hospice should take into account other programs for care that might be available, since hospice is not always the best option. For example, home hospice is poorly equipped to meet the needs of debilitated patients without informal caregivers who want to remain at home."[19]

It seems obvious that many dying patients need inpatient care: they have complex medical conditions, have often suffered numerous state-of-the-art cancer treatments, and are, after all, at the end of life. And yet, as we have seen, hospice limits access to inpatient care. Of course, economics is at the root of this bifurcation. Hospice care in the home is far cheaper than hospital care. Hospice as a movement in the United States took off only when Medicare coverage began and when insurance companies followed by offering similar coverage for those too young or too well-off to qualify for Medicare or Medicaid. It is to every insurance company's benefit to transfer dying patients from hospital to home and to shift the responsibility for care to family members. Insurance companies pressure doctors; doctors pressure patients and families. I will never forget one scene I witnessed on the cancer ward at my husband's hospital: a nurse pleading, "But she has no one to take care of her," and the doctor responding angrily, "She's discharged as far as I'm concerned." Home care provided by the family rather than professionals is cheaper than inpatient care of any kind. Many studies have shown that hospice, with its continual pressure to shift care from the medical system to family members and the patient himself, saves considerable money over hospital care.

During my husband's final weeks, my life devolved into a hectic and surreal whirl of activity in response to various demands from hospital administrators and hospice "liaisons" that I "do something," "put him in hospice," or otherwise find him a place in which to die. At that point, I held my job only by the grace of my employer as I had barely been to work for two months, having spent my time flying back and forth from our home to Houston, where my husband was barely surviving a failed surgery and, within days, the rapid metastasis of his cancer to liver, lungs, kidneys, bowels, and brain.

After my husband was air-ambulanced home (the Houston hospital seemed not to want him to die on their watch), I spent all my waking hours at the hospital or taking care of my daughter. Friends wanted to help, but they worked, had kids, and often had older family members who also needed help. In any case, no amount of informal help would have made it possible for me to manage his care. During the last month of his hospitalization, even hospital care seemed inadequate. I spent most of every day and some nights there, yet he was constantly in pain or in need, to the extent that the hospital staff could not keep up. I hired night "sitters" at $350 a night, yet discovered that they seemed to do little for him. If I called during the night, they did not answer his phone, and I could not even tell if they remained in the room with him as they were required to do. Meanwhile, I was frequently told that he should never be left alone. Given that the hospital could barely manage his care, I could not imagine how I could have done it at home.

Yet I was told by the cancer ward social worker as curious onlookers passed us in the hall, "If you don't arrange to take him home, I'll have him delivered to your front step. Then he's your problem." When I asked about inpatient hospice, she said, "Medicare won't pay for that." (This is actually not true: if a patient is covered by Medicare, hospice services, including inpatient care when authorized, will be covered.) When I pointed out that he had private health insurance and was not old enough to be on Medicare, she came back with "no insurance will pay for it." When I wondered how my daughter would handle seeing her father bleeding and incontinent, she sneered, "Well, she'll just have to adjust." When I asked how I would lift him if he fell, she said, "Just call 911." Mine was a situation particularly unsuited to in-home hospice care: No local family members, my only friends all from two-career families with children and plenty of problems of their own, my husband, a patient who needed twenty-four-hour care, had unpredictable bleeding and an active case of hepatitis B which I could not be immunized against (immunization takes ninety days and I did not have ninety days).

Given the confusing and stressful alternative universe I was trapped in, the online listservs became my refuge. There, I discovered that my situation was far from unique as numerous caregivers shared their strategies for staving off the unhelpful suggestions of hospital administrators and hospice promoters. "Just keep telling them that you're looking for a nursing home," said one. "They can't force you to take him home," said another.

Could my husband have experienced hospice's "good death" under any circumstances? The declining quality of hospital care and nursing shortages may make dying at home seem preferable to dying in an indifferent, even hostile, hospital. But, in part, the desire to die at home has been fostered by this very myth, the idea of the "good death." As Landace Woods puts it in words that seem more appropriate to hospice promotion than for a palliative-nursing journal: "Especially at end of life, patients should not experience suffering due to pain, shortness of breath, and other symptoms. . . . Although death is inevitable, the experience of a peaceful death is not."[20] Woods here assumes the universal possibility of the "good death," a death that with hospice's help, every patient can aspire to. In contrast, the more analytical Putnam suggests that the "good death" constitutes rhetoric rather than experience: "there tends to be an approved 'hospice story' of how to die. . . . The 'good death' experience is told and retold, and becomes what is expected and usual; it becomes routinized and objectified, acting as a symbolic vehicle and guide to future action. . . . These events become ritualized; rhetoric and powerful imagery work to reinforce shared meaning."[21] The idea of the good death has become part of a complex mythos throughout the hospice community, with many hospice volunteers believing that patients "see" family members who have predeceased them, that they are welcomed into the world of the dead, or that they voluntarily decide when to die based on who visits them and when.

True, "good deaths" do exist. During a "good death," a patient lies comfortably, preferably at home, surrounded by loved ones, pain controlled by opiates, other symptoms somehow invisible or at least unspecified. Closure is found, memories are shared, perhaps a last video is recorded. I have seen such deaths and they can occur in or out of hospice. My grandmother died such a death. Spending only a few days in the hospital at the end, she had time for reflection, talked of her loved ones, felt the presence of her husband of fifty years who had predeceased her. The family had flown in from around the country and her doctors, realizing that we could not leave jobs for more than a few days, were astute enough to increase her morphine on our last day, allowing her to shift from consciousness to unconsciousness and then drift into death while we were present. It was a good death. But it had nothing to do with hospice care and would have occurred in any setting that offered appropriate palliative care.

I thought of her death often during my husband's last weeks. It was obvious that he was going to die only with difficulty. In those final months, his condition was perilous: he rarely remained "stable" for more than a day or two at a time. He could not walk, use the toilet, or even manage the nurse's call button, which he seemed to confuse with the TV remote. Two or three times, he somehow managed to shift his body weight enough to fall, and on those occasions six to eight hospital staff would be mustered to raise him from the floor back to the bed. Once he was left on the cold hospital floor for hours while the staff tried to find enough people to help. Every few days he developed unexplained massive bleeding, bleeding that would be ejected all over the floor and, once, a complete wall of the hospital room. These late manifestations of imminent death would have occurred at home or in a hospice. Unpreventable, no matter what palliative care might have offered, they fly in the face of the hospice ideal of the "good death."

While he died in the hospital room, I spent a lot of time out in the hall being accosted by angry social workers, hospice liaison personnel, doctors, and nurses. "Why don't you take him home where your daughter can see him?" snapped one nurse, who worked part-time for a local hospice organization. She had been assigned to his case only recently and knew little about it, and suggested to him that if he didn't watch what he ate, he'd end up on dialysis, a ludicrous idea given that he had only a few days to live. Did I really need to explain, out in the hall, to someone I had just met, in front of people I would never know, that I had stopped bringing my daughter to visit only after my husband's symptoms had become so disturbing that even adult visitors were having nightmares?

I am not suggesting, of course, that our large urban hospital was a particularly desirable place to die. When my husband began to fail, he was placed in a room at the end of the corridor, as far from the nurses' station as it was possible to be. Nurses who less than a year earlier could be counted on to come in for a chat and to watch whatever game he found on TV would not look at me now. They never entered his room while I was there. But I could not be there twenty-four hours a day, so anyone who wandered in had access to him. Over time his cell phone, iPod, and other personal items disappeared. After his death, I was billed hundreds of dollars for long-distance charges on the hospital phone. It seems that someone had come into his room and used his phone while he lay in a coma. When I demanded an audit of the bill, the hospital accounting office said they would absorb the cost. Apparently, such things are common enough for billing offices to have developed a protocol. On the other hand, the room was more pleasant and private, if less protected, than our living room would have been; and if he fell, help was in the building, not a 911 call away. He could be bathed (it took four to six people), something I could not have managed at home even with a small staff. His doctors came to see him twice a day and did their best to keep him "comfortable" (an impossible task) and me informed.

Was he eligible for inpatient hospice? No one seemed to know. He might be eligible if his death was "imminent." But who would determine what "imminent" meant? During his last month, it seemed that every doctor, nurse, and social worker defined this differently and that the definition changed from day to day. One day a member of the medical team told me to find an inpatient hospice: "He's eligible now." I visited two that afternoon, but on my return to the hospital the next day, the same doctor said, "He's better today, so he's not eligible for inpatient hospice." When I asked exactly what "imminent" meant, one doctor told me "two weeks until death," a hospice worker said "one week," and then a third member of the medical team opined "a few days." In any case, ideas about the time of his impending death changed by the hour. Several times, I was called in to spend the night as death was "imminent," only to find him happily watching TV at 3:00 in the morning.

Meanwhile, I spent many hours researching our options, interviewing agencies who provided in-home nursing care, calling the insurance company and the hospital hospice liaison to try to get inpatient coverage so that my husband could be moved to a hospice facility. Could hospice provide, if not a good death, at least a better one? I did not know, but under pressure from the hospital, I visited local inpatient facilities. First the nursing homes with their sterile rooms and elderly patients tied to wheelchairs that lined the halls. Then the local inpatient hospice facility, an old school building with cramped rooms, all doubles. "Your daughter will be so much more comfortable visiting here than the hospital," I was told. But would she really? On my visit, the halls were noisy and crowded, the rooms with open doors seemed full of beds and people, crammed wall to wall. One poor young man writhed, tied into a reclining wheelchair, moaning incoherently, wearing only a loose diaper. I did not think this was a place to bring a child, even less one to bring my husband, who abhorred sharing a room with other patients and had consistently refused to do so throughout the two years of his treatment.

When I finally was able to tell the hospice liaison that I had found a nursing home and discovered that I could cash in his life insurance policy to pay for it (no thanks to any of the social workers), her face fell and she abruptly ended the session. She had been committed to moving my husband into home care, not into another institution. I did not see her again until twenty-four hours before he died, when she dropped by to say "looks like any time now." Along the way, there were hints that if pressed, the insurance company would pay for inpatient hospice: in one difficult phone call taken in a hallway at work, a "patient care representative" asked me detailed questions about my husband's condition. "Is his head wound bleeding? Does he have open sores that require treatment?" It seemed that she was trying to sort out how much of his care would require "skilled nursing" and how much nonskilled. Nonskilled would not be covered by insurance. Beyond what I could read into that phone call, information about such options was hard to find. Just recently, I spent a morning calling the insurance company again in an effort to find out exactly what the standard for inpatient hospice might be, what insurance companies might cover and might not. Five calls, two hours on hold, many transfers to numerous employees resulted in nothing. They were either unwilling or unable to answer these questions.

Eighteen hours before my husband's death, the insurance company called our oncologist to demand that he be moved to inpatient hospice. Although I did not know it, such late-in-life transfers fly in the face of hospice protocol. As Woods remarks, "Transferring patients who are actively dying and/or are not expected to live beyond the next 48 hours should be avoided."[22] By this point, my husband was on massive amounts of morphine for pain that still seemed agonizing. He could groan, his body tensed, struggling for every breath, but he could not talk except to mutter, "Help me." The suggestion that we ambulance him across twenty miles of potholed streets to the inpatient hospice facility took my breath away, but the social worker presented this as a matter of my convenience: "You won't have the long drive to see him," she said. Fortunately, our oncologist vetoed this plan.

In the end, my husband died at the hospital after his morphine was increased. He struggled for one breath after another, moaned, his body arched in agony. Our oncologist asked me repeatedly what I wanted to do. Did I want to increase the morphine "knowing the risks," he asked? Exhausted, I could not make this decision, rebellious proxy though I was. He issued the order. In less than five minutes, my husband's body relaxed for the first time in four days, then his breathing slowed, stopped. He died. This was not murder or even euthanasia, although many may think it so. Indeed, in palliative-care circles, such a result is covered by the rule of unintended consequences sometimes called the "doctrine of double effect."[23] Doctors who administer opiates to patients in pain, patients with terminal diseases, know that their patients may die. In our situation, they seemed quite sure of it. But they are protected from legal consequences under the rule.

Unintended consequences: the phrase stands in as an explanation for the medical system's failings, but also for hospice's failings, for the improbable claim that under hospice, patients can choose how they will die, for the consistent emphasis on hospice as an entity that provides care, and finally, for the claim that hospice offers a good death. When hospice was first imagined in the 1960s, no one could have predicted the current health-care crisis and the pressure it would place on hospitals to discharge patients who cannot be cured. Nor could the changes in family life wrought by the feminist movement be imagined. Those who originated the concept of hospice did not intend that patients would die accompanied only by desperate, traumatized family members unable to offer the care that could make them comfortable. They did not imagine a hospital staff that would threaten to put a dying patient out on someone's front steps. Nor did they expect hospice to stand in for skilled nursing care in cases where complex medical needs require it. Yet our experience and that of others, both those I know and those I came to know only through Internet chatrooms and listservs, suggest that these consequences are not uncommon.

Perhaps hospice should reconsider its promotional material. Perhaps hospice administrators should start fighting back, refusing to take patients without in-home support systems, refusing to cave in to inhumane insurance company demands, refusing in short to pretend to ideals that far too often cannot be realized in the managed-care world we live in today. Perhaps we all need to learn that hospice care, like hospital care, varies, that outcomes vary, and that neither the best hospital nor the best hospice can promise anyone a "good death."

NOTES

I would like to thank Paul T. Ruxin, Margaret Greaves, and Seth Lerer for reading and commenting on drafts of this essay. Any failure to execute their excellent suggestions is, of course, my own.

1. References to our local hospice Web site are to www.capitalhospice.org, last accessed September 22, 2008.

2. For the history of St. Christopher's and of Dame Cicely Saunders, see www.stchristophers.org.uk.

3. Constance E. Putnam, *Hospice or Hemlock: Searching for Heroic Compassion* (Westport, CT, and London: Praeger, 2002), 32–33, 36.

4. Beth Kiyoko Jamieson, *Real Choices: Feminism, Freedom, and the Limits of the Law* (University Park: Penn State University Press, 2001), 11.

5. Jay Katz, *Catastrophic Diseases: Who Decides What* (New York: Russell Sage, 1975); Joan Williams, *Unbending Gender* (New York: Oxford University Press, 2000), 15.

6. Sherwin Nuland, *How We Die: Reflections on Life's Final Chapter* (New York: Knopf, 1993), 228.

7. Robert S. Olick, *Taking Advance Directives Seriously: Prospective Autonomy and Decisions Near the End of Life* (Washington, DC: Georgetown University Press, 2001), 55.

8. Ibid., 59.

9. Ibid., 175.

10. Nuland, *How We Die*, 228.

11. Fiona Randall and R. S. Downie, eds., *The Philosophy of Palliative Care: Critique and Reconstruction* (Oxford: Oxford University Press, 2006), 75.

12. Putnam, *Hospice or Hemlock*, 33.

13. Ibid., 31.

14. Ibid.

15. Renee Royak-Schaler et al., "Family Perspectives on Communication with Healthcare Providers During End-of-Life Cancer Care," *Oncology Nursing Forum* 33, no. 4 (2006): 753–760, 757–758.

16. Reed Abelson, "A Chance to Pick Hospice and Still Hope to Live," *New York Times*, Business Section, February 10, 2007.

17. Joanne Lynn, "Why I Don't Have a Living Will," in *The Right to Die,* vol. 1, *Definitions and Moral Perspectives: Death, Euthanasia, Suicide, and Living Wills,* ed. Melvin I. Urofsky and Philip E. Urofsky (New York and London: Garland, 1996), 357–360, 358.

18. I have omitted the names of online posters, relatives, and friends to protect their identities.

19. David J. Casarett and Timothy E. Quill, "'I'm not ready for hospice': Strategies for Timely and Effective Hospice Discussion," *Annals of Internal Medicine* 146, no. 6 (March 2007): 443–449, 446.

20. Landace Woods et al., "Transitioning to a Hospice Program," *Journal of Hospice and Palliative Nursing* 8, no. 2 (2006): 103–111, 107.

21. Putnam, *Hospice or Hemlock*, 40, quoting B. McNamara et al., "The Institutionalization of the Good Death," *Social Science and Medicine* 39 (1994): 1501–1508.

22. Woods, "Transitioning to a Hospice Program," 110.

23. Putnam, *Hospice or Hemlock*, 87–88.

The Hospital Ethics Committee

Solving Medical Dilemmas

NATALIE R. HANNON

An eighty-three-year-old comatose woman, Mrs. J., came in to our hospital with a very poor prognosis. Although she was comatose, the staff became extremely attached to her. They were so attached that in the two months she was in the hospital, her skin never broke down and she never developed any bedsores. Her family, who lived in a distant state, would occasionally call to find out how she was doing. After two months, her daughter came to visit. The next day she brought in a living will signed by her mother. Mrs. J. had stated that if she had no hope of recovery and could no longer function, she would want to discontinue all treatment, including all food and water. The staff was very upset: "How could this daughter, who had not visited her mother for two months, take her parent off food and water?"

Should the hospital discontinue all treatment, including nutrition and hydration? This was an ethical dilemma. There was no right or wrong answer. Both yes and no were morally acceptable. The case went to the Hospital Ethics Committee, a standing committee that serves to clarify such dilemmas and offers recommendations to resolve them.

The hospital, from which I retired a few years ago, is in New York's inner city. Although not a major trauma center, it has an extraordinarily busy emergency room, which handles over one hundred thousand cases annually, including stab wounds, asthma, complications from diabetes, AIDS, and every other imaginable illness. The patient population is diverse, with Latinos from various countries, Western Africans, and African Americans. The staff is even more diverse, with ninety-eight different languages spoken.

The hospital's Ethics Committee is made up of physicians, nursing staff, a social worker, an administrator, a chaplain, and a member of the community, who was also a chaplain. I also sat on the committee. I was the director of training and staff development, responsible for all nonclinical training at the hospital. I have my doctorate in sociology and have received certificates in bioethics training from Georgetown University and a program conducted jointly by Montefiore Hospital (a major tertiary hospital in New York City) and Columbia University. The objective of the committee is to understand and clarify the medical dilemmas faced at the hospital, most of which are presented by the advanced technology, such as ventilators and feeding tubes, which keeps people from dying. After sorting out the issues by interviewing the parties involved in a particular case, including the physician, the nursing staff, the patient and the patient's family, the committee comes up with a recommendation.

The committee met with Mrs. J.'s daughter, who explained that she had wanted to visit but could not afford to take off from work and also had needed to save for a plane ticket. She had not sent the living will to the hospital because she wanted to see her mother before her mother died. We met with the physician in charge of the case, who stated that there was almost no chance that the woman would ever come out of her coma. We decided that the hospital should follow the patient's wishes as stated in her living will. We then met with the staff to tell them of our recommendation and offered to move the woman to a different unit. The staff refused this offer and said that they would take care of the woman until she died.

This was a relatively "easy" case since we knew what the patient's wishes were and the likelihood that Mrs. J. would ever recover was extremely small. Other cases were more difficult, particularly when the wishes of the patient were unknown.

During the seven years I sat on the Ethics Committee, many ethical dilemmas were raised, such as: Should life-saving treatment be given when the patient does not want it? Should the hospital discontinue artificial nutrition and hydration if requested to do so by the patient or the patient's health-care proxy? Should treatment be continued when it is futile? Should treatment be withdrawn although it may cause the patient's death? Should a patient be told the prognosis, even if the family is opposed to the physician doing so?

Fifty years ago there was no need for ethics committees. Without advanced surgical techniques, advanced intensive care units (ICU's), the ability to restart hearts after they stop, and similar procedures and advances, many of the dilemmas we are facing today did not exist. But it is not just the changing technology which has caused the ethical dilemmas; it is our changing attitudes and feelings toward physicians, as well.

Until the 1960s patients trusted physicians to do what was in their best interest, and patients did not question their physicians. What the physician recommended was invariably followed. When both physician and patient agree on a course of action, there is no ethical dilemma. In the 1960s, the physician-patient relationship changed, concurrent with the development of new medical technologies.[1] A number of factors contributed to this change: there was increasing specialization of medicine and patients were now treated by a variety of strangers rather than their local general practitioner; there was the feminist movement, which criticized the paternalism of male physicians and the medical establishment in general; there was the movement for patients' rights; and there was a realization of the fallibility of physicians.

Physicians had participated in and, in many cases, had led unethical research studies. The most well known was the Tuskegee Study of Untreated Syphilis in the Negro Male, which was conducted from the early 1930s to the 1970s. Poor, southern African American men who had syphilis were denied treatment so that the course of syphilis could be studied, despite the fact that the course of syphilis was known. The study was discontinued only because the story broke in the newspapers. Besides Tuskegee, there was exposé after exposé of other unethical medical studies. For example, patients at Willowbrook, a home for retarded children in Staten Island, New York, were infected with the hepatitis virus to study the infection; in Texas, Mexican American women participated in a double-blind experiment to see the effects of birth control pills, without the women's consent or knowledge. (All the women believed they were receiving birth control.)[2] These experiments led to congressional hearings in 1973, which were covered by the media. Many people began to feel that physicians were no longer to be trusted as a matter of course, resulting in the questioning of physicians' decisions by their patients.

The most significant ethical dilemma leading to the growth of ethics committees, though, was the Karen Ann Quinlan case. On April 15, 1975, Karen Ann Quinlan, a twenty-one-year-old woman, went into a coma. She was admitted to St. Clare's Hospital in Denville, New Jersey, and was placed on a respirator. In July, her father, Joseph Quinlan, signed a release to permit the physicians to turn off the respirator, which the physicians refused to do. They felt that to turn off the respirator would be an act of homicide. Joseph Quinlan then went to court to be appointed Karen Ann's guardian "with the express power of authorizing discontinuance of all extraordinary means of sustaining vital processes."[3] Karen's parents argued that she would have wanted to be removed from the machine; they reported that Karen Ann had discussed the fact that she would not want to be kept alive at all costs.

The judge of the Superior Court, Judge Muir, decided in favor of the hospital. He argued that Karen Ann Quinlan was still alive; she did not meet the Harvard criteria for brain death, and "there is a duty to continue the life assisting apparatus, if within the treating physician's opinion it should be done. . . . There is no constitutional right to die that can be asserted by a parent for his incompetent adult child."[4] He considered that to turn off the respirator would be an act of homicide.

Joseph Quinlan then appealed to the New Jersey Supreme Court, which overturned Judge Muir's ruling. One of the higher court's major concerns was the violation of Karen's right to privacy: "We think that the State's interest contra weakens and the individual's right to privacy grows as the degree of bodily invasion increases and prognosis dims. . . . It is for this reason that we determine that Karen's right of privacy may be asserted in her behalf, in this respect, by her guardian and family under the particular circumstances presented by this record."[5] Justice Hughes of the New Jersey Supreme Court decided that if there were no reasonable possibility of Karen ever becoming conscious, the life support systems could be removed without any civil or criminal liability. Karen Ann Quinlan was then weaned from the respirator. (She proceeded to breathe on her own and lived for an additional eight years.)

The Quinlan case became a media sensation, covered by news outlets across the country. The nation was thus made aware of the dilemmas occurring in hospitals on a daily basis, which were being resolved at the bedside by physicians and nurses. The public felt that there needed to be a better forum for guiding the decision-making process when patients and hospital staff disagreed.

Prior to Karen Ann Quinlan's case, there were precedents for turning to laypeople for making medical decisions: physicians had turned to the community in deciding who should have access to dialysis machines. When dialysis machines were first used, they were a very scarce resource and decisions had to be made as to who would get to use them—basically, decisions about who should live and who should die. Physicians did not want to make these decisions and so turned to the community. The first such committee, which came to be known as The Life and Death Committee, began in Seattle in 1962. It was made up of a minister, a housewife, an attorney, a banker, a politician, and a surgeon.[6] It was not until 1972, when Medicare funded dialysis, that these committees were dissolved.

In addition, in the Quinlan case, Justice Hughes took up a suggestion made by Karen Teel in the *Baylor Law Review* that physicians' decision-making responsibility for ethical dilemmas be shared by a committee made up of physicians, social workers, attorneys, and theologians. Teel believed that not only would these committees open a dialogue about medical decisions, but also they would diffuse the legal liability doctors might encounter when choosing to terminate treatments.[7]

By 1987, the American Hospital Association estimated that 60 percent of all acute care health-care facilities and 80 to 90 percent of major medical centers had bioethics consultants or committees.[8] Since 1992, the major accrediting body for hospitals, the Joint Commission on Accreditation of Health Care Organizations, has required that hospitals have a structure for addressing ethical dilemmas. This is the ethics committee.

When patients and/or patients' families and staff disagree on patient care, the ethics committee may be called on to resolve the dilemma. As discussed by bioethicist Brendan Minogue, ethics committees perform the following functions:

Continuously educate themselves and others on ethical issues and legal changes affecting ethical decisions

Write, review, and apply policies for the institution, such as the policy on the withdrawal of treatment, and educate the staff on these policies

Do case review, both retrospectively and prospectively

A retrospective case review is done to determine whether a case could have been managed better. It is for learning purposes and to see if policies need to be added or changed. Retrospective case review needs to be done with great sensitivity, so that the staff involved does not feel it is being blamed for handling a situation poorly.

With a prospective case review, the ethics committee is asked to make recommendations as to how a current case should be resolved. The ethics committee makes recommendations to the participants in a case; it does not have the authority to enforce these recommendations. However, it does have moral authority. The moral authority comes from the expertise of the committee, the perceived fairness of the committee, and the rationales given for the committee's decisions.[9]

The Ethics Committee I served on carried out the functions discussed above: we met on a regular basis to review cases retrospectively; to educate ourselves on any new issues through invited speakers and discussion of relevant articles; and to write and/or critique new policies regarding ethical issues. We also met on an ad hoc basis for prospective case review. Referrals were accepted from anyone involved in a patient's care, including the patient and the patient's family. We needed to reach consensus on our recommendations. Our goal, as defined by bioethicist Ruth Macklin, was to protect the rights and promote the interests of the patient.[10]

We followed the principles enumerated by Nancy Dubler, a well-known bioethicist at a major hospital in New York who has served on a number of bioethics think tanks:

The principle of "beneficence": medicine should promote the patient's welfare.

The principle of "proportionality": the risks and the benefits of a treatment must be weighed, and the treatment should be given only if the benefit outweighs the burden.

The principle of "respect for persons": patients should be treated as autonomous beings with the right to make their own decisions, and patients who cannot make choices for themselves need to be protected by others.

The principle of "justice": all persons, who are equal, should be treated equally.

The legal principle of "self-determination": adults who have the capacity to make decisions have the right to consent to or to refuse treatment, even if the result of that refusal is death.

The legal principle of "best interest": those who cannot decide have the right to have decisions made that maximize their welfare.[11]

Sometimes, cases came to us where we readily agreed on what was to be done, such as the case of Mrs. J. We knew what the patient's wishes were because of her advance directive and we knew that the law treated artificial nutrition and hydration as the same as any other treatment.

An advance directive lets health-care workers know patients' wishes regarding treatment if the patient is not capable of making a decision. There are two types of advance directives: a living will and a health-care proxy, or durable power of attorney. The living will specifies what treatment, if any, a patient would want given certain conditions; a health-care proxy or durable power of attorney appoints someone to make health-care decisions for the patient. Mrs. J. had an advance directive and we needed to follow that directive. Generally, such a case would not come to the ethics committee. But the staff was uncomfortable with the withdrawal of food and water, even though, in 1990, the U.S. Supreme Court had ruled, in the Nancy Cruzan case, that artificial nutrition and hydration were no different from any other medical treatments.

In 1983, Nancy Cruzan, a resident of Missouri, was in a car accident that left her in a persistent vegetative state; she could breathe, but she had no consciousness. She was maintained by artificial nutrition and hydration. Her parents requested that this be stopped, but the hospital refused since Cruzan had left no instructions concerning her wishes if she were in a comatose state. The Missouri Supreme Court upheld the Missouri law requiring "clear and convincing evidence" that a person would want the treatment to be discontinued and denied the parents' request to remove the feeding tube. On June 25, 1990, the U.S. Supreme Court, while upholding Missouri's right to require evidence that incompetent patients would have wanted treatment stopped, also ended the distinction between artificial nutrition and other medical treatments. (The Cruzans later found evidence to support their view that their daughter would not want to be kept alive in her condition. Nancy Cruzan was moved to another facility, where food and water were discontinued.)

Given the Cruzan case, and the advance directive that Mrs. J. had written, there was very little discussion on the Ethics Committee about removing food and water from Mrs. J. Although that removal was a very emotion-laden issue for the nurses who provided the day-to-day care, the Ethics Committee was abiding by Mrs. J.'s wishes and was following the law.

Making a recommendation in a case is much more difficult when patients cannot make decisions for themselves, for example when they have dementia or are comatose and have not written a health-care proxy or living will. In such cases, the ethics committee usually uses one of two standards which are related to autonomy and beneficence. The first is the "substituted judgment" standard. The ethics committee tries to figure out what the patient would have wanted, given her or his condition and talks to the patient's physician and family and friends. The other standard, the "best interest" standard, is related to beneficence. The ethics committee considers what would be in the best interest of the patient. It must weigh the burden versus the benefit of a treatment for the patient. Many times substituted judgment and the best interest standard coincide. When they do not, the committee would prefer to use the substituted judgment standard, by recommending what the patient's family says the patient would have wanted. However, sometimes it must question what the patient's family is saying concerning the patient's wishes, as in the following case.

Mrs. S. was an eighty-four-year-old woman who had suffered a major stroke. She was comatose, lying in the ICU, being kept alive on a ventilator. The physicians believed that this was futile. The prognosis was that the patient would never come out of her coma. She had no advance directive. Her physician said that Mrs. S. had told him several times that she did not want to live her life hooked up to machines. Her closest relative was her thirty-four-year-old grandson, who insisted that we keep his grandmother alive. He said that she would have wanted everything done for her and that she would not have wanted to come off the ventilator. The case was brought to the Ethics Committee. In our discussion we focused on what Mrs. S. would have wanted and what was in her best interest. There was another issue in this case, which was not verbalized: Mrs. S. was utilizing a scarce resource, an ICU bed. What about the patients waiting in the emergency room for such a bed? Although not mentioned, I know it was on some of our minds, including my own. But, given our respect for a patient's autonomy, if Mrs. S. wanted everything done to keep her alive, we would recommend that she stay on the ventilator.

Mrs. S.'s grandson repeatedly insisted that she would have wanted to be kept alive, and her physician stated the opposite: "Despite her age, she was a vital, lively woman, involved in her neighborhood and her church. Over the course of the years that I have been caring for Mrs. S., we would discuss what she would have wanted done to her if she could no longer function on her own. She said that she never wanted to be placed on machines."

We assumed that both the physician and the grandson were telling the truth; people may say different things to relatives than to physicians. What would therefore be in the woman's best interest? We argued this back and forth. If she had no hope for recovery, then some of us believed that recommending removal from the respirator was the right thing to do. Others argued that she had the right to remain on the respirator, if those were her wishes and her grandson's wishes. We decided to interview other players who had attended to Mrs. S. It was the social worker who provided the insight into the case. The grandson was unemployed and had been living off the grandmother's pension and social security. If she died, he would no longer be supported by her. We concluded that he was acting in his own best interest, not his grandmother's best interest. We recommended that the ventilator be shut off, and Mrs. S. died peacefully.

It is also difficult to come to a recommendation when the patients themselves disagree with the treatment advice, particularly when respect for self-determination and autonomy conflicts with the principle of beneficence. Mrs. R. was a fifty-six-year-old woman who was blind in one eye. She was admitted to the hospital with an infection in the other eye that was not responding to the oral antibiotics she had been taking. She was put on powerful IV antibiotics, but the infection persisted. The fear was that the infection would travel to her brain. The only alternative to the antibiotics was surgery to remove the eye. Mrs. R. refused to have it removed. When questioned about her decision, she would respond, "If God wants me to live, then He will cure me." She would not give permission for the surgery. The infectious disease specialist brought the case to the Ethics Committee.

Should the hospital take Mrs. R. to court to have her declared incompetent and force her to have the surgery? It was very difficult for us. The discussion centered on autonomy (the respect for persons and self-determination) versus beneficence (the patient's welfare should always be promoted), and on weighing the risks and benefits of Mrs. R. having the procedure. We also knew that, even if we decided that the surgery was in the best interest of the patient, we could not force her to have the surgery. In other instances such as this we would have turned to the family for guidance, but Mrs. R. was alone. As we discussed the case, it became clear that we wanted her to have the surgery, but none of us could find any reason that would allow us to recommend it. I remember one of the physicians saying what we were all thinking: "How can we let her die? If we don't force her to have the surgery, the infection will probably travel to her brain. We need to force her to have the surgery. Can we say that she is not capable of making a decision and take her court?" (Physicians may determine if a person is capable of making a decision; courts determine if a person is competent.) We decided we needed a psychiatrist to intervene. A psychiatrist interviewed the patient and reported back to us that Mrs. R. was not irrational in her decision and was totally capable of making decisions for herself. He found that Mrs. R. had very strong religious beliefs and her decision to put her life in the hands of God was totally consistent with her faith and her values.

Looking for other alternatives to try to convince her to have the surgery, the chaplain on the committee suggested that we speak to her minister about the situation. We all jumped on that idea. As it turned out, the minister agreed with Mrs. R. Instead of speaking with her about the surgery, he spent the time with her praying for her to get better. Unfortunately, since she was no longer getting any treatment, we could no longer keep her in the hospital. There was nothing we could do for her. She was discharged to a local skilled nursing facility. We never saw her again and we do not know what happened to her.

This was a very difficult case for the Ethics Committee because we knew that by respecting Mrs. R.'s right to make a decision, we would be allowing her to die.

In order to follow the principle of autonomy, patients must be given informed consent. Informed consent is not just signing a piece of paper which allows a procedure to be done. It also involves telling the patient the diagnosis, the treatment for the diagnosis and the risks and benefits for that treatment, and the alternative treatments and their risks and benefits. The patient must have the capacity to make the decision, understand what is being said, and make the treatment decision voluntarily. However, sometimes family members insist that the patient not be told their diagnosis, particularly in cases of cancer. This may be due to a number of reasons: cultural reasons; fear that the prognosis will lead the patient into a deep depression; or the relatives' reluctance to deal with their loved one's dying.

A case was brought to us by the daughter of a woman who was diagnosed with terminal cancer. Her mother, Mrs. C., had come in to the hospital for a hernia operation. When the surgery was done, the surgeon discovered that the woman had extensive cancer of the stomach, which was inoperable. Upon the daughter's insistence, the mother was not told of her diagnosis or prognosis. About three months prior to the surgery, the mother had lost a son to AIDS, and, of course, the daughter had lost a brother. The daughter believed that if her mother were told that she had cancer, Mrs. C. could not handle the diagnosis emotionally and would give up all hope. The mother, though, kept asking the staff why she wasn't being released from the hospital and why she wasn't feeling any better: "The operation should have made me feel better. What's wrong with me?" The staff hated lying to the patient or just making light of her questions. They asked the Ethics Committee for advice.

Despite the mandate of informed consent, we did not want to unduly upset Mrs. C. We decided that we first needed to talk with the daughter and that we also needed to get a psychiatric consultation for Mrs. C. It became apparent at the interview that the daughter was distraught about the situation and that she could hardly talk about her mother without sobbing. When the psychiatrist interviewed the mother, he found no reason to concur with the daughter's opinion. The mother was appropriately sad about her son, but seemed to be able to talk about her own feelings concerning dying and death. We came to the conclusion that the daughter did not want the patient told because the daughter, not the mother, could not handle the situation. What were we to advise?

Some on the Ethics Committee believed that since the hospital's first obligation is to the patient, the physician should talk with the mother. Others felt that this direct approach would be too hurtful to the daughter. Yet the mother needed to know. What we advised was that no one would go into the hospital room and tell the mother directly what was happening to her; but, if she asked the nurses or the physician about her condition, they would not lie. We explained to the daughter that if we continued to hold the truth from Mrs. C. we would have violated her right to informed consent, that Mrs. C. would realize the truth eventually since she was not improving, and that she could not get the care she needed if she did not know that she had cancer.

If we had believed that the patient would be harmed emotionally by obtaining informed consent, therapeutic privilege could have been invoked. However, this was not the case for Mrs. C. When we withhold a painful diagnosis and/or prognosis from a patient, we are taking away their right to make decisions concerning their own care. We are also participating in a charade in which we must avoid answering the patient's questions and lie to the patient about the treatments being given. Mrs. C. would not understand why she needed chemotherapy or other measures if she did not know the truth.

The next day Mrs. C. asked her nurse, "When am I going home? My doctor said my operation was a simple one, yet I'm still here after four days. Why aren't I getting better?" The doctor was paged; he went to Mrs. C.'s room and gently discussed what had been discovered during the surgery. The hospital arranged for Mrs. C. to get hospice care, which also provided support for the daughter.

Our decisions were even more difficult when we were faced with a cultural norm that gave the decision making not to the patient but to a husband or eldest adult son. As mentioned, the hospital has many patients from Latino and Western African countries. These cultures tend to be patriarchal. During my tenure on the Ethics Committee, I never came across a case where families insisted that decisions be made by the female in the family.

Sometimes, we did not know if a request to hide information from the female patient was due to cultural norms or family dynamics. We did not want to violate the patient's cultural values and norms; yet not telling a person their diagnosis led to an untenable situation in which the staff needed to keep up a façade. We also did not want to cause strife among family members. For these reasons, we trained physicians and nursing staff to ask patients if they would like anyone with them when the patient's situation is discussed. The patients were also asked if they would like to have someone help them make treatment decisions. This gives patients the opportunity to tell us that they would like someone else in the family to be the decision maker, or that they would not. We also educate the staff on when to ask patients these questions: that is, not in the presence of other family members.

Sometimes, a woman who is very quiet when her husband or other significant male relative is in the room says that she would like to make her own decisions when she is alone with the doctor or nurse. For example, the son of Mrs. T., an immigrant from Korea, told the staff not to tell his mother that she had terminal cancer, that in his country such a diagnosis would lead the patient to become very depressed and not want to live out her remaining days. When questioned by the staff, Mrs. T. told us that she knew her situation was very grave and she wanted to be told what was going to happen to her. But she also told us that we must request her son's wishes and pretend that she did not know that she had cancer. He would be alive after she died, and he needed to believe that he had acted in the best way he knew. We respected Mrs. T's wishes. This case was reminiscent of the "joke" about the husband who tells the doctor, "Please don't tell my wife she has cancer; she can't handle it," and his wife, who tells the doctor, "Please don't tell my husband that I have cancer. He can't handle it."

Cultural norms also make it difficult for many of our first-year residents who have been physicians in other countries to give their patients informed consent and to answer their patients' questions. Where they practiced prior to coming to the United States, the physician and the prescribed treatments were not questioned. As a result, we did a great deal of training with the new residents to educate them on issues such as autonomy and informed consent.

The neonatal intensive care unit (NICU) presents many unique ethical dilemmas and therefore will often have its own ethics committee. The NICU cradle is a very expensive, scarce resource. (The total cost of stays for premature babies in the NICU in the United States is over $13 billion. Although one in eight babies born end up in the NICU, these babies are responsible for almost half of the costs of infant hospitalizations.[12]) Ramifications of care may affect the infant's whole life. The substituted judgment standard cannot be used in these cases, since the patient is a baby, and it is difficult to use the best interest standard since conditions of the babies in the NICU are very fluid. There are also very specific laws regarding termination of treatment for infants. Of the Ethics Committee meetings I attended, I found the NICU Committee to be the most difficult. In the NICU, the committee must be especially sensitive to the needs of the parents. They have had what was expected to be a joyful event turn into a devastating one. Even when the care is defined as futile—that is, when the doctors agree that the baby cannot survive no matter what the treatment—we must give the parents time to come to this conclusion and time to say good-bye to the baby. Sometimes, it is the physicians and/or the nurses who want to continue treatment, because they see their job as saving infants' lives, and, many times, they have grown attached to the infants. Then, we allow the staff to say good-bye and discontinue treatment.

In cases in which the parents do not want to give permission for a treatment that would allow the baby to survive because of another condition, such as Down's syndrome, the Ethics Committee gets involved and may ask the courts to intervene. The courts will make the hospital the guardian of the baby and the life-saving procedure will be performed. But, the baby still goes home with the parents who do not want him or her.

There are times, however, when the outcome is a happy one. Baby Y. was born over three months prematurely. He weighed less than two pounds. Upon birth, he was given at most two weeks to live. The physicians felt that any attempt to treat Baby Y. was futile, but the parents, who had been trying to have a baby for a number of years, were adamant that the physicians and the hospital do all they could to keep the baby alive. The physicians agreed to continue treatment. At the end of three weeks, Baby Y. went into cardiac arrest. He was resuscitated at the family's request, but he continued to show no improvement. The physicians again requested that the treatment be terminated, and the parents refused. The social worker on the NICU asked for an ethics consultation.

The Ethics Committee met with the physicians involved, who explained their feelings: Baby Y. was not getting any better; the NICU resources could better be used for babies with a better prognosis; and more harm than good was actually being done to the baby. They also believed that if the baby did survive he would have multiple problems, such as blindness, stunted growth, and retardation.

We explained the feelings of the physicians to the parents. The family did not want to continue treating the baby if he was in pain and if he continued not to show any improvement. A decision was made to continue treatment for another week. If at the end of that time Baby Y. showed no improvement, the family agreed, treatment would be discontinued. A day after this decision the baby had a big turnaround. He increased in weight and became somewhat more responsive. Treatment was continued.

After two and one-half months, another decision had to be made. The baby had been on a feeding tube. The parents would try to feed him a few ccs through a bottle, but he could not seem to expend the energy to drink. The physicians wanted to implant the feeding tube, which the family objected to since they believed it was a risky operation. Again, the Ethics Committee was called in to help the physicians and the family come to an agreement, and one similar to the one regarding the termination of treatment was reached: a week was given to see if the baby could begin to eat on his own. Again, the baby came around. He was eating more at the end of the week; by the end of two weeks, he was drinking a full bottle. Although he still needed oxygen, the baby was released from the hospital after a total of four months in the NICU.

Follow-up: The baby is now two years old. He is being weaned from the oxygen. He is not blind, his growth is not stunted, and except for the weakness of his lungs, he seems to show normal and above normal developmental patterns.

Ethics committees serve a very important function in helping to resolve the issues surrounding modern medicine. Since there are no "right" answers, we try to sort out the issues and come up with the "best" answer. We also try to have all the involved parties, the patient, the family, and the hospital staff, come to some resolution about the dilemmas. Being in a hospital is generally an intimidating, frightening situation for the patient and the patient's family. When they disagree with the staff as to treatment, it is important to know there is a group of caring people who can help sort through their issues with sensitivity and compassion. We may not always come up with recommendations that make us happy, as in the case of Mrs. R., who refused to have the surgery on her eye, but we always try to respect the patients, while advising what we hope is the best resolution to the ethical dilemmas confronting them.

On a personal note, my experience on the Ethics Committee strengthened my belief that there is no one right way to die. How we die is an individual decision which must be respected by health-care workers. If a person wants everything done to be kept alive, including ventilators and feeding tubes, then we must follow that patient's wishes; if a person wants to shun such treatments, then we must respect that patient's wishes. I also believe that it is imperative to educate people about the importance of advance directives. Only with such a document can patients have their wishes known and met when they are dying.

NOTES

1. For an excellent discussion of this, see David Rothman, *Strangers at the Bedside* (New York: Basic Books, 1991).

2. Robert Veatch, "Experimental Pregnancy," *The Hastings Center Report* (June 1971): 2–3.

3. *Newsweek*, November 3, 1975.

4. Judge Robert Muir, "In the Matter of Quinlan," New Jersey Superior Court, 1975. In 1968, Harvard developed the following criteria for defining brain death: unreceptivity and unresponsivity; no spontaneous breathing (upon cessation of a respirator); no reflexes; a flat electroencephalogram (to be used as confirmatory evidence). Tests are to be repeated twenty-four hours later.

5. Justice Richard Hughes, "In the Matter of Quinlan," New Jersey Supreme Court, 1976.

6. Jon Marmor, "Insomnia, Teflon and Life Savers," September 1996, accessed March 5, 2008 at http://www.washington.edu/alumni/columns/sept96/back_pages0996.html.

7. Rothman, *Strangers*, 227–228.

8. M. L. Tina Stevens, *Bioethics in America: Origins and Cultural Politics* (Baltimore: Johns Hopkins University Press, 2000), ix.

9. Brendan Minogue, *Bioethics: A Committee Approach* (Boston: Jones and Bartlett, 1996), 5–6.

10. Cited in Nancy Dubler and David Nimmons, *Ethics On Call* (New York: Harmony Books, 1992), 3.

11. Ibid., 44.

12. March of Dimes, "Nation's Hospital Bill for Premature Births Is $13.6 Billion," November 18, 2003, accessed March 5, 2008, at http://marchofdimes.com/print-ablearticles/9564-10358.asp.

Ethical Principles for End-of-Life Decision Making

CANDACE CUMMINS GAUTHIER

The Principles of Health-Care Ethics

I trained as a philosopher, with a specialty in ethics, but my interest in health-care ethics started when I began teaching bioethics at the University of North Carolina–Wilmington twenty years ago. Over the years I have refined my thinking on the ethics of health care, particularly concerning end-of-life issues. I am convinced that we need to develop a more ethical way to deal with death and dying as individuals and as a nation.

We make moral judgments throughout our lives, deciding on certain courses of action and evaluating the actions of others based on our own sense of what is right or wrong. At those moments, ethical principles come into play. When these choices and actions concern medical treatment and health care, the most relevant ethical principles are the principle of beneficence, the principle of respect for autonomy, and the principle of distributive justice.[1] These principles were first presented in 1979 in *Principles of Biomedical Ethics* by Tom Beauchamp and James Childress, now in a sixth edition.[2] Tom Beauchamp is a philosopher at Georgetown University and James Childress is a theologian at the University of Virginia.

These principles are recognized and used by those who work in health-care ethics, even when they are being criticized, and are found in every Western health-care ethics text.[3] They will be known to health-care providers who have taken a course in health-care ethics, are interested in health-care ethics, or have been involved with a hospital ethics committee. I find these principles most useful as a way to think about and evaluate ethical issues involved in end-of-life situations, drawing our attention to elements of the situation that may have been unnoticed otherwise. I also like the fact that the principles create a shared language for the discussion of ethical issues.

As useful as the principles are in approaching ethical issues in health care, it is important to recognize that they may conflict with one another when health-care decisions need to be made. After explaining the principles, I will present fictional examples of end-of-life decision making to demonstrate how and why these principles might conflict. I will also make practical and, in some cases, controversial, recommendations for resolving these conflicts in a morally justifiable way.

The Principle of Beneficence

The principle of beneficence requires that health-care providers promote the patient's good, prevent harm for the patient, and do no harm to the patient.

In the context of health care, "good" usually refers to health, well-being, proper functioning, and life, while "harm" refers to disease, injury, impaired functioning, suffering, pain, and death. There may be different interpretations of what would be good or harmful for a particular patient with a particular medical condition. There may be times when continued life, for example a life accompanied by a great deal of suffering, is felt to be a harm to the person experiencing it and may even be considered to be worse than death.

Another complication with applying this principle is that most diagnostic tests and medical treatments have risks of side effects as well as potential benefits. Different people may judge the relative weights of possible benefits and risks in different ways. So, there may be disagreements about whether a particular test or treatment will cause more harm or more benefit and whether the possible benefits are worth risking potential harms. Only if the potential benefits for the patient outweigh the possible risks would a particular medical test or treatment be morally justified, on this principle.

The Principle of Respect for Autonomy

The principle of respect for autonomy requires that patients with autonomy (decision-making capacity) be permitted to exercise that capacity by making their own well-informed health-care choices. This principle allows the person who will actually experience the relevant goods and harms to make the decision to accept or reject them. Respecting the patient's autonomy includes veracity, so that patients should be given complete and truthful information about their medical conditions, all of the treatment options under consideration, and the expected progress of their illnesses.[4]

Respecting autonomy also requires voluntary informed consent for medical tests and treatments. The elements of voluntary informed consent are that (1) patients must be fully informed about the medical options offered to them, (2) they must understand the information given to them, and (3) their prior agreement must be given voluntarily, without deception, manipulation, or coercion.[5] The information that patients should receive prior to giving their consent includes the risks and benefits of the treatment under consideration and any alternatives, as well as the expected results of refusing all treatment options.

Just as patients with decision-making capacity must give voluntary informed consent for medical tests and treatments, they are also allowed to refuse these medical procedures. Imagine that a woman who is capable of making her own decisions refuses life-sustaining medical treatment, such as a ventilator or kidney dialysis, based on an understanding of complete and truthful information about these interventions that has been provided to her. Imagine, as well, that her decision is not being manipulated or coerced in any way. No one is appealing to emotions such as fear or guilt to talk her into accepting or rejecting this treatment and no one is putting pressure on her to make a particular choice. Here, the principle of respect for autonomy requires that she be allowed to refuse the treatment being recommended, even if this means she will die.

The Principle of Distributive Justice

The principle of distributive justice requires that health-care resources be distributed in a fair way among members of society. It is with this principle that the interests of society, for example to conserve scarce or expensive resources, are taken into consideration. The obvious difficulty with applying this principle is that it is unclear what a fair method of distribution would be. For example, one theory says that a fair way to distribute health-care resources would be to give them only to people who can pay for them. Others provide criteria such as need, merit, contribution to society, and the best use of resources.

Our society seems to have settled on a combination of criteria for the distribution of medical resources, including need; ability to pay; first come, first served; and the best use of resources. For example, anyone who needs emergency medical treatment must be cared for at all public hospitals. Once they are stabilized, it is legal for patients to be discharged if they are unable to pay and have no health insurance.

Another example of combining criteria comes from organ transplantation. Potential organ recipients are ranked in order of when they were placed on the list of those needing organs, as well as how badly they need an organ. However, in order to be placed on the list, patients must be able to pay for the transplant and they must be in overall good health, with sufficient social support, so that the donated organ will not be wasted.

The principle of distributive justice may be used to determine how many beds and nurses will be allocated to each service in a hospital, such as cardiac care, trauma care, and pediatrics, based on the relative costs and best use of these resources, as well as the needs of the community. Similarly, nursing home administrators may decide that they will not admit patients who require ventilators or feeding tubes, due to the high cost of providing these medical services.

Health-care institutions could also use this principle in comparing the costs of specific resources with the realistic benefits of their use for individual patients. This is unlikely at the present time, since there is an understandable reluctance on the part of hospital and nursing home administrators to be perceived as placing a monetary value on the lives of their patients. As the costs of health-care resources and the number of uninsured Americans continue to grow, we may reach the point, as a society, where we do need to make this kind of comparison.

Withholding and Withdrawing Medical Treatment

Many state laws that govern end-of-life decision making use the terms *withholding* and *withdrawing* in reference to life-sustaining medical treatment. "Withholding medical treatment" simply means that the decision is made not to initiate the treatment. Those who are conscious and capable of decision making may request a do-not-resuscitate (DNR) order if they are being cared for in the hospital or a nursing home. This is one method of authorizing health-care providers to withhold life-prolonging medical treatment. In this case what is being withheld is cardio-pulmonary resuscitation (CPR). The DNR order is written into the patient's medical chart and says that the patient is not to be resuscitated if the heart or lungs stop working. "Withdrawing medical treatment" refers to the situation when treatment is presently being provided and the decision is made to end or discontinue that treatment.

Both withholding and withdrawing life-sustaining medical treatment are legally permitted for patients capable of decision making and both are morally justified by the principle of respect for autonomy. Withholding and withdrawing medical procedures may also be justified by the principle of beneficence if the treatment being considered or provided would cause more harm than good for the patient. For example, a frail elderly patient at the end of life who receives CPR is not going to recover and leave the hospital and, moreover, is very likely to suffer broken ribs in the attempt to stop the dying process.

A Case of Withdrawing Medical Treatment: Mrs. Gregson

Mrs. Gregson is in the end stage of terminal cancer. The cancer has now moved into her lungs and she is on a ventilator for breathing. Although she is in a great deal of pain, Mrs. Gregson is conscious and fully capable of making her own decisions. Once she understands the extent of her illness and that she will not get better, Mrs. Gregson considers asking her doctor to remove the ventilator. When Mrs. Gregson's grown son and daughter come to visit her next, they express their concern for her suffering and feelings of dependence, but they also want her to continue to fight for her life. Mrs. Gregson replies, "I love you both and I don't want to leave you, but I'm not going to get better. Knowing that, what I really want is a peaceful death. I don't want to waste away in pain while this machine breathes for me. I want to die with dignity."

Mrs. Gregson's case is an example of a conscious and capable patient requesting the withdrawal of life-sustaining medical treatment, creating a conflict between the principle of beneficence and the principle of respect for autonomy. Considering death as a harm to be prevented and life a good to be promoted, the doctor may believe that beneficence requires that the ventilator be kept in place to preserve Mrs. Gregson's life. However, since

Mrs. Gregson is capable of making her own decisions and her informed choice is to have the ventilator removed, respect for autonomy requires that she be allowed to make this choice and that the ventilator be removed.

My opinion is that when patients are capable of making informed decisions about end-of-life medical treatment, they must be allowed to do so and their decisions must be respected, even if the decision is to refuse treatment and this will result in death. The doctor is also legally required to act according to a capable patient's wishes. Of course, complete and truthful information must be provided about the risks and benefits of any medical treatment and, in this kind of case, the emphasis must be on the expected results of refusing life-sustaining interventions.

Advance Directives

Advance directives allow capable patients to make their wishes about end-of-life medical treatment known in advance. They include a document, often called a living will, that allows doctors to withhold or withdraw life-sustaining procedures when the patient can no longer make medical decisions. Most states require that a patient be in a persistent vegetative state (with no cognitive function and no possibility of recovery) or have a terminal and incurable illness before this advance directive goes into effect.

Advance directives also include the power of attorney for health care, through which a health-care agent is appointed by a capable patient to make medical decisions when she is no longer able to make or communicate such decisions. The health-care agent is the legal representative of the patient and has the sole legal authority to make these decisions. In most states the health-care agent may authorize the withholding or withdrawal of life-sustaining medical treatment.

Both kinds of advance directives are supported by the principle of respect for autonomy. With the living will we can be reasonably confident that we know what the patient wanted in regard to life-sustaining interventions for certain medical conditions. With the power of attorney for health care we know, at least, whom the patient wanted to make these kinds of decisions.

Some have objected to the use of advance directives, arguing that the person who filled out these documents is not the same person as the one presently suffering from advanced dementia, a devastating stoke, or persistent vegetative state. They also argue that when we are not yet suffering from these kinds of conditions we cannot make an informed decision about what we would want if we had them. With these two arguments, opponents of advance directives are saying that we should not be allowed to make these kinds of decisions for our own future end-of-life care, even when we can, because they will not reflect our true wishes in the future.

I totally disagree with these arguments. If we are not qualified to make these decisions for our own future selves, then who would be? Even if we do, in some sense, become a different person as an Alzheimer's patient or in a persistent vegetative state, the earlier capable self is still the closest anyone could be to the later incapable self. Furthermore, the earlier and later selves still share the same body that will suffer and die one way or another, whatever we want to say about the person before and after the onset of the relevant medical condition.

In response to the argument about not knowing enough to be able to make an informed decision, I would point out that no one else could have this knowledge unless they, too, were in a persistent vegetative state or had advanced dementia. But, in those conditions, they wouldn't be able to make decisions for us, either. I maintain that we are each in the best position, of all possible candidates, to make these decisions for our own future medical treatment when we are conscious and capable of doing so. We each know our own tolerance for pain. We know whether or not we value length of life or quality of life more.

Advance directives may be challenged by physicians and family members who are not appointed as a health-care agent, based on the principle of beneficence. They may not want to let their patient or loved one die when this could be prevented with life-sustaining medical technology. However, both legally and morally, advance directives must be permitted to direct patient care at the end of life, based on the principle of respect for autonomy.

Because advance directives can be very different from state to state, those who are concerned about end-of-life medical treatment should find out what advance directives are available in their state and follow the instructions for making their wishes known in a legally recognized way. Most of these forms do not require a lawyer, but must be signed by two witnesses and/or a notary public.

A Case with Advance Directives: Mr. Benton

Mr. Benton has been diagnosed with advanced Alzheimer's disease. He is presently in a nursing home and is unable to chew and swallow enough for adequate nutrition. The doctor who is caring for Mr. Benton asks his wife if he had made any kind of advance directive that could be used to decide whether or not to initiate tube feeding. Fortunately, Mr. Benton had documented his wishes for end-of-life care in two ways and his wife was able to find copies of both of these documents. He had a notarized living will stating his desire not to have tube feeding or other life-sustaining treatments if he were in a persistent vegetative state or had a terminal and incurable illness. The living will does not apply to Mr. Benton's present condition, since Alzheimer's disease is not considered to be terminal (death expected within six months). However, Mr. Benton had also executed a power of attorney for health care, appointing his wife as his health-care agent.

Since Mr. Benton has severe dementia caused by Alzheimer's disease and this condition is covered by the power of attorney for health care in their state, the doctor caring for Mr. Benton must allow Mrs. Benton to make the decision about tube feeding. In this way, Mr. Benton's choice of who he wanted to make medical decisions for him is being respected so that the principle of respect for autonomy is being honored.

Surrogate Decision Making without Advance Directives

When a patient hasn't documented end-of-life wishes with an advance directive, family members should be permitted to make these decisions. Most states have a hierarchy, based on state statute or common law, that allows surrogate decision making, without a power of attorney for health care, by a legal guardian, spouse, and first degree relatives (parents and children), in that order.[6] Without an advance directive, such decisions should be made on the basis of information about what the patient would want or the patient's best interests.

Often, when we see a news report or read an article about a particular end-of-life case, we will discuss the case with our family, expressing our feelings about different medical procedures in different medical situations. We might say, "I never want to be kept alive on a ventilator or feeding tube if I'm not going to get better." This would be an example of information about a patient's wishes that could be provided in an end-of-life case.

Even without this kind of specific information, close family members may be able to determine what the patient would have wanted, based on knowledge of the patient's values and beliefs regarding things such as life, death, medical treatment, and hospitals. Surrogate decisions made in these two ways rely on the standard known as "substituted judgment." Employing this standard, the surrogate is making an informed judgment about medical treatment, as a substitute for the personal judgment of the patient, and is respecting the patient's autonomy.

When there is no advance directive and no one feels able to make an informed judgment about what the patient would want, the surrogate must make decisions about medical treatment based on what would be best for the patient, using the best interest standard.[7] This standard relies on the principle of beneficence and asks the surrogate decision maker to consider the harms and benefits of medical treatments for the patient. Some of the things that will need to be considered are the chances for survival and recovery, the quality of life that is expected for the patient, and the amount of pain and suffering the patient will have to endure.

I believe that the best people to serve as surrogate decision makers, even when the best interest standard is used, are still the patient's close family members, or intimate friends, when there is no family available. This is because these people may have insights into the ways in which their loved ones would be harmed or benefited by different medical interventions, for example, by a compromised quality of life or prolonged pain and suffering.

A Case without Advance Directives: Mrs. Wagner

Like Mr. Benton, Mrs. Wagner is in a nursing home with advanced Alzheimer's disease. Decisions need to be made about whether or not to initiate tube feeding. The doctor asks Mrs. Wagner's husband about advance directives and it turns out that she doesn't have either a living will or a power of attorney for health care. Because they never discussed the question of tube feeding at the end of life, Mr. Wagner is agonizing over this decision. In the end, he decides that this would not be the best thing for his wife. "It really won't change anything for her quality of life," he explains, "and it might even make it worse, if it causes her to suffer. Tube feeding also seems to be really invasive, to me. She might be frightened if we do this to her and can't explain why."

In most states Mr. Wagner would be legally permitted to make this decision for his wife, even if he has not been appointed her health-care agent.

Mr. Wagner doesn't know if his wife would have wanted tube feedings; thus, he must consider what would be in her best interests. He is particularly concerned about her quality of life and the extent of her suffering, since she is not going to improve. He is using the best interest standard and he is acting according to the principle of beneficence.

Ineffective Interventions

Some of the most difficult conflicts at the end of life arise around the question of ineffective interventions, or medical procedures that are unable to bring about a patient's recovery but can only postpone death. They may also impose burdens that outweigh any possible benefits for the patient. On the other hand, if an intervention is successful in relieving a patient's pain and suffering, then it is not ineffective.

Many hospitals have instituted what are known as "Ineffective Intervention Policies," according to which physicians are not required to provide interventions they determine to be ineffective, even if family members request or demand them. These policies may create a conflict between the principle of beneficence and the principle of respect for autonomy. Ineffective intervention policies appeal to the principle of beneficence, when physicians believe the interventions requested will cause more harm than good for the patient. Based on the principle of respect for autonomy, however, surrogate decision makers may argue that they should be permitted to make medical decisions for patients, if they are appointed as healthcare agents or have knowledge about what patients would want.

I strongly support these policies. Although I am an advocate of respect for patient autonomy, I think this principle should be limited to decision making about medical treatments offered by physicians. I believe that families must permit physicians, as the experts, to practice medicine according to their training and experience and should not demand interventions that physicians believe are ineffective.

Long-term tube feeding for those at the end stages of a terminal illness is an example of this. For long-term feeding, the tube is surgically placed directly into the stomach. This type of artificial nutrition will not cure the terminal illness or provide relief from pain and suffering. Long-term tube feeding has not been proven to have any survival benefit for those with terminal cancer.[8] Moreover, the complications of tube feeding include pain at the site of the surgery for tube placement, abdominal wall ulcers, wound infection, excessive bleeding, and penetration of the bowel.[9]

Often family members will ask for the surgical placement of feeding tubes because they are worried about the inability of the patient to take in sufficient calories at the end of a terminal illness. They are afraid that the patient is going to suffer and die from starvation. In reality, patients often voluntarily stop eating as their terminal illness advances. Physicians caring for terminally ill patients agree that conscious patients generally do not experience hunger or thirst and, if they do, are satisfied with small amounts of food and fluid or keeping the mouth moistened.[10] This is a natural and peaceful death in which the patient dies from the advancing illness and not from starvation.[11]

The principle of distributive justice and society's interest in conserving medical resources are also relevant when expensive resources are demanded for patients who will not benefit from them. Thus, I think family members should be informed of the financial costs of medical interventions when physicians believe them to be ineffective for the individual patient.

A Case of Ineffective Intervention and Family Disagreement: Mr. Stanley

Mr. Stanley has suffered a devastating stroke that has left him unresponsive and paralyzed on his right side. Test results show that, although he is breathing on his own, there is no chance of Mr. Stanley recovering consciousness or movement in the right side of his body. Mr. Stanley's physicians recommend that a do-not-resuscitate order be written and that a feeding tube not be inserted. Since his wife died ten years ago, Mr. Stanley has been living with his brother. Because Mr. Stanley has no advance directive, the doctor asks his brother to make these decisions. The brother believes that Mr. Stanley would not want feeding tubes in this condition. He also thinks Mr. Stanley would want to be allowed to have a natural death, without the violence of CPR. The decision is made not to implant feeding tubes and a do-not-resuscitate order is written on Mr. Stanley's chart. The next day Mr. Stanley's three children arrive from distant states. None of them has had much contact with their father since graduating from high school and moving away. However, they disagree with their uncle's decisions and they insist that a feeding tube be inserted and that their father be given CPR, if necessary.

This case is certainly tragic due to the lack of advance directives, the request for ineffective and invasive interventions for Mr. Stanley, and the disagreement between the members of his family, at the very time when they most need each others' care and support. I believe that Mr. Stanley's brother is in the best position to know what he would want and, thus, would be the best surrogate decision maker. The children have not kept in touch with their father and are not as likely to know what his wishes would be in this situation. According to most state laws, his children have the legal authority to make medical decisions for their father. Thus, the doctor must allow Mr. Stanley's children to make the decisions about feeding tubes and CPR.

Given their legal authority to be surrogate decision makers, the children will need truthful information about their father's condition and his poor prognosis for recovery and improvement. They need to be asked what they think their father would want, in the effort to honor the principle of respect for autonomy. If they are not sure about this, they need to be asked what they think would be in his best interests, using the principle of beneficence. The family needs to be told if the doctors involved believe feeding tubes or CPR would be ineffective interventions and they need to be told why.

Much of the anguish created by this situation could have been avoided if Mr. Stanley had used a power of attorney for health care to appoint his brother as his health-care agent. Then there would have been no legal question of who would be the surrogate decision maker. The children would still need to be informed about their father's medical situation, so that they could come to understand and, hopefully, accept the decisions their uncle had made.

Physician-Assisted Suicide

In October 1997, Oregon became the only state to permit physician-assisted suicide.[12] The Oregon Death with Dignity Act was approved by a state referendum in 1994 but was challenged in court. After a federal district court decision against the act was reversed by the Ninth Circuit Court of Appeals, another state referendum was held. The law was approved in this second referendum as well. According to this law, a state resident who is terminally ill (expected to die within six months), at least eighteen years of age, and capable of making and communicating health-care decisions is permitted to "obtain a prescription for medication to end his or her life in a humane and dignified manner."[13]

The patient must make an oral request, a written request, and a second oral request during a fifteen-day waiting period. The attending physician must determine that the patient has a terminal illness and make sure the patient is capable and has made the request voluntarily. The patient must receive information about her diagnosis and prognosis, the potential risks and probable results of taking the medication, and alternatives such as hospice care and pain control. The patient must also see a consulting physician who confirms the diagnosis and makes sure that the patient is capable and is making an informed and voluntary decision. If either of the physicians suspects that the patient is suffering from impaired judgment, a referral for counseling must be made.[14]

Physician-assisted suicide is controversial throughout the country. Philosophers have argued that allowing doctors to write a prescription to be used in this way violates the principle of beneficence. Edmund Pellegrino, for example, believes that assisted suicide "seems a peculiar kind of beneficence that extinguishes the beneficiary."[15] Law professor Yale Kamisar argues that such a policy could be misused so that vulnerable patients, such as the elderly, would be pressured into seeking this kind of help.[16]

I want to defend the Oregon Death with Dignity Act and the policy of allowing physician-assisted suicide under the limitations and requirements set out in that law. My first justification depends on the principle of respect for autonomy. The only patients who qualify for assistance with suicide are those who are capable of making health-care decisions, are fully informed, and have made repeated requests. Allowing terminally ill patients to obtain a prescription to end their lives at a time and in a manner of their own choosing seems no different to me than allowing patients to make decisions about when and how they will die by refusing life-sustaining medical technology. As long as two physicians are involved, making sure that the patient is fully informed, is not suffering from impaired judgment, and is not being coerced or pressured in any way, I think it is unlikely that vulnerable patients would be victimized by allowing physician-assisted suicide.

I also believe that physician-assisted suicide is justified by the principle of beneficence. Providing this kind of help promotes the patient's good by offering the security of knowing that when the physical and emotional effects of the illness become unbearable, the patient has a way to end his life with dignity. Physicians who are willing to do this are also preventing the harm of future suffering that will serve no good purpose, since the patient has an incurable illness. Although the principle of beneficence requires that physicians do no harm to their patients, it could be argued that, in this case, death is not harmful to the patient, who is suffering and asking for release.

It may also be possible to justify physician-assisted suicide with the principle of distributive justice. If a patient chooses an early death in the end stages of terminal illness, health-care resources that might have been needed by this patient may be provided to other patients. These may be patients whose illnesses are not terminal or those who have chosen to see a terminal illness through to its natural end.

Statistics from Oregon indicate that physician-assisted suicide is not used very often. Annual reports by the Oregon Public Health Division show that 292 patients died after ingesting the prescribed medication in the nine years after the law went into effect (1998–2006). We can also see from these reports that some patients who received a prescription did not use it, but died from their underlying illnesses. For example, in 2006, sixty-five prescriptions for lethal medication were written and only thirty-five patients died from taking the medication, while nineteen died from their illnesses, and eleven remained alive at the end of the year.[17] This may indicate that simply knowing they can end their suffering, if it becomes unbearable, provides a much-needed sense of security and control for terminally ill patients.

Active Voluntary Euthanasia

Active voluntary euthanasia occurs when a physician ends a patient's life, based on the patient's own request, with the motive of compassion. Active voluntary euthanasia differs from withholding or withdrawing life-sustaining treatment because, in this case, the patient is killed by a lethal injection, rather than allowed to die naturally. Active voluntary euthanasia differs from assisted suicide because, here, the physician kills the patient directly instead of prescribing a lethal medication the patient may take to kill herself. Active voluntary euthanasia is illegal in the United States. This is called "life-ending on request" in the Netherlands, where it is legal as long as certain guidelines are followed to ensure that the patient's request is informed and voluntary and that all efforts to treat the patient's pain have been tried.[18]

The arguments against active voluntary euthanasia are similar to those against physician-assisted suicide. Law professor Alexander Morgan Capron writes that providing patients with "a deadly substance to cause death" is forbidden according to the Hippocratic tradition of medicine.[19] Daniel Callahan, a philosopher, is concerned about the abuse of active voluntary euthanasia, were it to become legal, with the possibility that some patients would be killed without their "explicit permission."[20] Timothy Quill is a physician and an outspoken advocate of assisted suicide, yet he opposes the legalization of active voluntary euthanasia. He argues that with physician-assisted suicide the balance of power between physician and patient is "more nearly equal," while active voluntary euthanasia increases the physician's power and "the risk of error, coercion, or abuse."[21]

My own view is that active voluntary euthanasia is morally permissible and should be legalized, with requirements similar to those in the Oregon Death with Dignity Act. My justifications, here, are the same as those for the Oregon law. I believe one of the purposes of medicine is to relieve suffering, particularly when healing is no longer possible, based on the principle of beneficence. It is also true that some patients who are in unbearable pain are not able to take pills; something more than assisted suicide will be needed to relieve them of their suffering. I also think the patient should be the one to decide when that suffering has gone on long enough, based on the principle of respect for autonomy. However, because of the controversial nature of active voluntary euthanasia, physicians should not feel pressured to do this for their patients. Combining these ideas, my position is that if a physician is comfortable with ending a patient's life in this way and the patient asks for active euthanasia, I think it should be allowed, again, with all of the safeguards of the Oregon law.

The Terri Schiavo Case and Final Thoughts

The case of Terri Schiavo illustrates the importance of making our end-of-life wishes known with an advance directive. Schiavo suffered a cardiac arrest in February of 1990. Her husband, Michael, was appointed as her legal guardian because she did not have an advance directive. She was diagnosed as being in a persistent vegetative state a year later. After numerous rehabilitation efforts, Michael asked that his wife's feeding tubes be removed in 1998. Schiavo's parents opposed this request and challenged Michael's authority to make medical decisions for her. A series of court decisions all agreed that Michael had the authority to request the removal of his wife's feeding tubes. The Florida Senate and House of Representatives, the governor of Florida, the

U.S. Congress, and the president all tried to intervene to keep Schiavo alive. Finally, in March 2005, Schiavo died after her feeding tubes were removed.[22]

From an ethical perspective, Michael Schiavo's decision to have his wife's feeding tubes removed was justified by the principle of respect for autonomy since he testified that his wife had said she did not want to be kept alive on life support. Schiavo had made similar statements to her brother and sister-in-law. This decision could also be justified by the principle of beneficence since keeping Schiavo alive artificially with no chance of a return to consciousness could be considered harmful to her, especially with the risks of long-term tube feeding. According to the principle of distributive justice, the continued use of feeding tubes in this case would never be effective in bringing about Schiavo's recovery and could be described as a misuse of medical resources.

With Michael Schiavo as his wife's legal guardian, her parents had no legal standing to challenge his decisions about her medical care. The courts all recognized this and decided accordingly. Moreover, there was no ethical justification for the involvement by members of the executive and legislative branches of government in this case, as no interest of society could possibly have been served by keeping Schiavo alive. What was essentially a private medical decision was turned into a media circus and a public spectacle for primarily political ends. And all of this could have been avoided if Schiavo had made her wishes for end-of-life treatment known in a living will and named her husband as her health-care agent in a power of attorney for health care.

My recommendation is that all those involved in end-of-life decision making be fully informed about the risks and benefits of treatments recommended by health-care providers, as well as the expected outcomes of the refusal of all treatment options. I maintain that capable patients must be permitted to make their own medical decisions, even if these will result in death. I believe that capable patients should be allowed to seek the means to end their own lives, when death is imminent, as permitted in the Oregon Death with Dignity Act. I also support the legalization of active voluntary euthanasia, with requirements similar to those of the Oregon law.

When patients are no longer able to make their own decisions, surrogate decision makers must be permitted to make decisions about end-of-life care, based on their appointment as a health-care agent or their relationship with the patient. The surrogate decision maker should be allowed to refuse medical treatment if this is what the patient would want or is in the patient's best interests. These decisions should be based on truthful and complete information provided to surrogate decision makers including the expected progress of the illness and the expected results of refusing treatment.

Finally, health-care providers should not be pressured into providing medical interventions they believe will not be effective in meeting reasonable goals for their patients and, most importantly, will cause suffering at the end of a patient's life, when the ultimate outcome is unlikely to be changed. This may include long-term tube feeding for patients in a persistent vegetative state, those with an incurable and terminal illness, and those in advanced stages of Alzheimer's disease.

The ethical dilemmas and conflicts that often arise at the end of life could be greatly reduced if all of us made our wishes for end-of-life care known to our loved ones. If we do not want to be kept alive with medical technology when we cannot recover, we should execute a living will. This would eliminate much of the anguish that family members experience when they do not know and cannot guess what their loved ones would want. Most importantly, we should appoint someone we trust to be our health-care agent in a power of attorney for health care, so that this person can express our wishes when we can no longer do so. These documents would provide physicians with the legal authority to end life-sustaining treatments they may already feel ambivalent about providing and would give us the peace and comfort of knowing that we will end our lives in a way we have chosen for ourselves.

NOTES

1. These principles are best described in Tom L. Beauchamp and LeRoy Walters, *Contemporary Issues in Bioethics*, 6th ed. (Belmont, CA: Wadsworth-Thomson Learning, 2003), 21–26.

2. Tom L. Beauchamp and James F. Childress, *Principles of Biomedical Ethics* (New York: Oxford University Press, 1979).

3. Critics of the principles approach to health-care ethics include the casuists, following Albert Jonsen and Stephen Toulmin, who argue that the principles need to be supplemented with the particulars of the moral situation, and the particularists, such as Jonathan Dancy, who argue that ethical analysis should be based only on concrete details, without the use of principles. Virtue theorists, like Edmund Pellegrino and David Thomasma, want to see the virtues of the health-care provider included in health-care decision making. Alisa Carse, representing the ethics of care, claims that the principles approach ignores the emotions and relationships of those faced with making moral decisions. Communitarians, such as Daniel Callahan, are critical of the principle of respect for autonomy, in particular, because it emphasizes the individual and ignores responsibilities to others and to the common good.

4. Tom L. Beauchamp and James F. Childress, *Principles of Biomedical Ethics*, 6th ed. (New York: Oxford University Press, 2009), 288–289.

5. Tom L. Beauchamp and LeRoy Walters, *Contemporary Issues in Bioethics*, 2nd ed. (Belmont, CA: Wadsworth, 1982), 170–172.

6. Most states do not allow same-sex partners to make these decisions unless they are named as the patient's health-care agent in a power of attorney for health care.

7. These standards were developed and applied in a series of end-of-life legal decisions beginning with *Superintendent of Belchertown State School v. Saikewicz* (Supreme Judicial Court of Massachusetts, 1977) and continuing through *In the Matter of Claire Conroy* (New Jersey Supreme Court, 1985). They have since been incorporated into the ethics of surrogate decision making.

8. M. Molly McMahon et al., "Medical and Ethical Aspects of Long-Term Enteral Tube Feeding," *Mayo Clinic Proceedings* 80 (2005): 1461–1476, 1469.

9. McMahon et al., "Medical and Ethical Aspects," 1463.

10. Ibid., 1462.

11. Ibid., 1462.

12. Editors' note: After this essay was submitted, Washington State passed a referendum (in November 2008) to allow physician-assisted suicide. This law closely resembles that adopted in Oregon.

13. *Oregon Death with Dignity Act*, 127.800.

14. *Oregon Death with Dignity Act*, 127.800–127.850.

15. Edmund D. Pellegrino, "The Place of Intention in the Moral Assessment of Assisted Suicide and Active Euthanasia," in *Intending Death: The Ethics of Assisted Suicide and Euthanasia*, ed. Tom L. Beauchamp (Upper Saddle River, NJ: Prentice-Hall, 1996), 163–183, 169.

16. Yale Kamisar, "Are Laws against Assisted Suicide Unconstitutional?" *Hastings Center Report* 23 (1993): 32–41, 39.

17. "Summary of Oregon's Death with Dignity Act—2006," Public Health Division of the Oregon Department of Human Services, www.oregon.gov/DHS/ph/pas//docs/year9/pdf<http://www.oregon.gov/DHS/ph/pas/docs/year9/pdf.

18. Margaret Pabst Battin, *Ending Life: Ethics and the Way We Die* (New York: Oxford University Press, 2005), 49–53.

19. Alexander Morgan Capron, "Euthanasia in the Netherlands: American Observations," *Hastings Center Report* 22 (1992): 30–33, 32.

20. Daniel Callahan, "When Self-Determination Runs Amok," *Hastings Center Report* 22 (1992): 52–55, 54.

21. Timothy E. Quill, *Death and Dignity: Making Choices and Taking Charge* (New York: W.W. Norton, 1993), 159–161.

22. C. Christopher Hook and Paul S. Mueller, "The Terri Schiavo Saga: The Making of a Tragedy and Lessons Learned," *Mayo Clinic Proceedings* 80 (2005): 1449–1460.

Life or Death

Who Gets to Choose?

CHERYLYNN MacGREGOR

"Seeking death and accepting death when it arrives are very different matters."

–Eric Cohen, "What Living Wills Won't Do"

The word *euthanasia* comes from the Greek root meaning "good death."[1] There are two types of euthanasia: 1) passive euthanasia, which involves the withholding of life-sustaining treatment; and 2) active euthanasia or physician-assisted suicide, which involves the patient taking a lethal dose of medication to hasten death.[2] Trying to determine what a "good death" is, and who has jurisdiction over one's life to make those decisions, has been at the core of all major discussions involving euthanasia. Historically, there has been controversy involving end-of-life choices, clearly indicating that there are no easy answers to these complex dilemmas.

Why would someone request euthanasia? Usually the answer to this question involves someone's quality of life being compromised by intolerable pain, the failure or futility of treatment options, or patients feeling like they are a burden to their families.[3]

The first situation in which someone may request euthanasia relates to the issue of pain. Patients who have been diagnosed as terminally ill may have a slightly better chance of receiving pain medication, but even they are at risk of not receiving enough. There are several reasons that pain management is so inadequate:

Government sanctions for physicians: Doctors can be accused of excessively prescribing pain medication and receive punishment ranging from a reprimand to jail time for doing so.

The war on drugs: Since the Reagan administration in 1982, the obses-
sion with drug regulation has applied not only to illegal street
drugs, but to prescription drugs as well. Patients have become
afraid to take medication for fear of addiction and the pharma-
cies are afraid to stock certain medications because abusers
may rob them.

Inadequate education of physicians: Doctors are not extensively
trained in pain management. Death is viewed as a failure;
therefore, end-of-life care is given little attention in medical
schools.

Cultural beliefs: There are many cultural reinforcements that speak
to the issue of pain. The idea that pain builds character is
embedded in religious, gender, political, and media attitudes.

Insurance regulations: It is very difficult to standardize pain treatment as every case is different and every patient has his/her
own pain threshold. Medicare patients must be enrolled in a
hospice program to have pain medications covered. For
Medicaid patients, doses and services are limited, as well as
closely monitored, for "medical necessity and appropriateness"
Like government sanctions, the expectations of these govern-
ment-funded programs may lead doctors to underprescribe
pain medications.[4]

A second reason that patients or family members often request euthanasia is that they want an end to failed or futile treatments. Technological
advances, beginning in the 1960s, have prolonged life beyond previous
measures.[5] But having the modern technology creates the dilemma for the
physician and family members as to whether these measures should be used.
Despelder and Strickland argue "that 'what can be done, should be done'
increases the likelihood that technological fixes will be tried even when success or cure is unlikely."[6] In earlier times, when technology wasn't as
advanced, or was only used in heroic cases, life-sustaining decisions may
have been less complex and obligatory. Nature was allowed to take its course
because that was the only option available.[7] Many physicians today feel they
would be violating the Hippocratic oath by not using any or all measures
available to prolong the patient's life; but at what cost? Other health-care
professionals who deal with end-of-life issues on a daily basis recognize that
not all treatments are beneficial. They use the term QALY (quality-adjusted

life years), referring to the measuring of quality of life versus quantity of life. Many patients opt to cease or forego life-sustaining treatments, choosing a better quality of life for a shorter amount of time rather than living more years in a compromised condition.[8]

A third situation in which patients may ask for euthanasia involves their belief that they are a physical, emotional, or financial burden to their families. Extra stress may be put on caregivers as they try to meet the daily needs of the person who is sick.[9] Based on earlier arguments, one can imagine how horrific some medical conditions would be without pain medication, and how expensive medications can be. Along the same lines, extraordinary technology sometimes requires extraordinary capital to fund its use. It is understandable that patients may refuse further treatment due to the exorbitant costs.

What happens when a patient does request euthanasia? Dr. Suresh Reddy, who works at M. D. Anderson Cancer Center in Houston, Texas, described the way their Palliative Care Unit helps those who request euthanasia. Staff ask the patients specifically why they want to die if they request euthanasia. If it's because of being in too much pain, then more or different pain medication is ordered. If they are having financial problems paying their medical bills and feel like a burden to their families, then social services are contacted to assist them.[10]

These solutions sound simple enough; however, they may not be available or feasible for everyone. First, M. D. Anderson is a major medical center with a large budget for patient treatment. Few other hospitals have these resources for their patients. Even with unlimited resources, not all pain can be medicated, not all life-sustaining treatments are beneficial, and people may continue to feel they are a burden, so euthanasia may still be requested.

In the United States, there is only one state that allows for active euthanasia, or physician-assisted suicide, and that is Oregon. The Oregon Death with Dignity Act was passed by voters in 1994, and confirmed in 1997. It states that "to qualify for physician-assisted suicide, a patient's terminal condition must be verified by two physicians, two witnesses must certify the decision is voluntary, and the patient must wait for fifteen days before the request can be granted" The doctor is allowed to provide only the prescription for the drugs, and is prohibited from administering the lethal medication.[11]

For twenty-seven years, polls have shown that Californians support the right to physician-assisted suicide. A statewide poll taken in 2007 found 70 percent of adults in favor of the latest legislative attempt to approve active euthanasia, the California Compassionate Choices Act (AB 374). This bill, based on the Oregon Death with Dignity Act, allowed terminally ill adults the option of taking lethal doses of medication to end their lives. The author of AB 374, Assembly member Patty Berg, built numerous safeguards and standards into the bill protecting against wholesale eugenics of populations, which the bill's opponents claimed would result from it. The stipulations of the bill were as follows:

1) the patient must be a terminally ill adult with less than six months to live;
2) the patient must be a resident of California;
3) the patient must make an informed decision based on all information and options given by his or her attending physician;
4) the patient cannot be coerced by family or an outside party;
5) the patient must be evaluated by a secondary physician who confirms the attending physician's diagnosis and prognosis;
6) the patient must be mentally capable;
7) the patient must make two oral requests for the lethal prescription, and one written request that must be witnessed by two individuals;
8) there are two waiting periods (15 days after the first oral request before the written request is made, and 48 hours after the second oral request before the prescription is given);
9) the patient can change his or her request at any time;
10) the patient must self-administer the prescription; no one else can administer the medication to the patient;
11) no doctor would be forced to participate in this program;
12) anyone who violated the provisions of the act would be prosecuted; and
13) both physicians would submit detailed reports to the Department of Health Services.[12]

The California Compassionate Choices Act had to pass the Assembly floor by June 8, 2007, to get to the Senate in time for consideration. Despite all the regulations and public support of the bill, the "lawmakers declined to bring AB 374 to a vote" on June 7, 2007. A spokesperson for the coauthor of the bill said that "the people are there, and the politicians aren't."[13]

Perhaps no other name is as synonymous with physician-assisted suicide as that of Dr. Jack Kevorkian. In 1999, Kevorkian was convicted of second-degree murder in Michigan for administering lethal medication to terminally ill patients. Kevorkian not only practiced active euthanasia in a state that disallowed it, but he also administered the medication himself, which is prohibited even in Oregon. On June 1, 2007, Jack Kevorkian was released from a Michigan prison after serving eight years of his ten-to-twenty-five-year sentence. Although he will no longer participate in administering lethal medication or counsel patients on how to commit suicide, Kevorkian has vowed to continue to be an advocate to allow physician-assisted suicide in terminally ill patients.[14]

One of the most controversial cases regarding active euthanasia occurred after Hurricane Katrina devastated New Orleans, Louisiana, on August 29, 2005. A local doctor and two nurses were accused of murdering patients by administering lethal doses of morphine and Versed on the third day after the disaster. On July 18, 2006, nurses Lori Budo and Cheri Landry and Dr. Anna Pou were arrested for the murder of four patients (between the ages of sixty-one and ninety-one years old) who had been housed on the Life Care floor at Memorial Hospital in New Orleans. The doctor and nurses, along with other Louisiana doctors, claimed that due to the horrific conditions in the hospital after Katrina, the act should be considered a mercy killing. According to Dr. Pou, "There was no air conditioning and windows were broken by nurses to seek relief from temperatures that peaked at 110 degrees. With the heat came the stench of human waste. There was no water. The telephones did not work. Food was limited. At night it was pitch black. Nurses fanned patients. Ventilators did not work. Patients were at risk of dying from dehydration. . . a rumor spread that no organized rescue was coming."[15]

Louisiana Attorney General Charles Foti presented evidence that classified the act as murder. Foti stated that "medical doctors—including two pathologists, a coroner, an oncologist who specializes in palliative care and a bioethicist—were consulted. These respected professionals gave opinions that the manner of death was homicide."[16] He proposed that none of the patients gave consent for such an act, adding that having a DNR (do not resuscitate) code on their files did not qualify as an approval to give the lethal drugs. None of the patients had been prescribed the morphine and Versed before September 1, which raised suspicion about why it was administered at that time. The families of the victims protested that none of them was considered terminally ill, and all could have lived many more years. The defense proposed that perhaps those arguments would be warranted under ordinary circumstances, but the scenario described after Katrina was anything but ordinary.[17]

Many health-care professionals and attorneys have argued that the "battleground conditions" after Katrina called for and justified "battleground decisions" in the hierarchy of treatment and resources. However, bioethicists such as Charles Lugosi claimed that this case "marks a major shift in American medical practice by expanding the frontier from killing consenting dying patients whose lives are deemed to be not worth living to killing non-consenting patients whose unhealthy lives are deemed to be not worth saving."[18] On July 24, 2007, a grand jury refused to indict Dr. Pou and the two nurses previously charged with murder. However, the patients' families are still pursuing lawsuits.[19]

After reviewing the turmoil surrounding active euthanasia, one might assume that passive euthanasia, or the withholding of treatment, invokes a less volatile debate. Although passive euthanasia is permissible by law, by no means does this legal allowance result in easy or uniform decisions. Many times, family members, physicians, and the courts disagree on what is the best treatment for the patient. When disagreements occur, the state or federal courts intervene to determine a solution.[20]

One of the first cases to address passive euthanasia was that of Karen Ann Quinlan in 1975. She was a twenty-one-year-old woman who went into a coma after taking Valium and drinking alcohol. Her parents fought the medical staff to disconnect her respirator when it became clear her condition was not improving, but the hospital staff refused to disconnect the equipment, claiming that would result in her murder. In the mid-1970s, medical malpractice suits were on the rise. This occurrence could have played a role in the staff's decision regarding the Quinlan case in that they were trying to avoid possible legal ramifications."[21] When Quinlan's father petitioned to the New Jersey Supreme Court, it exercised Quinlan's Fourteenth Amendment right to liberty.[22] The court acknowledged that Quinlan was not benefiting from the ventilator; therefore, it could be removed. Quinlan was disconnected from the ventilator in May 1976 and transferred to a nursing home, where she died nine years later. Aside from the Quinlan case being one of the first to capture public attention, it also contributed to the debate surrounding the concept of "substituted judgment," which asks the family to relay or imagine what the patient would have wanted done if they could speak for themselves.[23]

Another pivotal case regarding passive euthanasia was that of Nancy Cruzan. Cruzan, twenty-five, was in a car accident on December 11, 1983, which left her with severe brain damage due to oxygen deprivation. She was placed on a feeding tube to artificially sustain her life. After five years, Cruzan's parents wanted to remove the feeding tube because it was evident her condition would never improve.[24] The hospital staff refused, so the case went to the courts. The initial trial court heard the testimony of Cruzan's roommate, who stated that she wouldn't have wanted to be kept alive this way. This seemed to be enough for the trial court to rule in favor of removing the feeding tube, based on the precedent of substituted judgment. However, the Missouri Supreme Court later reversed this, saying the testimony was inadequate in establishing the patient's wishes. The U.S. Supreme Court sided with the Missouri Supreme Court in the reversal.[25]

Cruzan's parents were tasked with producing "clear and convincing evidence" of Nancy's wishes. The parents produced three new witnesses to testify in state court that her wish was to not be kept alive by artificial means. This time, the courts felt the testimony provided "clear and convincing evidence," and they, along with the Missouri Supreme Court, ruled in favor of removing the feeding tube. Nancy Cruzan's feeding tube was removed on December 15, 1990, and she died eleven days later.[26]

The importance of the Cruzan case was that it established the criteria for informed consent by the patient in regard to refusal of medical treatment. The case stiffened the evidence required of the proxy in order to speak on the patient's behalf. According to law professor Darren Mareiniss, "the United States Supreme Court in Cruzan established the doctrine that error in choosing to continue life is preferred over error that brings about death, and thus requires a high standard of evidence for proxy decision-making about withholding treatment."[27]

The most recent case to attract nationwide attention to the issue of passive euthanasia was the Terri Schiavo case. Due to medical complications from bulimia, Schiavo suffered a heart attack in 1990, which left her in a persistent vegetative state requiring a feeding tube for survival. In 1998, her husband, who was her guardian, petitioned to have her feeding tube removed, based on the argument that she was not getting better and would not have wanted to live in that way. The parents of Schiavo contested this action.

Unlike the Quinlan and Cruzan cases, in which there was a general consensus among family members for the removal of life-sustaining measures, the Schiavo case was further complicated by the opposing views of her husband and her parents. In Florida, where Schiavo resided, proxy decision making for incapacitated adults falls to the spouse first, then the children, then the parents. The trial court allowed for the removal. However, Schiavo's parents appealed the ruling, saying that her husband's decision was guided by being romantically involved with another woman and that he stood to gain financially from the death of his wife. The parents also claimed that because of her devout Catholic upbringing, Schiavo would not have wanted the removal of her feeding tube. In 2001, the Florida appellate courts agreed that the feeding tube could be removed. Several more appeals occurred in the next two years.[28]

The Schiavo case gained mass media attention in 2003. Doctors gave their expert opinions that, contrary to popular belief, feeding tubes do not benefit the patient, and that that would be true especially in this case.[29] Professor of law Edward Larson cites the consensus of many experts by saying that "in the annals of medicine, virtually no one has regained consciousness after being in a persistent vegetative state for as long as Schiavo, and no one has ever done so without suffering severe, permanent physical and mental impairment."[30] In spite of this medical advice, the public, along with celebrities and politicians, protested the removal, calling it murder and "starving Terri to death."

Florida Governor Jeb Bush placed a stay on the removal orders by the lower courts. However, in 2004, the Florida Supreme Court viewed this action as a violation of the separation of powers.[31] Schiavo's feeding tube was removed on March 18, 2005.[32] On March 21, 2005, President Bush signed into law the bill Congress had newly passed to allow federal jurisdiction over Schiavo's case. However, the federal courts refused to intervene, and therefore reinsertion of the feeding tube was denied. Schiavo died on March 31, 2005. Emotions were somewhat tempered when autopsy results revealed that "Schiavo had been beyond hope of recovery... she had irreversible brain damage, was blind, and couldn't respond to visual stimulus" (contrary to what Schiavo's parents had argued).[33]

The biggest contribution of the Schiavo case was that it sparked nationwide discussion of the importance of letting one's wishes be known before a tragedy occurs. The legal mechanism for doing so is the living will (also called the physician's directive). Had the three aforementioned women each had a living will, perhaps the legal struggles could have been avoided.

However, there are two potential problems with relying on one's living will to alleviate the disputes like the ones mentioned above. First, usually a living will is written in such general terms that the conditions may not apply to a specific end-of-life situation when it arises. No one can predict all possible circumstances and options for the future.[34] Second, a living will is only as good as the family and friends who uphold it. Optimally, the family members would adhere to the patient's requests, even if in direct conflict with their own wishes.

By now, the reader may be wondering why I would be interested in this topic and how I have come to this knowledge. One may assume it is because I have taught a course entitled "Death and Dying" for eleven years. However, I wouldn't have been elected to teach the course if not for my personal background. I have (not had) a neuromuscular disease called myasthenia gravis, which landed me in a wheelchair eighteen years ago. My condition was getting worse, leading doctors to speculate that I would be on a respirator within the year, and that I'd be dead within two years after that. I fully understand the need for a living will, because I was telling anyone who would listen that I did *not* want to live in a compromised condition by artificial means. I have always been very active, and the thought of "just existing" was a fate worse than death. Friends would ask if I was afraid to die. My response was simply, "No, I'm afraid to live this way!" I am very fortunate that through the combination of Western and Eastern medicine I have been allowed to live much longer than expected. Although I am mobile and breathing well today, there are absolutely no guarantees for tomorrow.

Clearly, I am emotionally invested in end-of-life choices regarding my own health issues. However, the true motivation for writing this article comes from my grandparents' experiences. The historical accounts of the aforementioned cases are adequately chronicled for the general public to read. But the countless personal tragedies regarding end-of-life choices that were not honored by surviving family members are poorly documented. The following stories portray the consequences when the patient's specific wishes are violated.

My grandparents were married for sixty-five years. At age fifty, my grandfather became very ill with tuberculosis. Because of the disease, he had a considerable portion of his lungs removed. He survived forty more years. No, he didn't just survive, he *lived*! He was forced to take early retirement after the TB, so he bought land and became a farmer. I never knew that he was old because he never acted like it. He built me a tree house, where we would have lunch. At age eighty, he was still playing ball with my daughter. He taught me the value of living life to the fullest.

In the last nine years of his life, he developed emphysema. His breathing was very difficult, and he could no longer do the things he loved to do. This once vibrant man was confined to sitting in a chair inside all day. After years of suffering physically and emotionally, he stopped eating, didn't want to take his medication, and refused to use his oxygen. He was sending the message loud and clear that he was sick and tired of being sick and tired. He made his wishes known by drafting a living will stating that if anything should happen, not to resuscitate him.

In August 1995, my grandfather fell unconscious. My grandmother panicked and called 911. The paramedics are in the business of saving lives. Ignoring his living will, my grandmother asked the paramedics to revive my grandfather. Almost immediately, my grandmother knew that she had violated my grandfather's wishes; however, her decision was already implemented. My grandfather was placed on life support from August until November. Not only did the family watch my grandfather suffer, but we also watched my grandmother suffer because she knew he didn't want to be kept alive by machines. Every day, she would tell him that she loved him, and apologized to him that she had made a bad mistake. She could not bring herself to ask the doctors to disconnect my grandfather's life support, so we waited. The only consolation came when I asked a nurse if anything could be done to end this suffering. She responded that if my grandfather's heart stopped, they would move very slowly to attend to him. There was some semblance of peace knowing that the health professionals recognized the situation. My grandfather passed away on November 12, 1995.

In October 2002, my ninety-two-year-old grandmother showed symptoms of having a mild stroke. She insisted on staying at home and not being taken to the hospital. She made it clear that she didn't want medical attention and that she preferred to die at home. Although it was emotionally difficult, I honored those wishes and stayed with her through the night at her house. I didn't want to make the same mistake that she had made with my grandfather seven years before.

The following day, another family member came to the house so I could go in to work. I soon discovered that my grandmother had been taken to the hospital. She had a second, more severe, stroke four days later. The second stroke left her without speech, incontinent, and semi-paralyzed. My grandmother prided herself on her words. She didn't have a formal education, but she studied the dictionary to be able to use educated language. She was left with no words. A modest and independent woman, she was left having total strangers change her diapers as if she were a child. Much as had happened to my grandfather, the very essence that defined her was compromised. The tortured, desperate look in her eyes spoke volumes to being a prisoner in her own body. Our family was pressured by the medical staff to approve the use of a feeding tube that, thankfully, was unanimously denied by our family. Because of the family member's earlier decision to take her to the hospital, my grandmother's wishes weren't honored—she never went back to her home. My grandmother passed away in an unfamiliar place, almost seven years to the day after my grandfather's death. In both of my grandparents' cases, their quality of life had been severely compromised. How and where they wanted to die had been ignored.

Why are the wishes of patients—like my grandparents—violated? People in our culture have been conditioned in various ways to believe that they need to "do" something when a relative becomes severely ill or close to death. Perhaps this comes from an emotional attachment to the patient, as in Terri Schiavo's parents' case or in the case of my grandparents. Family members may be coerced or guilted to change their mind by health-care professionals, spiritual advisors, or legal consultants who don't agree with the requested treatments or nontreatments.[35]

Medical staff may be prompted to "do" something for fear of being charged with malpractice or accused of murder. Courts may err on the side of life versus death, even if the life choice is not in the best interest of the patient, as in the Quinlan, Cruzan, and Schiavo cases. Politicians may feel they are "doing" their duty by refusing to pass legislation to allow active euthanasia.

Perhaps the most compelling motivation affecting end-of-life choices involves societal pressure. Religious doctrine considers euthanasia murder. Therefore, even withholding available treatment is viewed unfavorably. Equally as powerful is the media portrayal of high-profile cases such as Schiavo's and the one from New Orleans discussed above. Hearing accusatory language such as *murder* and *starving her to death* could certainly guide one's decisions against euthanasia.

In order to get beyond the previous problems surrounding end-of-life decisions, all participants in the dynamic must accept responsibility for their part. The patients must make their wishes known through a living will or physician's directive. An estimated 20 percent of people have living wills.[36] This means that 80 percent of people don't. The living will serves as an autonomous voice of the dying person giving "clear and convincing evidence" that they maintain jurisdiction over their own bodies.

The family members must have the strength to respect the patient's wishes, even if those are in opposition to their own personal wishes. The doctors must recognize that saving lives should not necessarily be done at any cost. If treatments are worse than the condition, yielding no benefit, then they should be withheld if that is requested.[37] Doctors should reevaluate euthanasia in regard to the Hippocratic oath and realize that in many cases death *is* the "best treatment" in the patient's view.

The legal system drives the actions of all of the participants in end-of-life decisions. Laws need to be revised so that doctors can prescribe the pain medication patients need. Enabling doctors to adequately prescribe pain medication would help patients who choose to live, and those who choose to die, do so more comfortably. Legislation that will allow patients more end-of-life choices is also needed. If politicians are not going to pass euthanasia legislation, then they need to provide funding for doctors and hospitals to model after the M. D. Anderson Cancer Center in offering end-of-life resources. The legal system needs to respect the difficult decisions that families may be forced to make, instead of ruling against them. Most importantly, the patient's autonomy to determine his or her own "good death" should be honored. Until further legislation approves active euthanasia, "seeking death" may still be illegal, but shouldn't it be the patient's decision through the living will to "[accept] death when it arrives"?

NOTES

The epigraph to this chapter is from Eric Cohen, "What Living Wills Won't Do," in *Dying, Death, and Bereavement*, ed. George Dickinson and Michael Leming (Dubuque, IA: McGraw-Hill, 2007), 139.

1. Margaret Battin, *The Least Worst Death* (New York: Oxford University Press, 1994), 113.

2. Lynne Despelder and Albert Strickland, *The Last Dance* (Boston: McGraw-Hill, 2005), 235.

3. Timothy Quill, "Doctor, I Want to Die. Will You Help Me?" in *Dying, Death, and Bereavement*, ed. George Dickinson and Michael Leming (Dubuque, IA: McGraw-Hill, 2007), 139.

4. Beth Weinman, "Establishing a Constitutional Right to Pain Relief," *Journal of Legal Medicine* 24 (2003): 495–539.

5. Norman Cantor, "Twenty-five Years after Quinlan: A Review of Jurisprudence of Death and Dying," *Journal of Law, Medicine, and Ethics* 29 (2001): 182–196.

6. Despelder and Strickland, *The Last Dance,* 232.

7. David Moller, *Confronting Death* (New York: Oxford University Press, 1996), 37.

8. Despelder and Strickland, *The Last Dance*, 130.

9. Quill, "Doctor, I Want to Die. Will You Help Me?" 109.

10. Suresh Reddy, personal communication, M. D. Anderson Cancer Center Palliative Care Unit, September 7, 2007.

11. Institute of Government and Public Affairs, University of Illinois, www.igpa.uiuc.edu (accessed 2007). Editors' note: After this essay was submitted, Washington State passed a referendum (in November 2008) to allow physician-assisted suicide. This law closely resembles that adopted in Oregon.

12. Frank Russo, "California Compassionate Choices Act, AB 374, Passed by Assembly Judiciary Committee," *California Progress Report,* March 28, 2007.

13. www.caforaidindying.org.

14. Kathleen Gray and Tamara Audi, "Assisted-Suicide Advocate Kevorkian to Be Released; 'Out of Business' but Plans to Keep Publicizing Issue," *USA Today,* May 30, 2007.

15. Charles Lugosi, "Natural Disaster, Unnatural Deaths: The Killing on the Life Care Floors at Tenet Memorial Medical Center after Hurricane Katrina," *Issues in Law and Medicine* 23 (2007): 71–85.

16. Charles Foti, "Katrina Was No Excuse," *USA Today,* July 27, 2007.

17. Lugosi, "Natural Disaster, Unnatural Deaths," 73.

18. Ibid., 77.

19. Mary Foster, "No Indictment in Katrina Hospital Deaths," Associated Press, July 24, 2007.

20. Cohen, "What Living Wills Won't Do," 138.

21. Alan Meisel, "Quality of Life and End-of-Life Decision-Making," *Quality of Life Research* 12 (2003): 91–94.

22. Cantor, "Twenty-five Years after Quinlan," 183.

23. Meisel, "Quality of Life and End-of-Life Decision-Making," 92.

24. Edward Larson, "From Cruzan to Schiavo: Similar Bedfellows in Fact and at Law," *Constitutional Commentary* 22 (2005): 405–417.

25. Darren Mareiniss, "A Comparison of Cruzan and Schiavo," *Journal of Legal Medicine* 26 (2005): 233–260.

26. Larson, "From Cruzan to Schiavo," 408.

27. Mareiniss, "A Comparison of Cruzan and Schiavo," 246.

28. Ibid, 237.

29. David Orentlicher and Christopher Callahan, "Feeding Tubes, Slippery Slopes, and Physician-Assisted Suicide," *Journal of Legal Medicine* 25 (2004): 389–409.

30. Larson, "From Cruzan to Schiavo," 406.

31. Mareiniss, "A Comparison of Cruzan and Schiavo," 241.

32. Larson, "From Cruzan to Schiavo," 406.

33. Andrea Stone, "Schiavo Autopsy Results Reach a Divided Congress," *USA Today*, June 16, 2005.

34. Cohen, "What Living Wills Won't Do," 138.

35. Wesley Smith, *Culture of Death* (San Francisco: Encounter Books, 2000).

36. Cantor, "Twenty-five Years after Quinlan," 189.

37. Battin, *The Least Worst Death*, 103.

Empowering Patients at the End of Life

Law, Advocacy, Policy

KATHRYN L. TUCKER

Imagine you have a cancerous tumor growing in your neck that continues to grow even after surgery, radiation, and chemotherapy, and is spreading cancer throughout your body.

Imagine that the surgery required removal of most of your tongue, so that you can barely swallow or speak, cannot eat, and are often choking on secretions.

Imagine that you had to have a tube surgically implanted into your stomach to provide nutrition and hydration.

Imagine that the tumor has eaten through the flesh of your neck and there is a seeping, open wound, with foul-smelling emissions.

Imagine that this tumor causes severe pain, in addition to all the other symptoms, and that you must choose between taking enough medicine to control the pain and accepting the loss of alertness that accompanies such sedation, or remaining in pain but with your alertness intact.

Imagine that you have been told that the location of the tumor makes it highly likely that as it grows it will breach the large artery in your neck and you will bleed to death. Imagine that your life, until now, has been one in which you enjoyed a good deal of control and autonomy.

If you were in this situation, would you know what options were available to you?

Options for the Seriously Ill

In every state, patients who are seriously ill or dying are entitled to aggressive pain management. Guidelines for treatment of pain associated with terminal illness have proliferated.[1] Medical organizations establishing standards or guidelines for pain treatment include the World Health Organization, the American Pain Society, the American Medical Association, the Agency for Health Care Policy and Research, the Federation of State Medical Boards, and the Joint Commission on Accreditation of Healthcare Organizations (JCAHO).[2] These guidelines all indicate the importance of pain management as an element of medical treatment. For instance, the *Model Guidelines for the Use of Controlled Substances for the Treatment of Pain* state that the "principles of quality medical practice dictate that . . . people . . . have access to appropriate and effective pain relief. . . . The Board encourages physicians to view effective pain management as a part of quality medical practice for all patients with pain, acute or chronic, and it is especially important for patients who experience pain as a result of terminal illness."

If a clinician fails to provide adequate pain management, a patient or the patient's survivors can file a complaint with the state's medical board or bring a lawsuit for monetary damages.[3] A number of such complaints and cases have been brought in recent years, bringing much needed attention to this problem. Some patients will find that taking enough pain medication to obtain relief requires that they surrender more consciousness than they are willing to, and will opt to be in pain rather than insensate. Other patients will welcome the relief of pain, despite the surrender of consciousness. The choice should be left to the patient, not made for the patient by the healthcare provider.

If pain cannot be brought under control with conventional pain management, an aggressive therapy known as palliative sedation, also referred to as terminal or total sedation, is an option. This involves a physician inducing unconsciousness via intravenously administered medication and withholding artificial nutrition and hydration until death ensues days or weeks later. The patient is kept unconscious the entire time and is unaware of pain or other distressing symptoms.[4] The choice for palliative sedation has been recognized in law by the U.S. Supreme Court and in U.S. medical practice and offers an option some patients consider acceptable.[5] For others it might seem barbaric to linger in this way.

Sometimes a medical care provider has personal, moral, or religious beliefs that impede his or her willingness to provide the care a patient chooses. For example, a significant number of physicians are opposed to palliative sedation for personal reasons and do not tell patients about or offer this option.[6] It is interesting to note that a survey of physicians showed that almost 100 percent would choose this if they were dying of Chronic Obstructive Pulmonary Disease (COPD), yet only 1 percent tell their patients about it.[7]

These conflicts are increasingly common because of the consolidation of health-care facilities involving the merger of Catholic and secular facilities.[8] Catholic health-care facilities are subject to the Ethical and Religious Directives for Catholic Health Care Services (the ERDs), promulgated by the National Conference of Catholic Bishops in 1995, and revised in 2001 (4th edition). A number of these directives may undermine a patient's ability to control end-of-life care, including:

24. ... a Catholic health care institution will make available to patients information about their rights to make an advance directive. The institution, however, *will not honor an advance directive that is contrary to Catholic teaching.*

28. ... The free and informed health care decision of the person or the person's surrogate is to be followed *so long as it does not contradict Catholic principles.*

55. [Dying patients] should also be offered the appropriate medical information that would make it possible to address *the morally legitimate choices* available to them.

58. There should be a *presumption in favor of providing nutrition and hydration to all patients,* including patients who require medically assisted nutrition and hydration, as long as this is of sufficient benefit to outweigh the burdens involved to the patient.

59. The free and informed judgment made by a competent adult patient concerning the use of withdrawal of life-sustaining procedures should always be respected and normally complied with, *unless it is contrary to Catholic moral teaching.*

61. ... Since a person has the right to prepare for his or her death while fully conscious, he or she should not be deprived of consciousness without a compelling reason. ... *Patients experiencing suffering that cannot be alleviated should be helped to appreciate the Christian understanding of redemptive suffering.* [Emphasis added.][9]

However, as recognized by the U.S. Supreme Court in *Cruzan v. Mo. Dept. of Health,* 497. U.S. 261 (1990), patients in every state have the right to direct the withdrawal of life-sustaining interventions, including a feeding tube supplying artificial nutrition and hydration. Those caring for patients who choose to refuse, or direct the withdrawal of, such treatment should provide supportive comfort care in the days or weeks that follow until death ensues. Hopefully, such patients have been informed about and enrolled in hospice care, which is available for patients with life expectancy of six months or less.[10] Hospice providers are specially trained in caring for terminally ill patients and are expert in providing pain and symptom management.[11] A patient's right to choose this course is well recognized in both law and medicine. Even if a patient is not dependent upon a feeding tube and has the ability to consume food and fluid by mouth, the option to voluntarily stop eating and drinking is available.[12]

A number of federal and state court cases address the right to choose to forgo, or direct the withdrawal of, feeding tubes or other life-prolonging types of care, and thereby bring about death. The courts considering such cases have based their decisions on principles of autonomy, privacy and liberty.[13] Medical practice also supports a patient's decision to choose this course. For some this will be satisfactory. For others, the slow, inexorable deterioration to death may seem barbaric.

Confronted by certain suffering and death in the near future due to cancer, you might determine that the cumulative burden is intolerable. You might want a prescription for medication which you could consume to bring about a peaceful death—at home, in bed, surrounded by loved ones. This option is not affirmatively made legal in any state other than Oregon.[14] If you want such a prescription and live outside Oregon, you may or may not find a physician willing to provide one, as discussed below.

An Additional End-of-Life Option

If you live in Oregon and are diagnosed with a terminal illness, with a prognosis of less than six months to live, and are mentally competent, you could ask your physician for a prescription for medication which can be self-administered to bring about a peaceful death. This is legal in Oregon under the Death with Dignity Act (Dignity Act) and has been since 1994. Oregon's law has survived a series of attacks brought by opponents in court, by federal legislators, and by the former United States attorney general.[15] All such attacks have failed and the law remains intact.

Under the Dignity Act, you would need to follow a strict set of procedures to establish that you are eligible to obtain the medications. A physician must determine that you have less than six months' life expectancy; you must make multiple requests, waiting at least fifteen days between the first and last request; you must establish that you are capable to make medical decisions for yourself; and you must be informed of palliative-care options such as hospice, if you are not already receiving such services.[16] If all of these procedures are followed, and you are deemed eligible by the physician to obtain the life-ending medication, an Oregon physician can provide a prescription for such medication.

The terminology used to refer to a physician's prescribing medications that can be self-administered to bring about a peaceful death has evolved. In the past, the term *physician-assisted suicide* was used. Yet, the Dignity Act explicitly states: "Actions taken in accordance with Oregon Revised Statutes (ORS) 127.800 to 127.897 *shall not, for any purpose, constitute suicide, assisted suicide*, mercy killing or homicide, under the law" (emphasis added). When this was pointed out to the Oregon Department of Human Services (DHS), which reports on the Dignity Act, an official there acknowledged "[it] probably has not been correct for us to be using this language all along."[17] Accordingly, the DHS has since rejected the term "assisted suicide" in describing deaths under the Dignity Act.

Health policy organizations such as the American Public Health Association (APHA) have also addressed the terminology issue, recognizing the importance of using accurate language to describe care options and rejecting use of the term *suicide* or *assisted suicide* when discussing the choice of a mentally competent, terminally ill patient to seek medications that he or she could consume to bring about a peaceful and dignified death.[18]

Mental health professionals readily appreciate that "suicide" and the choice of a dying patient to hasten impending death in a peaceful and dignified manner are starkly different from a mental health perspective. Profound psychological differences distinguish suicide from deaths under the Dignity Act. As one psychiatrist recently summarized the differences:

> The term "assisted suicide" is inaccurate and misleading with respect to the DIGNITY ACT. These patients and the typical suicide are opposites:
> - The suicidal patient has no terminal illness but wants to die; the DWD patient has a terminal illness and wants to live.

- Typical suicides bring shock and tragedy to families and friends; DWD deaths are peaceful and supported by loved ones.
- Typical suicides are secretive and often impulsive and violent. Death in DWD is planned; it changes only timing in a minor way, but adds control in a major and socially approved way.
- Suicide is an expression of despair and futility; DWD is a form of affirmation and empowerment.[19]

The American Psychological Association points out: "It is important to remember that the reasoning on which a terminally ill person (whose judgments are not impaired by mental disorders) bases a decision to end his or her life is fundamentally different from the reasoning a clinically depressed person uses to justify suicide."[20] Medical organizations and legal experts also recognize that the terms *suicide* and *assisted suicide* are inappropriate when discussing the choice of a mentally competent, terminally ill patient to seek medications that he or she could consume to bring about a peaceful and dignified death.[21]

Over the decade that aid in dying has been legal in Oregon, roughly thirty terminally ill patients a year have gone through the process, obtained and taken the medication, and died peacefully. Those present at these deaths report that the patient was enormously relieved to be able to make this choice. On a date chosen by the patient, loved ones may gather around for a final good-bye. The patient consumes the medication, soon becomes drowsy, falls deeply asleep, and after a short period of time ceases to breathe.[22] The long road from diagnosis to curative treatment to palliative care to death has ended on terms acceptable to this patient. More patients obtain the medication than go on to use it; some fraction each year get the medication, put it in the medicine cabinet, feel comforted to know it is there, and never take it.[23]

Oregon collects a great deal of demographic data about the patients who choose to use the Dignity Act. The data show that most patients choosing to obtain life-ending medications have cancer.[24] The next most common condition is ALS (Lou Gehrig's disease). Patients using the law are insured, well educated, and receive comprehensive pain and symptom management, typically through hospice services.[25] The data show that the concerns that opponents voiced before the law was passed have not materialized. Opponents had argued that such a law would be forced on the uninsured, the poor, minorities, or disabled persons. The evidence is that this has not happened.[26]

A number of unexpected developments were observed in Oregon after the Dignity Act took effect: Referral of patients to hospice care and physician enrollment in continuing education courses on how to treat pain and symptoms associated with terminal illness increased dramatically.[27] Oregon now has the highest hospice enrollment rate in the nation. It is likely that physicians want to ensure that no patient makes use of the Dignity Act due to inadequate pain and symptom management, and this galvanized both the increase in hospice referrals and physician efforts to learn more about treating pain and symptoms.

If You Do Not Live in Oregon

What if you do not happen to live in Oregon, yet still want to obtain medication that you could take to bring about a peaceful death? In this case you would have to resort to the underground.

It is well known that terminally ill patients across the nation ask their physicians, and most often their cancer doctors, for aid in dying.[28] Many physicians agree to help.[29] In this situation there are no safeguards or procedures to follow, as there are in Oregon. In a murky legal environment, many physicians decline to assist, even if they would do so if the practice were legal.

Researchers have found that outside of Oregon, complications are more likely due to covert, unsanctioned, and unregulated practice.[30] For example, there is greater chance of an extended time until death after consuming lethal medications if the practice is unregulated or unsanctioned.[31] In addition, the stress and anxiety for the patient and family is much higher when no physician can legally be involved to counsel the patient and family and provide a prescription.[32]

When patients do not feel able to discuss the desire for aid in dying with their physicians, or cannot find a physician willing to provide it, the patients may seek assistance in hastening death from a family member or loved one. Unfortunately, these incidents often involve a violent means to death, such as gunshot. Cases of this nature appear with some frequency in the newspapers. For example, in March of 2005, headlines in Connecticut newspapers detailed the death of John Welles, who was dying of prostate cancer and asked his friend Huntington Williams to clean and hand him his gun so he could self-inflict a fatal gunshot wound.[33] Deaths like these are not peaceful or dignified. The situation for a patient seeking aid in dying outside of Oregon is reminiscent of the situation faced by women seeking to terminate unwanted pregnancies when abortion was not legal.

Some patients in this situation have sought relief in court. In the mid-1990s, groups of terminally ill patients and physicians who treated such patients brought lawsuits in the states of New York and Washington, arguing that the patient had the right to choose aid in dying under the guarantees of liberty and privacy of the U.S. Constitution. I represented these patients and physicians in these lawsuits.

These patients were dying of cancer, AIDS, and heart failure. They had all sought curative therapy, but all had come to the point where a cure was not an option and they faced certain death due to their illness. These patients valued their autonomy and felt strongly that the decision to control their final days was deeply personal and involved their most deeply held values and beliefs. In these cases, state laws criminalizing "assisted suicide" were challenged, to the extent that they prohibited doctors from providing medications to competent dying patients that the patients could use to hasten death if they so chose.[34] Liberty and equality guaranteed by the Fourteenth Amendment of the U.S. Constitution formed the basis of the claims.[35] Two federal courts of appeals, including the Ninth Circuit sitting en banc, agreed that statutes preventing patients from exercising this option were unconstitutional.[36] The Supreme Court reversed these decisions, but left the door open to both future legislative reform and a future successful constitutional claim (*Glucksberg* case).[37]

The opinions, both majority and concurring, invited legislative reform. The majority opinion stated: "Throughout the Nation, Americans are engaged in an earnest and profound debate about the morality, legality, and practicality of physician-assisted suicide [sic]. Our holding permits this debate to continue, as it should in a democratic society."[38]

Justice Souter's concurring opinion stated an explicit preference for legislative action in this area. He wrote that "[t]he Court . . . should stay its hand to allow reasonable legislative consideration," and that "the legislative process is to be preferred."[39] Similarly, Justice O'Connor's concurrence demonstrated her concern that state legislatures be given the first opportunity to address the issue: "States are presently undertaking extensive and serious evaluation of physician-assisted suicide and other related issues. In such circumstances, the . . . challenging task of crafting appropriate procedures for safeguarding . . . liberty interests is entrusted to the 'laboratory' of the States. . . ."[40]

In support of the patients and physicians in these cases, many citizens of Washington and New York shared their stories in a brief filed with the Supreme Court, detailing the suffering of loved ones who did not have access to medications that they could self-administer to hasten death when their dying process became intolerable.[41] Countless citizens began the discussion about aid in dying in the wake of the publication of these stories.

Dozens of briefs were filed on both sides by those interested in the outcome. Groups supporting the patients included the American Civil Liberties Union, Americans United for Separation of Church and State, the Older Women's League, and the American College of Legal Medicine. Groups opposing the patients included the Catholic Church, many so-called right-to-life groups, some disability groups, and the American Medical Association.

When the cases were presented to the U.S. Supreme Court, there was no data to inform the question of whether a legal practice of aid in dying would pose a risk to patients or populations deemed vulnerable. Many of the opponents claimed that such a risk would arise. The Court was influenced by this lack of data and, while acknowledging the possibility that it would find such a right in the future, it urged the states to grapple with the issue first.[42]

In the course of these cases' movement through the courts, a tremendous amount of public education and debate was stimulated on both improving the end-of-life care and a dying patient's right to choose to hasten impending death by self-administering medications prescribed by a physician for this purpose.[43] This discussion took place in newspapers and in academic conferences and publications. Medical, nursing, bioethics, health policy, and hospice programs all brought new attention and resources to this issue. Programs to improve end-of-life care proliferated throughout the country. A tremendous amount of funding was funneled through these programs, and no doubt the awareness levels of the importance of good end-of-life care increased among health-care professionals and the public.

At the time the cases were considered by the Supreme Court, the arguments made by those opposed to aid in dying were focused primarily on the contention that if aid in dying were legal, patients would be put at risk. Arguments were advanced that the uninsured, the poor, the disabled, or

minorities, all deemed to be vulnerable populations, would be disproportionately encouraged to make this choice. As discussed above, ten years'
experience in Oregon shows no evidence of this. Now, with the Oregon experience providing data on how aid in dying actually works, observers are con-
cluding that laws like Oregon's Dignity Act can safely be supported and ought
to be passed elsewhere. For example, the American Medical Women's
Association and the American Public Health Association have adopted policy supporting passage of Oregon-type aid-in-dying laws.[44]

Public support for aid in dying is strong. Polls routinely show 70 percent
of American citizens favor passage of laws similar to Oregon's. A poll released
by the Pew Research Center in January 2006 found that 60 percent of
Americans "believe a person has a moral right to end their life if they are suffering great pain and have no hope of improvement," an increase of nearly
20 percentage points since 1975, and 53 percent "believe a person has a
moral right to end their life if suffering from an incurable disease."[45] A Harris
poll published in January 2002 found that 65 percent of respondents support
legalization of the right to aid in dying and 61 percent favored implementation of a version of the Dignity Act in their own states.[46] Another group of
studies found that between 63 percent and 90 percent of people with a terminal illness support a right to physician aid in dying and would like to have
the option available to them.[47] In California, surveys in February 2005 and
February 2006 found that 70 percent of California residents support the idea
that "incurably ill patients have the right to ask for and get life-ending medication."[48] Organizations advocating for civil liberties, seniors, and patients
actively support passage of such laws. Certain religious groups, most notably
the Catholic Church, and some disability groups continue to zealously
oppose passage of such laws. The vocal, well-funded opposition from aid-in-
dying opponents has succeeded, until recently, in limiting the legal practice
to the State of Oregon.

Citizens in Washington invoked the initiative process in 2008, as was
used in Oregon, to pass an aid-in-dying law. In the initiative process a
measure is placed on the ballot and voted upon directly by citizens, does
not need legislator support, and is not subject to the legislative process.
The measure was approved in the November 2008 election, making
Washington the second state in which aid in dying is a legal option.
Another way aid in dying could become legal in a state would be if a case
like *Glucksberg* were brought to a state high court, asserting that a state

constitution provides greater protection than does the federal. Florida and Alaska state courts have decided cases of this sort, both declining to find state constitutional protection extended to this choice. Another such case was filed in the State of Montana in 2007, brought by two terminally ill individuals, four Montana physicians, and the group Compassion and Choices, claiming that the Montana Constitution's guarantees of privacy, liberty, and dignity protect the choice of aid in dying (*Baxter v. Montana*).[49]

The case filed in Montana has at least two significant advantages over the previously brought state cases. First, Montana's state constitution is broader and more protective of individual choice and includes a unique explicit protection of individual dignity. Second, the Montana court will consider the issue with the benefit of a decade of experience in Oregon, which shows there is no harm to patients, physicians, or society when this choice is available. The Oregon experience undermines the argument about risk that the state is likely to advance.[50] A Montana Supreme Court opinion recognizing a state constitutional right in this arena would have persuasive influence in other courts considering the issue in the future.

On December 5, 2008, District Court Judge Dorothy McCarter issued summary judgment to plaintiffs, holding that the state constitution's individual dignity clause and the Constitution's "stringent" right of privacy are "intertwined insofar as they apply to plaintiffs' assertion that competent terminal patients have the constitutional right to determine the timing of their death and to obtain physician assistance in doing so." The court said that "the decision as to whether to continue life for a few additional months when death is imminent certainly is one of personal autonomy and privacy." The right of personal autonomy encompassed in the right to privacy and the right to dignity "mandate" that a mentally competent, terminally ill patient has the right to decide to end his or her life, and to obtain lethal drugs prescribed by a physician, according to the court. The "fundamental" right to die with dignity is constitutionally protected in Montana and "necessarily incorporates the assistance" of a doctor, the court said. The court concluded that the state can address its interests in preventing potential abuses while allowing patients to choose to die with dignity by adopting safeguards.

The state has appealed. The state sought a stay of the lower court ruling, pending review by the Supreme Court; this request was denied. Plaintiffs have reason to be optimistic that the lower court will be affirmed. In *Baxter*, plaintiffs acknowledged that the state could act to protect legitimate state interests with narrowly tailored regulation. The district court agreed that the state could do this.

At this time it does not appear that any legislation governing aid in dying will be passed in the 2009 legislative session. It is important to keep in mind that while the provisions of Oregon's law might offer ideas on possible regulation, any such regulation would need to meet constitutional scrutiny. Neither Oregon nor Washington courts have considered the question of whether their constitutions protect a citizen's right to choose aid in dying. The situation in Montana is quite different; the question for any measure regulating aid in dying in Montana is whether the measure would impose an undue burden on the exercise of a right recognized as protected by Montana's constitution. If so, the measure ought not be enacted, or if enacted it would be vulnerable to challenge.

It is likely that through one of these avenues other states will soon legalize the choice of aid in dying. A fraction of dying patients, even with excellent pain and symptom management, confront a dying process so prolonged and marked by such extreme suffering and deterioration that they determine that hastening impending death is the least bad alternative. Passage of aid-in-dying laws harms no one and benefits both the relatively few patients in extremis who make use of the option and a great many more who would draw comfort from knowing it is available, should their dying process become intolerable to them. The question, finally, is simply this: is a state sufficiently compassionate to allow the choice of aid in dying to terminally ill, competent patients who are receiving sufficient end-of-life care but are still suffering?

NOTES

1. See, e.g., A. Jacox, D. Carr, and R. Payne, "New Clinical Practice Guidelines for the Management of Pain in Patients with Cancer," *New England Journal of Medicine* 330 (1994): 651; David Joranson, "State Medical Board Guidelines for Treatment of Intractable Pain," *American Pain Society Bulletin* 5, no. 3 (May/June 1995).

2. World Health Organization, *Cancer Pain Relief* (1986). American Pain Society, "Quality Improvement Guidelines for the Treatment of Acute Pain and Cancer Pain," *Journal of the American Medical Association* 274 (1995): 1874. W. T. McGivney et al.,

"The Care of Patients with Severe Chronic Pain in Terminal Illness," *Journal of the American Medical Association* 251 (1984): 1182. Agency for Health Care Policy and Research (AHCPR), "Acute Pain Management: Operative or Medical Procedures and Trauma Clinical Practice Guideline" http://www.ahrq.gov/clinic/medtep. acute.htm (accessed February 18, 2000) and *Clinical Practice Guideline No. 9: Management of Cancer Pain*, Publication 94–0592(1994). "Model Guidelines for the Use of Controlled Substances for the Treatment of Pain," *Federation of State Medical Boards* (2004); Federation Bulletin: *Journal of Medical Licensure and Discipline* 85 (1998): 84. JCAHO, *Comprehensive Accreditation Manual for Hospitals: The Official Handbook (CAMH)* http://www.jcaho.org/standard/pm_ac.html (accessed May 31, 2000).

3. For an example of one such case, see Tanya Albert, "Doctor Guilty of Elder Abuse for Under-treating Pain," *American Medical News*, July 23, 2001.

4. Z. Schuman et al., "Implementing Institutional Change: An Institutional Case Study of Palliative Sedation," *Journal of Palliative Medicine* 8, no. 3, 666 (2005); B. Lo, "Palliative Sedation in Dying Patients," *Journal of the American Medical Association* 294 (2005): 1810–1816.

5. *Washington v. Glucksberg*, 521 U.S. 702 (1997); Schuman et al., "Implementing Institutional Change: An Institutional Case Study of Palliative Sedation."

6. Farr A. Curlin et al., "Religion, Conscience, and Controversial Clinical Practices," *New England Journal of Medicine* 356 (2007): 593.

7. J. Lynn and N. Goldstein, Advance Care Planning for Fatal Chronic Illness: Avoiding Commonplace Errors and Unwarranted Suffering," *Annals of Internal Medicine* 138 (May 20, 2003): 812–18.

8. See http://www.mergerwatch.org/hospital_mergers.html; see also, Religious Coalition for Reproductive Choice, *Report on the Medical Right* (2007).

9. See generally, Robert McClory, "A Question of Last Rights: What If a Catholic Hospital Doesn't Respect Your Wishes?" *Chicago Tribune*, October 21, 2007.

10. Medicare provides a hospice benefit, designed to provide comfort care, pain relief, and emotional and spiritual support to individuals with a terminal illness, generally in a home setting. United States Government Accounting Office, "End-of-Life Care: Key Components Provided by Programs in Four States," GAO-08-66 (December 14, 2007), http://www.gao.gov/new.items/d0866.pdf?source=ra (accessed January 15, 2008).

11. Information about hospice is available on the Web site of the National Hospice and Palliative Care Organization, www.nhpco.org; see generally, G. Gazelle, "Understanding Hospice—An Underutilized Option for Life's Final Chapter," *New England Journal of Medicine* 357 (2007): 321–4.

12. See, e.g., J. Schwartz, "Exploring the Option of Voluntarily Stopping Eating and Drinking within the Context of a Suffering Patient's Request for a Hastened Death," *Journal of Palliative Medicine* 10 no. 6 (2007): 1288–1297.

13. See, e.g., *Cruzan v. Mo. Dept. of Health*, 497 U.S. 261 (1990); *Bouvia v. Superior Court*, 225 Cal Rptr. 297 (1986).

14. Or. Rev. Stat. §§ 127.800–.995 (2005). Washington passed a similar measure in the November 2008 election, see infra.

15. See Kathryn Tucker, "U.S. Supreme Court Ruling Preserves Oregon's Landmark Death with Dignity Law," *NAELA Journal* 2, no. 2 (2006): 291–301.

16. Or. Rev. Stat. §§ 127.800–.995 (2005).

17. Kevin B. O'Reilly, "Oregon Nixes Use of Term 'Physician Assisted Suicide'," amed-news.com, November 6, 2006 (quoting Katrina Hedberg, a DHS Public Health Division medical epidemiologist). See http://www.oregon.gov/DHS; http://www.ama-assn.org/ amednews/2006/11/0606/prsc1106.htm.

18. APHA policy, "Patient Self Determination at the End of Life" (adopted October 2008), http://www.apha.org/advocacy/policy/policysearch/default.htm?id=1372.

19. E. J. Lieberman, Letters to the Editor, "Death with Dignity," *Psychiatric News* 41 no. 15 (August 2006): 29.

20 Brief of Amicus Curiae Coalition of Mental Health Professionals, WL 1749170 at 17, *Gonzales v. Oregon*, 126 S. Ct. 904 (2006) (No. 04–623); see also Rhea K. Farberman, "Terminal Illness and Hastened Death Requests: The Important Role of the Mental Health Professional," *Professional Psychology: Research and Practice* 28 (1997): 544; Smith and Pollack, "A Psychiatric Defense of Aid in Dying," *Community Mental Health Journal* 34 (1998): 547.

21. See, e.g., American Medical Women's Association Position Statement on aid in dying; American Academy of Hospice and Palliative Medicine (AAHPM) Policy on Physician Assisted Death, adopted February 2007, available at http://www.aahpm. org/positions/suicide.html (rejecting the term *physician assisted suicide* as "emotionally charged" and inaccurate); James Dallner, "Death with Dignity in Montana," *Montana Law Review* 65 (2004): 309, 314–315; ; and, for an extended discussion of the importance of language in framing discussion in this context, Kathryn Tucker, "Patient Choices at the End of Life: Getting the Language Right," *Journal of Legal Medicine* 28 (2007): 305–325.

22. For a detailed account of one such death, See D. Colburn, "She Chose It All on the Day She Died," *Oregonian*, September 30, 2007 (profiling the death of Lovelle Svart, who was terminally ill with inoperable, metastatic lung cancer, and who chose to make use of the Dignity Act).

23 Ibid. See also, *Death with Dignity Act Annual Reports*, Oregon Department of Human Services, http://oregon.gov/dhs/ph/pas/ar-index.shtml.

24. Ibid.

25. Ibid.

26. Margaret P. Battin et al., "Legal Physician-Assisted Dying in Oregon and the Netherlands: Evidence Concerning the Impact on Patients in 'Vulnerable' Groups," 33 *Journal of Medical Ethics* (2007): 591–597.

27. See, e.g., Linda Ganzini et al., "Oregon Physicians' Attitudes about and Experiences with End-of-Life Care Since Passage of the Oregon Death with Dignity Act," *Journal of the American Medical Association* 285 (2001): 2363; Melinda A. Lee and Susan W. Tolle, "Oregon's Assisted Suicide Vote: The Silver Lining," *Annals of Internal Medicine* 124 (1996): 267.

28. H. Starks et al., "Family Member Involvement in Hastened Death," *Death Studies* 31 (2007): 105–130.

29. Ibid.

30. Ibid. When patients must go underground for medical care, the risk of encounter-
ing a provider who does not practice competent, ethical medicine is greatly
increased. The most well known back-alley provider for patients seeking control
over their own death may be Jack Kevorkian, the Michigan pathologist who
assisted patients with chronic and terminal conditions to end their lives, often in
the back of an old Volkswagen van. Kevorkian was ultimately convicted of homicide in the death of Thomas Youk. After serving part of his prison sentence,
Kevorkian was granted parole and released on June 1, 2007.

31. Starks et al., "Family Member Involvement."

32. Ibid. The authors of this study recommend that for patients outside of Oregon,
support be sought from Compassion and Choices, a national advocacy group supporting a full range of end-of-life choices, including aid in dying. www.compassio-
nandchoices.org.

33. Cara Rubinsky, "Connecticut Case Puts Spotlight on Assisted Suicide," Associated
Press, March 5, 2005.

34. It should be noted that in these cases, it was assumed that these laws could reach
the conduct of a physician prescribing medications for this purpose; this is a
rather large assumption and a compelling argument could be made that such conduct is simply outside the scope of such statutes. As I have noted, there is an
emerging consensus that it is inaccurate to refer to the choice of a mentally competent, terminally ill patient to seek to hasten death as "suicide"; thus it can be
persuasively argued that a physician prescribing medications for such a patient
does not "assist suicide."

35. These cases have been the subject of extensive commentary. A terms and connec-
tors search conducted in December 2007 for the *Glucksberg* cite in the Westlaw
Law Reviews and Journals Database yielded 1,555 cites; a similar search with the
Quill cite yielded 456 citations.

36. See *Compassion in Dying v. Washington*, 79 F.3d 790 (9th Cir. 1996) (en banc), *rev'd
sub nom. Glucksberg*, 521 U.S. 702; *Quill v. Vacco*, 80 F.3d 716 (32d Cir. 1996), *rev'd*, 521
U.S. 793.

37. The fact that the door was plainly left ajar by the *Glucksberg* court decision distin-
guishes the *Glucksberg* ruling from *Bowers v. Hardwick*, 478 U.S. 186 (1986), and the
two decisions ought not be considered of a kind. But see Brian Hawkins, "Note,
The *Glucksberg* Renaissance: Substantive Due Process since *Lawrence v. Texas*,"
Michigan Law Review 105 (2006): 409, 411 (arguing *Glucksberg*'s restrictive approach
to due process is alive and well).

38. 521 U.S. 702, 735 (1997).

39. *Glucksberg*, 521 U.S. at 789 (Souter, J., concurring) and at 788.

40. Ibid. at 737 (O'Connor, J., concurring) (citations and internal quotation marks
omitted).

41. Brief of the Surviving Family Members in Support of Physician-Assisted Dying as
Amicus Curae in Support of Respondents, *Glucksberg*, 521 U.S. 702 (No. 96–110),
1996 WL 722032.

42. *Glucksberg*, 521 U.S. at 789 (Souter, J., concurring).

43. See Carol M. Ostrom, "Physician Survey: Suicide Aid Should Be Legal," *Seattle Times*, July 14, 1994; Brian Willoughby, "Suicide Debate Draws 80," *The Columbian*, August 9, 1994; "State's Medical Association Repeats Support for Reform," *The Columbian*, September 26,1994; Carol M. Ostrom, "End-of-Life Issues Prove Perplexing—'Right to Die' Raises Legal Questions," *Seattle Times*, October 1, 1994; Carol M. Ostrom, "State ACLU Proposes Assisted-Suicide Law," *Seattle Times*, November 16, 1994; Peter M. McGough, Letter to the Editor, "Physician-Assisted Suicide—Most Patients Are Unaware of Their Treatment Options," *Seattle Times*, November 28, 1994; J. B. Deisher, Letter to the Editor, "Living and Dying—Suffering That Precedes Death Should Be the Real Enemy," *Seattle Times*, December 20, 1994; "Study: Terminally Ill Fear Loss of Independence," *The Columbian*, April 11, 1996; Nancy L. Purcell, Op-Ed, "Coming to Terms with How We Treat 'The End of Life,'" *Seattle Times*, December 5, 1996; Robert A. Free et al., Op-Ed, "Compassion, Dignity In Dying—Terminal Patients Turn to Family When Living Becomes Unbearable," *Seattle Times*, January 12, 1997; Charlotte B. Hammond Suquamish, Letter to the Editor, "Right to Die—Support for Assisted Suicide," *Seattle Times*, January 17, 1997.

44. AMWA position statement, "Aid In Dying" (adopted September 9, 2007), www.amwa-doc.org/index.cfm?objectId=242FFEF5-D567-0B25-585DC5662AB71DF9; APHA policy, "Patient Self Determination at the End of Life."

45. Pew Research Center for the People and the Press, "More Americans Discussing—and Planning—End-of-Life Treatment: Strong Public Support for Right to Die," news release, January 5, 2006, http://people-press.org/reports/pdf/266.pdf, at 8.

46. Humphrey Taylor, "2-to-1 Majorities Continue to Support Rights to Both Euthanasia and Doctor-Assisted Suicide," press release, Harris Interactive, January 9, 2002, http://www.harrisinteractive.com/harris_poll/index.asp?PID=278 (last visited October 19, 2007).

47. Andrew I. Batavia, "The Relevance of Data on Physicians and Disability on the Right to Assisted Suicide: Can Empirical Studies Resolve the Issue?" *Psychology, Public Policy, and Law* 6 (2000): 546, 553 (citing William Breitbart et al., "Interest in Physician-Assisted Suicide among Ambulatory HIV-Infected Patients," *American Journal of Psychiatry* 153 [1996]: 238, 240, and Brett Tindall et al., Letter to the Editor, "Attitudes to Euthanasia and Assisted Suicide in a Group of Homosexual Men with Advanced HIV Disease," *Journal of Acquired Immune Deficiency Syndrome* 6 [1993]: 1069).

48. Mark DiCamillo and Mervin Field, "Continued Support for Doctor-Assisted Suicide," press release no. 2188, Field Research Corp., March 15, 2006, http://www.field.com/fieldpollonline/subscribers/RLS2188.pdf, at 2.

49. *Baxter v. Montana*, No. 2007–787, Lewis and Clark County District Court.

50. For a full discussion of Montana law and how such a claim might fare, see Kathryn L. Tucker, "Privacy and Dignity at the End of Life: Protecting the Right of Montanans to Choose Aid-in-Dying," *Montana Law Review* 68 (2007): 317–333.

Dying Down Under

From Law Reform to the Peaceful Pill

PHILIP NITSCHKE AND FIONA STEWART

"My quality of life is still good but it would give me great peace of mind to know that I could end it should the situation change and with something that would be peaceful (e.g., Peaceful Pill) and less traumatic for my family and friends than the means now available (plastic bag). I also consider that it is my right to do so without interference from church or state. Realising this will take time, money and a lot of work. One day we may live in more enlightened times and reason will prevail."
–Betty, seventy-two years old, retired business owner, Western Australia

In Australia, voluntary euthanasia (VE) has attracted a consistent 70 percent support among the Australian community for the past forty years. Yet where public policy is concerned, governments of all political convictions have done little to address this growing social need.

As one who has been working in the field of end-of-life choices in Australia for over a decade, I [Nitschke] have been privileged to witness the benefits an end-of-life law can bring to the terminally ill, while feeling helpless and frustrated at the plight of those left behind.[1] Unlike the terminally ill, who have the benefit of significant advances in palliative care to reassure them that their passing will not be traumatic, the well elderly have very little at all. And the more frail a person is, the less able she or he will be to organize the end for themselves.

In most jurisdictions in the post-industrial West, suicide remains legal, while assisted suicide can attract the most savage of penalties. In some states of Australia, assisting a suicide can attract life imprisonment, the harshest penalty the state can exact. The point of this paradox is awful in its stark reality.

In this essay I provide a personal, historical account of my involvement in the right-to-die movement over the past decade. From the heady days of the world's first voluntary euthanasia law to the innovative work of my non-profit organization, Exit International, ten years later in developing a home-made Peaceful Pill, I document my travels from law reform advocate to Do-It-Yourself (DIY) activist, noting along the way that there is no more important human right for the coming decades than deciding when and how we will die.

Falling Feet First into Voluntary Euthanasia

In mid-1995, when the chief minister of the Northern Territory (NT) first proposed his voluntary euthanasia law, I was working as a physician operating an after-hours home medical service. Like most people in the Northern Territory at that time (and Australia today), I thought that was a brave idea. I was surprised that such an innovative and ground-breaking piece of public policy was being proposed in Darwin, since the Northern Territory is hardly a place known for its forward thinking, let alone social liberalism. In too many ways, attitudes in the Northern Territory are reminiscent of hard-line attitudes of the southern United States in regard to both crime and race. Our Australian version of being tough on law and order means we have manda-tory life sentences for murder and regressive and discriminatory race poli-cies, which do little for the indigenous (majority) population of the north.

With the vision of Chief Minister Marshall Perron, the Northern Territory had an opportunity to lead the world on end-of-life choices. Yet within days of the announcement, the medical profession declared its oppo-sition to the bill with a statement by the head of the NT branch of the Australian Medical Association (AMA), a right-to-life advocate, Dr. Chris Wake. Wake said that "killing patients is not a proportional or proper response to terminally ill situations."[2] He went on to add that "AMA mem-bers will have nothing to do with the drug protocols and the like necessary to enact the legislation."[3] The message from the medical profession was that they would wreak havoc on the legislation, no matter what the people or the politicians wanted.

Why the vitriol? I wondered. What was it that the AMA was so afraid of? And what about the patients? What do seriously ill and dying patients want? Did the AMA ever ask them? My imagination was ignited. I felt the AMA was out of line. They had no right or role in dictating end-of-life choices to the Australian community. So while I had certainly never voted for Perron's conservative Country Liberal Party—indeed I had stood as a Greens candidate in the 1995 Federal election—I felt his proposal had merit. And I was annoyed that the AMA would deny Territorians this type of legislative approach to this sleeping social issue.

Throughout my life, including during my medical career, I had hardly heard the word *euthanasia* mentioned. While I was in medical school in the mid-1980s the issue never raised its head. But, probably like most people in society, I had a clear view on what I would want my end-of-life choices to be. The idea of the medical profession coming along and attempting to use its power to impose its view on the issue I found breathtakingly arrogant. Even though I had only been a physician for only a few years, this was the worst example I had seen of the profession's insufferable paternalism. I resolved to set myself apart from the AMA and show that they did not speak for all Territory physicians.

The Rights of the Terminally Ill Act

On July 1, 1996, the Rights of the Terminally Ill (ROTI) Act became the world's first voluntary euthanasia law.[4] ROTI was passed in the Northern Territory Parliament by just one vote. That vote was from the Aboriginal member for Arnhem, Wes Lanhupuy. The bill indeed received support from all corners of the Northern Territory.

The ROTI Act was a cautious, carefully written piece of legislation. While it might have been radical in that it allowed for the world's first case of medically assisted voluntary euthanasia, the act was relatively conservative in that it applied only to those who were terminally ill (as opposed to the seriously ill). The act also had many stipulations and even more safeguards.

To qualify to use the act, a person had to be over eighteen years of age and, in the treating physician's opinion, "suffering from an illness that will, in the normal course and without the application of extraordinary measures, result in the death of the patient." This is to say that the person had to be terminally ill and "experiencing pain, suffering and/or distress to an extent unacceptable" to that person. To prove that this was the case, the patient had to consult three medical professionals in addition to his or her own treating physician. And there was a mandatory forty-eight-hour cooling-off period applied, once all consultations and paperwork were completed.

In regard to the consultations (which were the responsibility of the treating physician), the first had to be performed by a psychiatrist in order to certify that the person was not "suffering from a treatable clinical depression in respect of the illness." The second needed to be carried out by a "medical practitioner who holds prescribed qualifications, or has prescribed experience, in the treatment of the terminal illness from which the patient is suffering."

A further stipulation involved the patient consulting a palliative-care specialist. The act stated that there could be no "palliative care options reasonably available to the patient to alleviate the patient's pain and suffering to levels acceptable to the patient." This final safeguard ensured that people could only qualify under the act if there were no palliative-care options *acceptable to* them. This stipulation was designed to ensure that no one would request VE simply because they could not access palliative care. Rather, the two had to go hand in hand.

And finally, the person did not need to be a long-term resident of the Territory to access the act. A late amendment to the act gave the NT coroner the role of watchdog over the implementation and monitoring of the legislation.

The form we include here, *"Request for Assistance to End My Life in a Humane and Dignified Manner Form,"* reproduces the wording of the paperwork that was required to be completed by the patients and their physicians. In terms of the specific action that would cause death, the ROTI Act stated that a medical practitioner could prepare, administer, and give a lethal substance to a patient. This same person provides "the assistance and/or is and remains present while the assistance is given and until the death of the patient." This meant that while the physician did not have to administer the lethal drug, she or he did have to be present at the death. After the death of the patient, the same medical practitioner had to sign the death certificate and then report the death to the coroner by forwarding the death certificate and the patient's medical records as they related to the terminal illness and death of the patient. This was to be done as soon as possible after a death.

Request for Assistance to End My Life in a Humane
and Dignified Manner Form

I, _____, have been advised by my medical practitioner that I am suffering from an illness which will ultimately result in my death and this has been confirmed by a second medical practitioner.

I have been fully informed of the nature of my illness and its likely course and the medical treatment, including palliative care, counselling and psychiatric support and extraordinary measures that may keep me alive, that is available to me and I am satisfied that there is no medical treatment reasonably available that is acceptable to me in my circumstances.

I request my medical practitioner to assist me to terminate my life in a humane and dignified manner.

I understand that I have the right to rescind this request at any time.

DECLARATION OF WITNESSES

[This form was then signed and dated in front of the patient's own physician who then completed their section.]

I declare that—

   (a) the person signing this request is personally known to me;

   (b) he/she is a patient under my care;

   (c) he/she signed the request in my presence and in the presence of the second witness to this request;

   (d) I am satisfied that he/she is of sound mind and that his/her decision to end his/her life has been made freely, voluntarily and after due consideration.

Signed: Patient's Medical Practitioner

[The signature of another medical practitioner was also required.]

I declare that—

   (a) the person signing this request is known to me;

   (b) I have discussed his/her case with him/her and his/her medical practitioner;

   (c) he/she signed the request in my presence and in the presence of his/her medical practitioner;

> (d) I am satisfied that he/she is of sound mind and that his/her deci-
> sion to end his/her life has been made freely, voluntarily and
> after due consideration;
>
> (e) I am satisfied that the conditions of section 7 of the Act have
> been or will be complied with.
>
> Signed: Second Medical Practitioner

In summary, the ROTI Act confirmed the right of a terminally ill person to request assistance from a medically qualified person to voluntarily terminate his or her life in a humane manner. Furthermore, it provided procedural protection against the possibility of abuse of the rights recognized.

Why the Northern Territory of Australia?

While the Northern Territory of Australia is hardly a place known for social liberalism in our country, on this one occasion the Territory's government showed remarkable insight and vision. I am often asked, "Why the Territory?" and this is what I say:

The Northern Territory is a unique place in Australia. In watching the enactment of VE bills elsewhere in the world since 1997, I have come to realize that certain ingredients are required for the successful passage of a law on VE. Quite remarkably, in the mid-1990s in Darwin, we had all that was needed.

At the time of the ROTI Act, the Northern Territory was led by a charismatic politician who was prepared to stand by his beliefs. More than this, though, Marshall Perron was a popular and well-known local identity. His long involvement with Darwin gave him unique insight into the Territory psyche. A politician from the conservative side of politics, he could provide leadership on VE that would reinforce the fact that the issue is beyond party politics, left or right.

A second factor in the initial success of the ROTI Act in the Northern Territory Parliament is that there is no upper house. This makes the passage of legislation more efficient. The government of the day is all the more powerful when the checks and balances of the house of review of the traditional Westminster system are absent. This was the case in 1995 in the Territory and it worked in voluntary euthanasia's favor.

A third factor that helped get the ROTI Act through is that the Northern Territory was, at the time, the least religious place in Australia, with 18 percent of the population considering themselves to have "no religion." This compared to a national average of 12 percent. Territorians were also the most likely people to leave the religion question in the census unanswered.[5]

Finally, the Northern Territory has a mindset that is different from everywhere else in Australia. In this part of the world, car license plates contain words like *Frontier, Barra Country* (Barra for the fish barramundi), and *Outback*—words that conjure up Territory fact and myth. It should come as no surprise that Crocodile Dundee found fame in the mangrove swamps of the Northern Territory. And this is the point. Territorians can be rough, rugged, and cynical as hell about the gentrified south of Sydney and Melbourne. In some ways, the Territory welcomed a VE law precisely because no one else had one. No other Australian state or territory was tough enough to find a legislative way to deal with this political hot potato.

The First Death in Darwin

While the ROTI law lasted only nine months before a conscience vote in the Federal Australian Parliament successfully overturned it, four of my patients used the law to achieve dignified, peaceful deaths. All of them with family were able to die surrounded by those they loved and those who loved them back. A fifth patient, the nurse Esther Wilde, qualified to use the law (her paperwork was in order) but ran out of time in the days immediately preceding Easter when the Australian Senate voted the law down.

The first person to use the Rights of Terminally Ill Act was local man Bob Dent, who was dying of prostate cancer. On that fateful day (September 22, 1996), I found myself at Bob's house. His wife, Judy, had invited me over for lunch. Bob said he wanted to die at about 2 p.m.

As I ate my lunch I realized I couldn't swallow, my mouth was so dry. And my shirt was dripping with sweat, yet it wasn't even hot. I realized it was the stress. My responsibility was huge and I was on my own; this brand-new law had to work. I couldn't suddenly say to Bob, "Ah, let's do this tomorrow." The lethal injection could not fail and Bob's death had to be as peaceful and as dignified as the circumstances would allow.

Bob Dent died using the "Deliverance Machine." The machine consisted of a laptop computer connected to a syringe driver. This device allowed patients to self-administer lethal drugs. When the reservoir of the syringe was filled with a lethal drug, such as Nembutal, and an intravenous line was connected to the patient, the person self-administered the drug. The Deliverance Machine restored the balance, placing the patient's family in that person's immediate physical space, and leaving me, the medical practitioner, to retire to the corner of the room.

I invented the Deliverance Machine after the ROTI Act was passed because I did not want to be the one holding the syringe that would lead to the death of another person. Like many other physicians, I do not believe this is our role. However, unlike some other physicians, I do not have any selective adherence to the Hippocratic oath. My commitment stems from the belief that, in many circumstances, the physician has no role at all. Dying need not be a medical experience.

On this occasion (and three others after it) I inserted the cannula into the patient's arm and the laptop computer started its program. The Deliverance Machine asked Bob his three final questions:

1. Are you aware that if you go ahead to the last screen and press the "Yes" button, you will be given a lethal dose of medications and die?
2. Are you certain you understand that if you proceed and press the "Yes" button on the next screen that you will die?
3. In 15 seconds you will be given a lethal injection . . . press "Yes"' to proceed.

Bob completed the questions and the tick, tick of the drug administration started. As Judy took Bob in her arms, he went quickly to sleep, dying a few minutes later. The Deliverance Machine is now on display at the British Science Museum in London, a relic of Australia's brief lead in what is now end-of-life choices history.

The Overturning of the Rights of the Terminally Ill Act

On March 26, 1997, the Australian Parliament passed the Private Member's Bill of the staunchly Christian Member of Parliament Kevin Andrews. At this point, the Rights of the Terminally Ill Act became legislative history. Like countries such as the United States, Australia has an active Christian Right. Unlike in the United States and other countries, the ability of this lobby to influence public policy is disproportionate to its representation in the Australian community.

In the 2006 Australian Census, 54 percent of Australians considered themselves Christian. This compares with a 2001 figure in the United States of 76 percent. In Australia there has long been overwhelming community support for a voluntary euthanasia law. Yet as soon as the ROTI law was passed by the Northern Territory Parliament, the religious Right across the political spectrum swung into action, organizing themselves to ensure that this act had a short life. It was amazing that the ROTI law lasted long enough for my four patients to make use of it.

The Legislative Regime around Dying

As an active participant in the administration of this ground-breaking right-to-die law, I had increasing reservations about the fundamental inequality and unfairness implicit in the legislative approach to when and how we die. As instruments of the state, laws create the framework that determine, among many other things, when and how dying is experienced. In my opinion, however, the existence of a law can be as undermining as it is empowering for those who use it. As legal theorists and others have noted, a law is often a means of reinforcing control over an individual, rather than a way of freeing them to make their own decisions.[6] Far from protecting a person's end-of-life right to self-determination, the law can be prescriptive, enforcing a rigid set of rules in the form of hoops through which patients and their families must jump.

In the Northern Territory I was witness to the problematic nature of end-of-life legislation. I am often asked, "Did the ROTI law grant decision-making power to the person who wanted to die?" In the four cases I have to answer yes, but only once those four people had been approved by the medical profession. Rather, under the ROTI law, it was the physicians who became the arbiters and gatekeepers of a rational, adult Australian's wish to die. In the scenarios I witnessed, the patient became dependent upon the opinion of the expert(s) and at the mercy of the physicians' professional opinions. In the Darwin experience, the law projected an "illusion of freedom," while the individual's rights and choice were significantly and consistently undermined.[7]

In Darwin in 1996, a person could access the ROTI law only under a strict set of guidelines (what some might call safeguards). The patient had to be suffering from an illness that would result in death, but the patient could not be depressed, even though depression could be considered a natural and normal consequence of experiencing a life-threatening disease; and the patient had to have exhausted all *acceptable* treatment and palliative-care measures. The fact that the ROTI law exacted such criteria made objects of people in that to use the law one first had to be ordered, checked, regulated, and controlled. This proscription became most obvious in the case of the third person to use the law, a man known only as "Bill."

Bill's Story

Dying of stomach cancer, Bill had undergone a long period of hospitalization, surgery, and palliative care before he came into my care. Bill was canny enough by this stage to know that what lay ahead of him was further deterioration. He told me he had "had enough of dying."

Like the patients before him, Bill had a considerable amount of paperwork to complete before he would qualify to make use of the law. First, he needed the signatures of a medical specialist, a psychiatrist, and a palliative-care physician. While he had no trouble getting two of these (Bill's own surgeon unreservedly signed off one of the forms and his palliative-care physician the other), finding a psychiatrist was a little harder.

After much ringing around, we found one who said he would have a consultation with Bill to see if he was depressed or otherwise psychiatrically ill. Things boding well, the required documentation would then be complete. The only problem was that the psychiatrist would not come to the hospital to see Bill. Rather, this dying man had to attend the psychiatrist's private consulting rooms. For most people, such a visit would not have been a problem, but Bill was distressed at the prospect. He was, after all, very sick, and he was scared the psychiatrist might find him depressed and not sign the paperwork. Bill kept putting the visit off, hoping he might "cheer up."

Finally, Bill had to face seeing the psychiatrist, and we made the visit together on the day that Bill had chosen to die. An ambulance was arranged to take Bill from the hospital to the psychiatrist's, and then on to his home, where he wanted to die. Bill was too weak to walk; he needed a wheelchair and considerable assistance.

Upon his arrival at the consulting rooms, the receptionist insisted that a "first visit form" be completed. It was more than five pages long. The process was grueling. Bill could hardly sit in the wheelchair, let alone answer questions. I protested to the receptionist, pointing out that completing the form was surely not necessary, given that the visit would be Bill's last, and that he planned to die in two hours' time. The receptionist stood her ground; the protocol would prevail.

What would also prevail was the up-front consulting fee. I protested again; surely payment could be made later? But no, $200 was needed at once or nothing was going to happen. Bill searched his bag; he had only $40. So while he sat in the wheelchair, in his hospital gown and with his small overnight bag on his lap, I made a dash to the car to collect my checkbook. I still have the stub for that $200 check, undoubtedly the most important payment of Bill's long life.

When the psychiatric assessment finally began, it took far less time than the arduous completion of the preliminary paperwork. Thankfully, the psychiatrist did sign the form that would allow Bill to die. That same afternoon Bill eased into the afterlife to the soundtrack from the British TV series *The Choir*. A month later, two of Bill's friends hired a small plane and sprinkled his ashes over Darwin Harbour just as he had requested. The ROTI legislation eventually worked for Bill, but no one should have been subjected to that form of psychiatric assessment when so desperately ill.

It was my experience, not only in the death of Bill, but also with the other three people who used the Northern Territory law, that started me thinking that there has to be a better way. Ten years later and I remain unconvinced that a law based on degrees of illness—and hence arbitration by the medical profession—is the solution to our end-of-life decision-making legislative needs.

Not only does such a law risk excluding people whose suffering may be similar, if not more extreme, than those with a "terminal" illness, but it also fails people who wish to have control over their time and place of death but who may be perfectly healthy for their age. Given the increasing lifespan of those who live in the industrialized West, a law based on terminal illness alone will inevitably fail to address the needs of an increasing minority of people who say they have had "good innings but now is the time to go."

Lisette's Story

In 2004, Janine Hosking made the documentary film *Mademoiselle and the Doctor*, which chronicles the final months of the life of seventy-nine-year-old French academic Lisette Nigot, who had retired to Perth in Western Australia. Like the character of Maude in the 1972 movie *Harold and Maude*, Lisette had decided that eighty years of age was her cut-off point: "I'm going to be eighty in a couple of months, and that's the limit I had given myself. I decided long ago that I would not become too old. At that time I didn't really know what too old might be. But lately I have said, you know, that's enough. I want to go and I decided that, okay, I'm going to be eighty, that's a good age. I don't want to be in my eighties . . . I don't take to old age very well."[8]

For Lisette, the right to die was a given, yet there is no legislation anywhere in the world that would have allowed her assistance—even in the form of information. Lisette was acutely aware that this legal omission was forcing her hand, forcing her to leave sooner than she would otherwise have done if she had the assurance of being able to seek assistance when and if it were required. Perhaps, quite wisely, Lisette knew that going early would be the only way that she could be guaranteed of not losing her ability to make the ultimate decision herself. "I don't like the deterioration of my body . . . I don't like not being able to do the things I used to be able to do . . . and I don't like the discrepancy there is between the mind which remains what it always was, and the body which is sort of physically deteriorating. Perhaps my mind will go and I would hate that. And certainly my body will go and I wouldn't be very happy with that either. So I might as well go while the going is good."[9]

A highly organized woman, Lisette Nigot wanted to know fully about her end-of-life options. While she knew there was no law for people like herself, she nonetheless thought it her right to access end-of-life information. Lisette sought out and obtained the best drugs she could. The old-fashioned barbiturates Soneral and Seconal were her choice, and it took her years to stockpile them. But what Lisette needed and what she wanted from me was information about lethal amounts and the drugs' shelf life.

I answered her questions bluntly. I gave her the facts and in doing so put myself at risk of allegations of assisting a suicide. Despite several attempts by the medical establishment to have me deregistered as a physician, the courts are yet to rule on cases that provide clarity to the very gray legal issues of suicide, assisted suicide, and the role of information therein.

Lisette was an important patient to me. She was the first person to call my bluff as a physician who thought that he knew better than the patient. Finally, Lisette had enough of me and my protestations that she should live. She told me to stop "patronizing" her. I was mortified to hear her allegation that I had become the type of physician I despised. Lisette noted that I preached one thing in theory—that people of sound mind have a right to end their life at a time and place of their choosing—and another in practice. As a medical practitioner, I was still taking it upon myself to "know best," treating this well person as a "patient."

Upset, but also indignant that Lisette had begun to see me that way, I took a step back and stopped trying to frustrate and thwart her plans. That was very hard to do. I really liked Lisette—this gutsy, intriguing, vivacious woman from another generation—and I didn't want her to leave.

On November 22, 2002, Lisette Nigot suicided. The front-page headline of the *Sydney Morning Herald* the next day read, "She Didn't Want to Turn 80." Speaking on ABC radio, Dr. Bernard Pearn-Rowe, then president of the Australian Medical Association in Western Australia, was particularly vocal about her actions. When the host asked if there was anything Pearn-Rowe would have done as a physician to help Lisette, he replied, "If she had been a patient of mine . . . I would relieve any suffering . . . [and] I would help [her] move into some kind of institution. . . . It is very sad that this lady could see no future."

Upon her death, Lisette left a friend a handwritten note. In it she had said, "Please tell Philip that it took more than an hour to swallow those 200 capsules." And she added, "I do hope I will get there. There must an easier way." And there must be.

The Shift in Paradigm to DIY Dying and the Peaceful Pill

The late Dutch Supreme Court Judge Huib Drion was the first person in the world to call openly for the introduction of a pill that would provide a peaceful, pain-free death at a time of a person's individual choosing—a pill that is orally ingested and available to "most" people.

In 1991, Huib Drion wrote a letter to the editor of the Dutch newspaper *NRC/Handelsblad*. In that letter he bemoaned the fact that while his elderly physician friends would know what to do and how to access the right drugs when the time came, as a retired judge he did not. Drion questioned the logic of why he should not have the same knowledge and the same ready access to a peaceful death as his friends.

In writing the letter, Drion opened a can of worms. His ideas struck a chord among readers and generated hundreds of letters in response. It seems there was something to be said for Drion's innocent-enough question.[10] Why should older people of sound mind be denied end-of-life choices to enable their suicide just because they do not share the knowledge and the privileges of physicians or vets (both of whom have access to the best Peaceful Pill, the barbiturate Nembutal)? All people, he argued, should have the right to die at a time of their choosing. A pill would confer this power. He wrote: "Elderly and often ailing people realize that, at some time in the future, they will find themselves in an unacceptable and unbearable situation which only can get worse, never better. A pill to end life at one's own discretion would solve the problem. Not a pill for now, but for the unforeseeable future so that the end can be humane."[11]

Thus the concept of an accessible and reliable pill was born, a concept highly relevant to older people *and* those terminally ill. And just as the contraceptive pill broke new ground for women's reproductive rights in the 1960s, so the Peaceful Pill is quietly revolutionizing the quality of life and death for other groups (e.g. the elderly) within our community.

Implicit in Dion's call for a pill that would be accessible to all is the concept of universal access. Devoid of any qualifying criteria—other than old age—the approach advocated by Drion stands at odds with legislative reform in the area of end-of-life choices all around the globe.

In the Netherlands, for example, to qualify to use the law a person must be experiencing extreme unrelievable suffering. In Oregon and Washington, the only states in the United States where end-of-life choice legislation exists, the person must be "terminally or hopelessly ill." In Switzerland—the only place in the world that allows foreigners to receive an assisted suicide—the organization Dignitas only accepts people who are "terminally ill" or who have "an incurable disease" or who are in a "medically hopeless state." In none of these places can well, older people legally ask for assistance to end their own lives at a time or place of their choosing. While suicide is legal, obtaining the means to a peaceful, dignified passing—particularly if barbiturates are being sought—is illegal and can incur significant legal penalties in most jurisdictions.

Defining a Peaceful Pill

In our book *The Peaceful Pill Handbook*, we define a Peaceful Pill as "a pill or drink that provides a reliable, peaceful, pain-free death at a time of a person's individual choosing; a pill that is orally ingested and available to 'most people.'"[12] With this definition in mind, one drug group or family

fulfils the important criteria. While there are many drugs that *might* provide a peaceful death when desired, it is the old-fashioned barbiturate
sleeping drugs that can be relied upon to do so.

In 2003, when Exit International was considering the feasibility of developing a homemade Peaceful Pill, we surveyed the membership of our organization. In undertaking this work, Exit became the first Australian end-of-life
choices organization to poll our members' attitudes about various end-of-life
approaches. The aim of this survey work was to establish a research agenda
for the organization for the coming decade.[13]

In the Australian (and even international) context, Exit International is
one of the foremost organizations to concentrate on the *practicalities* of self-
deliverance over law reform. Our research and development priority involving the development of a Peaceful Pill needed to be tested against the
priorities of the members of the organization, whose donations underwrite
our activities.

Among the key findings of this research was the strong preference stated
by the 1,163 respondents to the survey for a Peaceful Pill. Eighty-nine percent
reported that if a Peaceful Pill were available they would prefer to use it over
a plastic bag, a gas like carbon monoxide, or other less reliable prescription
drugs. The reasons included "reliability" (88 percent), "ease of use" (85 percent), and the "dignity" (86 percent) that a Peaceful Pill would afford.

Since this survey work, Exit International has actively pursued the development of a Peaceful Pill with several small groups of elderly Australians setting out to make their own Nembutal-like substance. To date, our attention
has been almost exclusively upon the barbiturate family of drugs. These were
the sleeping drugs commonly used in the 1950s to cause death, drugs that
were used by Marilyn Monroe, Judy Garland, and Jimi Hendrix. These drugs
are a) easy to administer—they are usually taken as a small drink that
requires little preparation; b) reliable—when taken in overdose they do not
fail; and c) provide a dignified, peaceful passing—the person dies in his or
her sleep. It is Nembutal that is used around the world where voluntary
euthanasia and assisted suicide are legal. It is the drug used in the
Netherlands, Belgium, Switzerland, and Oregon. It was also the drug used in
the Northern Territory for that short period back in 1996.

In Australia, barbiturates have long since been removed as sleeping
agents from physicians' prescribing schedule. While in the United States
some barbiturates are still technically available from physicians, it is clear

that their prescription is neither commonplace nor standard medical practice. After all, why would any physician prescribe for insomnia a drug dangerous in overdose when there are many better modern, safer alternatives?

At the current time, the most reliable place where a person may obtain
the useful barbiturate Nembutal is Mexico, where the drug is marketed as a
veterinary anesthetic agent to be used either during surgery on an animal or
in the course of animal euthanasia. A single 100 ml bottle of Nembutal
(sodium pentobarbital) with a standard concentration of 60 mg/ml, contains
6 gm, which is an amount suitable for one person. This product currently
retails for around US$30 and is widely available at veterinarian supply shops
throughout Mexico. While the purchase of Nembutal is legal in Mexico, its
importation into countries like the United States and Australia is not, and
detection could result in significant fines or a possible jail sentence.

For elderly people who don't wish to travel to Mexico, there are fewer
choices on offer. This is why Exit has sought to actively facilitate groups of
our elderly members intent on making their own Peaceful Pill. The most
recent development in this project has been the use of a converted-coffee-
pot pressure-reacting vessel for the synthesis. The methodology has been
called "The Single Shot," as the quantity made is enough for one person
only.[14]

While the activities of the Peaceful Pill manufacturing groups remain
highly illegal (in some Australian states the manufacture of barbiturates can
attract a jail sentence of twenty years), other information-based approaches
to the promotion of end-of-life choices have also attracted the ire of the
Australian government. The conservative government of Prime Minister
John Howard (with the support of the opposition—the center-left Australian
Labor Party) worked actively for over a decade to prevent elderly and seriously ill Australians from accessing information about their end-of-life
choices.[15]

Censorship in Australia

In a 2007 *Quarterly Essay* article, "His Master's Voice: The Corruption of
Public Debate Under Howard," David Marr argued that the current regime of
censorship in Australia began with the overturning of the Northern
Territory's Rights of the Terminally Ill Act in 1997. "Moral campaigns advance
in this country by plugging every hole," he wrote. "Once the fundamental

decision is accepted—in this case, overturning the Northern Territory law—every act of censorship that follows is represented as merely tidying up and blocking loopholes. Euthanasia remains a crime in all jurisdictions: the borders are sealed, the internet is cleansed; phones are silenced; and Hansard (the official parliamentary record) is censored. When the Office of Film and Literature Classification allowed adults to buy and read [Nitschke and Stewart's] *The Peaceful Pill Handbook*, pressure was immediately brought to bear on the Attorney-General, Philip Ruddock, to plug a gaping hole. He needed little persuasion."[16]

In recent years in Australia, the federal government has moved regularly and in systematic fashion to prevent adult Australians from having access to a voluntary euthanasia law and, more recently, to information about end-of-life issues. (Unlike countries such as the United States, Australia has no right to free speech in its Constitution. As a result, censorship, as an arm of state control, can and is brought to bear.) The first of the so-called gaps to be plugged concerned Australian customs law.

In 2001 the Howard government tightened regulations amending the Australian Customs Act in regard to the type of information and equipment that could be brought in and out of the country. This change led to a ban on printed information about voluntary euthanasia methods being imported or exported either by mail or on one's person.

Five years later, the same government turned its attention to the Internet with the Suicide Related Materials Offences Act (2006), which bans discussion of voluntary euthanasia methods on the Internet, e-mail, telephone, and fax. Penalties for infringement range from a fine of $110,000 for individuals and $550,000 for organizations. The result of this new legislation is that adult Australians can no longer discuss—even privately—end-of-life issues using one of these carriage services. In countries such as the United States, Canada, and even the United Kingdom (as part of the European Union), such laws would be unconstitutional, but not in Australia.

More recently, the federal government has taken to book banning. In January 2007, the Literature Review Board—a quasi-governmental body that oversees the classification of books, films, and video games—voted unanimously to ban *The Peaceful Pill Handbook*. The reason given was that the book "instructs" in matters of crime.

In a hearing that seriously lacked "natural justice" (e.g., our defense lawyers were never allowed to see the submission of the attorney general and hence the nature of the allegations being made against the book and in favor of why it should be banned), the term *instructs* was never interrogated. Despite an earlier decision that allowed the book's sale to adults aged eighteen years and over, the board ruled that by presenting case studies of Australians visiting Mexico and bringing Nembutal back into Australia or groups intent on manufacturing their own Peaceful Pill, it could be argued that the book was instructing in matters of crime. The same argument was successfully applied to the descriptions in the book that related to the tidying up of a death scene (e.g., the removal of equipment) so the death is thought to be natural rather than by assisted suicide. Ironically, a description of tidying up to disguise a suicide is also contained in Derek Humphry's 1991 book, *Final Exit.* That *Final Exit* remains classified as able to be sold in Australia only serves to highlight the political climate and the selective nature of the Howard government's targets when end-of-life issues are concerned. Derek Humphry is of no concern to the Australian government; we only wish the same could be said of our good selves. We remain heartened that despite the government's best efforts, the Internet continues to allow Australians (who choose to break the law) the ability to obtain *The Peaceful Pill Handbook* (e.g., at peacefulpillhandbook.com and amazon.com).[17] And like most customs services, Australian customs lacks the resources to intercept every package or monitor every electronic download. Some routes to information simply cannot be closed down.

Looking Back, Looking Forward

While there were many flaws (e.g., the nature of the illness-based qualifying criteria) with the Rights of the Terminally Ill Act—as there are with all laws that attempt to enshrine end-of-life rights—it is the attack on Australians' freedom of speech that is most objectionable. The Big Brother attitude of government in Australia—an attitude detectable in both the conservative party (Liberal Party of Australia) and liberal party (Australian Labor Party)—keeps our country looking backward, hoping vainly that elderly and seriously ill Australians will remain silent about their unmet needs.

But this is wishful thinking indeed if the baby boom generation is taken into account. This large population cohort has been on the cutting edge of social change since the 1960s. Throughout our adult lives, we have borne witness to such fundamental social changes in a broad human rights agenda as women's rights, including contraception and reproductive choices, no-fault divorce, indigenous people's land rights, and gay rights. It is now only a matter of time and good government until the issue of when and how we want to die becomes another of a growing list of human rights in the industrialized West. Meanwhile, Australians will continue to speak out. Oh, and we suspect Qantas would tell us that flights to Mexico have never been so popular.

NOTES

1. Editors' note: The "I" in the first part this essay refers to Philip Nitschke; the "we" in the second part refers to Nitschke and Fiona Stewart. The colleagues and partners collaborated throughout on the authorship.

2. "Australian medical, church groups challenge euthanasia law." Reuters, June 18, 1996, at http://www.aegis.com/news/re/1996/RE960673.html.

3. A. Toulson, "AMA Pledge to End Right to Die," *Northern Territory News*, May 31, 1995.

4. Since the 1940s, suicide has been decriminalized in Switzerland under Article 115 of the Swiss Penal Code. In the Netherlands voluntary euthanasia falls under the Termination of Life on Request and Assisted Suicide (Review Procedures) Act 2002. In Belgium, the relevant law is the Belgium Act on Euthanasia of May 28, 2002. In Oregon physician-assisted suicide (but not euthanasia) is permitted under the Death with Dignity Act of 1997. Editors' note: After this essay was submitted, Washington State passed a referendum (in November 2008) to allow physician-assisted suicide. This law closely resembles that adopted in Oregon.

5. *Australian Social Trends* 1994, ABS Catalogue no. 4102.0 (Canberra: Australian Bureau of Statistics, 1995).

6. J. C. Batlle, "Legal Status of Physician-Assisted Suicide," *Journal of the American Medical Association* 289, no. 17 (2003): 2279–2281.

7. A. R. Idol and J. D. Kaye, "The Discursive Positioning of People Who Are Terminally Ill in Terms of Power: A Parliamentary Debate on Voluntary Euthanasia," *Australian Psychologist* 34, no. 3 (1999): 188–197.

8. *Mademoiselle and the Doctor*, directed by J. Hosking (Sydney: Ikandy Films, 2004).

9. Ibid.

10. I. Dikkers, "Special Drion Pill," *Magazine of the Dutch Voluntary Euthanasia Society (NVVE)* 28, no. 1 (January 2002), at http://www.nvve.nl/english/info/summaries/summo2–1.htm.

11. Ibid.

12. P. Nitschke and F. Stewart, *The Peaceful Pill Handbook* (Waterford, MI: Exit International US, 2007), 30.

13. A four-page paper survey was mailed to 2,600 Exit members and a response rate of 45 percent was achieved. Of the 1,163 members who participated, 47 percent were male and 53 percent female. The median age of participants was seventy-two years and most were retired (77 percent). Around half of all respondents had been

members of Exit or another voluntary euthanasia organization for five or more years. Participants were from all states and territories of Australia. Four percent were from overseas. Fifty-five percent of participants reported their health as "very good," with a third saying their health was "fair." Eleven percent said their health was "poor," with 3 percent reporting a terminal illness.

14. A short film of this project has been posted on the video Web site YouTube at: http://www.youtube.com/watch?v=o8we89neDUo.

15. John Howard was prime minister of Australia from March 1996 to December 2007.

16. D. Marr, "His Master's Voice: The Corruption of Public Debate Under Howard," *Quarterly Essay* 26 (Melbourne: Black Inc Books, 2007).

17. Since the completion of this essay, the Australian government has been testing mandatory internet filtering that will block access to the book's site for all Australians.

Ageism and Late-Life Choices

MARGARET CRUIKSHANK

A sizable body of work on ageism has been published in the past fifteen years, but ageism's impact on a wide range of late-life and dying issues hasn't attracted the attention it deserves, either from academics or from community-based workers who deal with elderly persons. One reason may be that ageism in employment or in the media has seemed more obvious or important to those studying its impact. Or perhaps the health-care or socio-logical perspectives have simply led those who study late life and dying away from the more political implications of ageism. Community-based workers and academics may even unconsciously hold ageist attitudes themselves.

Whatever the reasons, if ageism is as pervasive as gerontologists and others believe it is, this form of prejudice bears directly on subjects such as health care in late life, suicide, and the experience of dying. In fact, these experiences cannot be fully understood without an analysis of ageism's overt forms and more subtle manifestations.

What Is Ageism?

One reliable definition says that ageism consists of 1) antipathy, caused by misconceptions, misinformation or myths; 2) avoidance; and 3) discrimi-nation.[1] This form of prejudice shows itself both in attitudes toward old people and in actions that demean or harm them. Ageism exists not only in the beliefs or behavior of individuals but also within social structures. Noted gerontologist Robert Butler, who coined the word *ageism*, compared it to racism and sexism.[2] The analogy is obviously apt, although it compares life-long identities to one that individuals have for only part of their lives. Moreover, ageism will, potentially, affect everyone: whites do not usually become victims of racism or men of sexism, while anyone can live long enough to become a target of ageist stereotypes. Alex Comfort, a British gerontologist and sexologist, described ageism as the belief that those who are old "become people of a distinct and inferior kind, by virtue of having lived a specified number of years."[3]

Contemporary language reveals this bias. Many derogatory terms designate elders, including old goat, fossil, old bag, deadwood.[4] Formerly reserved for males, *geezer* now covers both sexes, and the terms for women are particularly harsh: *shrew, crone,* and *hag,* for example. Linguists have named and study "elderspeak," a response to perceived incompetence on the part of old people that is marked by a slow rate of speaking, simple sentence structure, repetitions, a demeaning tone, and, in an extreme form, baby talk.[5] Stereotypes of old people as impaired and curmudgeonly evoke such patronizing speech.

Population aging may intensify ageism if young and middle-aged people resent benefits for an increasingly large number of elderly persons in their midst. This irrational fear of an aging population can be stirred up by conservative economists and politicians in order to defend extreme proposals for reducing benefits to citizens over sixty-five, such as raising the age for full Social Security benefits to seventy. Such a change would greatly harm people of color and the poor, many of whom do not live as long as seventy. Economic crises may also lead to the scapegoating of elderly Americans if the costs of Social Security and Medicare are not seen in the light of the lifelong economic contributions made by those now old. Talk of entitlements encourages bias toward elders; a more accurate, less judgmental, term for benefits they receive is *deferred compensation.*

Ageism has deep roots in a culture that defines those in late life by their biology: they are, thus, the sick. As a result, that same culture lacks health promotion programs to encourage old women and men to maintain their physical and psychological well-being and believes that old citizens need to be managed. Not surprisingly, negative media images, derogatory jokes on birthday cards, assumptions that older adults cannot learn new skills, and insulting references to their memory loss—all ageist practices—emotionally distance the majority from those who have lived past seventy or seventy-five years.

In a particularly virulent form, ageism attributes ugliness to old bodies, especially to old women's bodies. Hidden from view except in medical settings, censored in mass media, old bodies are judged shameful. The absence of images of naked old bodies, including female bodies, deprives those not yet old from knowing what old bodies look like, a deprivation both aesthetic and psychological. This absence makes late life seem alien or frightening.

Internalized Ageism

Internalized racism, sexism, and homophobia may be offset to some degree by the social movements of civil rights, women's liberation, and gay/lesbian liberation, whereas old persons have no comparably large movement to encourage pride and group identity.[6] Thus, internalized ageism may be a more damaging psychological problem than other forms of prejudice that we apply to ourselves.

An example of internalized ageism is when long-term-care patients settle for inadequate care because they see their decline as an inevitable consequence of aging, something they must simply accept without complaint. "This propensity to accept less, and hence to demand less, is . . . . interpreted as some form of coping, but the propensity really reflects ageism." In addition, discharge planners and case managers may only suggest nursing homes for future care rather than take the time to explore other options with the patient.[7]

Internalized ageism keeps elders from accurately assessing their capabilities and then rationalizing others' unfair treatment of them. Denying one's age by scorning senior centers, for example, as some seniors do, requires mental gyrations to exempt themselves from a group others assume they belong to. Age passing, or pretending to be younger than one is, is a form of internalized ageism. Being taken for "not old" can be flattering, but requires deception, and the frequently heard statement "Nothing has changed but my body" requires self-deception. Perhaps the only safeguard against internalized ageism is a double consciousness that lets elders see how others regard them (negatively, perhaps) and yet maintains their own high self-regard. Their "survivorhood" can be a source of pride that deflects ageism directed at them.

How Ageism Works

In our culture, ageism works in various ways, as the preceding and following examples demonstrate. It compromises the quality of life for elders, inhibits their freedom to make choices, hastens or downplays the significance of their deaths, and may contribute either to suicide itself or to social attitudes that accept late-life suicide as natural, even desirable.

Internalized ageism can have significant consequences. The quality of life for elders can be greatly affected by their interactions with the health-care system. Numerous studies have shown that medical students hold stereotypical views of elderly patients, that, for example, they are disagreeable and ineffective and a drain on health-care resources. Older patients are rarely a focus of study in medical schools, and "one of the few exposures that a medical student may have to elders is during the dissection of a cadaver."[8] Moreover, most medical students do not see geriatric medicine as a desirable career. And medical workers may not recognize their own entrenched ageist attitudes, such as distancing themselves from elderly patients judged hard to talk to. Such distancing functions as a "protective mechanism" shielding them from those who are near death.[9]

Doctors use the same ageist language as the general population. Anecdotal evidence reveals that doctors use ageist slogans such as GOMER (get out of my emergency room) for elderly patients they deem undeserving of attention. Old crock is not confined to medical settings, of course, and commonly used terms such as geezer (mentioned above), old fart, and biddy, indicate that doctors are not unique in expressing age bias and that some caregivers' attitudes toward elderly patients will be disrespectful. An annoying habit of some medical workers is to greet an obviously old woman with, "How are you today, young lady," a patronizing attempt at humor that signals to an old woman that her age is seen as a deficit. Caregivers also often infantilize older people. When the Canadian writer and painter Mary Meigs depended on caregivers, she wrote in her journal that she resented being disciplined by them. Meigs recognized that only children and old people are disciplined and wrote that she missed the autonomy she had enjoyed into her eighties.[10]

Another quality-of-life issue relates to rationing health care to elders. Proposals to ration health care have been advanced with the implied but unstated notion that people over eighty or eighty-five are less valuable citizens than others. In fact, former Colorado governor Richard Lamm actually said that old people have a "duty to die and get out of the way."[11] A response to this blatant ageist bias is to insist that older people contribute in many ways to the common good, by volunteering, for example, and that they differ greatly in health status. Even if all were infirm or confined to bed, limiting their health care would be wrong.

Canadian philosopher Christine Overall concludes that she would have a duty to die if she had a highly contagious, deadly disease likely to cause others to die; but she argues against any moral or political proposition that elderly people are "social liabilities" unentitled to continued life.[12] Medical professionals who see elderly patients as social liabilities cannot provide the same level of respectful care they would afford middle-aged and young patients. If they believe that an injured or ill elderly person cannot fully recover *because* of age, they may not be completely attentive to her or his needs.

Ageism Inhibits Choices

An unrecognized form of rationing health care is the strong encouragement of old people to file advance directives for health care. Rosalie Kane and Robert Kane, she a social worker and he a physician, point out that signers of advance directives "effectively sign away their rights to future care on the presumption that living in the states of dependency that might result would be intolerable. Researchers have found, however, that many people who in theory would decline care can in fact live quite well under the same conditions they feared." Families of elderly patients may overlook that fact that many of these patients want treatment even if it will be uncomfortable or require stays in intensive care.[13]

Although advance directives are praised for encouraging autonomy for elderly persons, they may not always have this effect. Some elderly who do want active care, such as resuscitation, may be subtly coerced into forgoing this possibility by relatives who speak strongly in favor of advance directives. The cost of care may also motivate relatives, but the idea that old people should die to reduce medical costs signifies "deep, naïve, and unquestioned ageism" by unfairly seeing old patients as undeserving of such medical attention.[14]

Long-term care itself provides examples of age bias. In 2007, violations of federal health and safety standards were found in more than 90 percent of nursing homes, a fact that illustrates the low social status of these residents. Aside from overt ageism, subtle forms exist as well. Staff may use baby talk, for example, or call residents by their first names regardless of their wishes. Other examples of "elderspeak" are speaking to an old person with exaggerated slowness or shouting.[15] This behavior has consequences. Staff who infantilize nursing home residents are more likely than other workers to abuse residents psychologically.[16]

Long-term-care recipients differ significantly from other consumers because they may not know themselves what their needs are and because they have do not have a variety of choices. "Their very lack of consumer sovereignty makes them vulnerable to institutional pressures to cut costs by lowering aspects of quality that are hard to measure," according to Nancy Folbre in *Science* magazine.[17] At a time when many caregivers are poorly paid and nurses overworked, sensitivity to this power difference and conscious resistance to ageism may be unusual.

Suicide or Choice in Dying among the Elderly

Even though depression and old age are associated, it is important not to draw too close a link between aging and depression and the choice of suicide.[18] Many factors motivate people to kill themselves. Moreover, a person who has suffered from depression for many decades may find this disease alleviated in late life, through new medications, talk therapy, or a deepening sense of life's pleasures. Assuming old people, in general, have much to be depressed about is ageist and ignores the great diversity among people over sixty-five and especially over eighty, when hardy women and men exhibit great differences from those whose health is failing.

The phrase "altruistic suicides" is used to describe old people who want to relieve their relatives of a burden.[19] In fact, however, old people are seen as "much more burdensome than most of them actually are," and this automatic assumption about them is "extremely ageist."[20] Child care, which may be just as demanding, is not usually seen as a burden, for example.

The suicide of a terminally ill elderly person differs from that of one not so close to death. Noted writer Carolyn Heilbrun, author of the Amanda Cross murder mysteries, literary criticism, and a collection of personal essays, *The Last Gift of Time: Life Beyond Sixty*, killed herself at age seventy-seven. She was not depressed, according to her family, although she had previously written about the fact that she would choose to die when she felt she had lived long enough. Some feminists lamented the loss of a pioneering feminist literary scholar while others praised her "agency" in deciding when and how to die.

In the only conversation I had with Heilbrun, by phone, two years before her death, she expressed great annoyance at not being quoted by writers who told her they admired her books. She included me in this offending group, although I had quoted her approvingly, albeit briefly, in *Learning to Be Old: Gender, Culture, and Aging.* Clearly, Heilbrun felt underappreciated. Was that a temporary mood, I wondered later, or a deeply felt resentment? If the latter, could it have contributed to her suicide? I vacillate between regretting the choice that has deprived readers of future Heilbrun books and respecting her unconventional decision.

In the case of one suffering intolerable pain, the choice of suicide in late life seems rational. At the same time, greater tolerance today for suicide and assisted suicide may reflect prevalent ageism if a dependent life is viewed as not worth living. In this case, "suicide is viewed as an inexpensive solution to increasingly expensive older adult health care."[21] It is ageist to regard the suicide of an eighteen-year-old as more tragic than the suicide of an eighty-year-old, for example. In her excellent book *The Fountain of Age*, Betty Friedan argued that a focus on the "right to die" is too narrow. She urged a broader discussion of all of the services and supports beyond medical care that are geared to maintaining vital health, autonomy, and participation in life until the end. [22]

Death and Dying

In Hurricane Katrina, 1,300 people died, some in appalling circumstances. Many victims were old and poor. Graphic television images of dead bodies heightened our horror at the disaster. Because the majority of those killed were black, the ageist implications of this tragedy have not been as prominent as the racial dimensions. It is difficult to determine which social disadvantage was the greatest factor in their deaths—race, poverty, or old age. But clearly their advanced age made many victims particularly vulnerable.

Too close a link between aging and death overlooks the fact that some persons attain their highest degree of development—artistic, intellectual, social, or altruistic—late in life. "The more accomplished a person becomes in expressing uniqueness, the more absurd death may seem as an annihilation of the irreplaceable individual," according to ethicist, gerontologist, and nursing professor Sally Gadow. She also observes that, when elderly persons are vulnerable, they will accept from the people around them, their relatives and doctors, "an external view of the naturalness of their death." Thus they may be pressured into feeling their time is up, that they should accept the inevitable, even through they are very much alive. Gadow concludes that the relationship between aging and death can only be determined by the individual.[23]

The families of the elderly patients killed by British doctor Harold Shipman accepted these deaths as natural, even though, in most cases, the victims had led active, relatively healthy lives. Eighty percent of his victims were women in their seventies and eighties who lived alone and whom Shipman killed with injections of diamorphine. Relatives and another doctor became suspicious. In 2000, Shipman was found guilty of the deaths of 15 patients, and perhaps over 250 more, between the years 1975 and 1998 during his practice in Todmorden, West Yorkshire, and Hyde, Greater Manchester. In 2004 he hanged himself in his prison cell. But the fact that he got away with these murders for so long indicates that people expect the elderly to be vulnerable and ill, whether or not they are.

A 2007 study of intensive care units across the country revealed that doctors often withheld life support for terminally ill patients who had no surrogates, without knowing the patients' wishes.[24] Death with dignity should mean not only that the caregivers, families, and doctors treat the dying person respectfully by determining his or her wishes and paying close attention, but also that the dying person feel completely worthy of the best possible end-of-life care.

The Terminal Patients Right to Know End-of-Life Options Act became law in California in September 2008. As a result, patients in that state now have a legal right to information from their doctors, upon request, about hospice, palliative care, refusal of life-prolonging treatments, and the choice to refuse food and water with the intention of hastening death. Doctors are not required to volunteer information on these subjects, to avoid undue influence over patients.[25] To a layperson, there appears to be a difference, however, between reminding terminally ill persons that hospice is available and telling them that refusing food and water will hasten their deaths. If a person has not previously thought about declining food and water, the suggestion could be misheard as an instruction.

Betty Friedan urged resistance to being hooked to machines beyond the point at which life is meaningful, adding, however, that we must also resist letting our end be delayed or hastened "by church or state or doctors or even our own families, for motives of their own profit or convenience."[26] Friedan's strong words remind us that a dying person's best interests and the interests of others may collide. Neither profit nor convenience belongs at a deathbed. Even with pure motives and kind hearts, relatives may inadvertently control the final hours of a loved one.

Another kind of end-of-life story, one in which a woman deliberately prepares for her death and thoughtfully shares the entire process with her family and friends, is documented in *Living Consciously, Dying Gracefully* by Minneapolis writers Nancy Manahan and Becky Bohan.[27] Their book, interweaving Diane Manahan's journal, letters, photographs, and friends and family's memories of her, describes the ways their sister-in-law, Diane, took charge of her last years when breast cancer that had been in remission returned and metastasized. A holistic nurse and teacher of nursing who relied on both complementary and traditional medicine, Diane used her experience to help her students become better nurses. She made detailed plans for her life celebration and the handling of her remains. When Diane died, at age sixty, her family washed her body, brought it to a crematorium, and there took part in rituals designed to help them accept the finality of her death. To a degree that is most unusual in our culture, Diane Manahan controlled her dying and death.

As a gerontologist, I often insist on a sharp separation between the topics of aging and death to emphasize that aging is an important subject in itself. I do this to highlight our special field, but my insistence may mask discomfort with the subject of death and reveal a wish to distance myself from it. While I encourage dealing with age in ways that raise our consciousness and increase our comfort level with the topic, I may inadvertently pay too little attention to death and dying, for example by excluding them from my aging courses.

Gender Issues

Because women outlive men and tend to have more illness in late life, they are more likely to be targets of ageism than men. Even more significant is the fact that women experience appearance-based denigration to a far greater degree than men. One of the biggest obstacles to women's complete self-acceptance in late life is the judgment that loss of attractiveness (by conventional norms) is a tragic fact of life rather than a cultural prejudice that can be examined critically and repudiated. Few women in this culture can regard even their midlife bodily changes with complete equanimity. Some women over sixty or sixty-five may feel great pressure to choose cosmetic surgery to disguise the fact that their faces have changed. They may then willy-nilly present faces that do not match an aging neck or hands, or the "angel wings" of fat hanging down from upper arm bones. The hoped-for escape from age prejudice may be thwarted, in other words.

Since self-sacrificing behavior is part of female socialization, especially for women now over seventy, an ill elderly woman may request assisted suicide not only to save her family money but also to spare them "the sight of an unaesthetic deterioration."[28] Concern about her appearance then becomes her most pressing concern as she faces death.

Disentangling discriminatory treatment based on gender from that based on age is difficult, but women who have never before consciously encountered sexism may find late in life that they have lost the respect they once took for granted, just as aging beauties discover as early as midlife that heads no longer turn when they enter rooms.

When ethnicity is considered along with age and gender, isolating forms of discrimination becomes even more difficult. A Latina, for example, may be triply disadvantaged in a health-care setting, by her sex, her ethnicity, and her age, while at home she may be seen as powerful. Recent work on women's aging demonstrates that class, gender, and ethnicity create significant differences among women who share the designation "old."[29]

Audiotapes of interactions between male doctors and elderly women patients reveal another gender issue: frequent interruptions from the doctors and a devaluing of the women's concerns.[30] Whether or not this study is representative, most doctors today have little time to treat the often complex or multiple ailments of elderly patients, no matter how good their intentions, and doctors are far more likely to have older female patients than older male patients since seventy-five percent of elders over eighty-five are female.

Another sign of age bias affecting women disproportionately is that the rate of hip replacements is lower in the United States than in many Western European countries.[31] While this figure includes both women and men, since women live longer, one can safely say that Western European women are more likely than American women to get a hip replacement. This fact suggests that the mobility and well-being of older U.S. women should be a higher priority and deserves close attention when health-care reform is enacted.

In general, neither the study of women's health nor the treatment of women in the United States has been as good as that of men's health and men.

Conclusion

Ageism has been called a psychological and social disease of epidemic proportions.[32] Those over sixty have heard ageist messages all their lives, messages probably less muted than racist or sexist ones. And no matter how sturdy the self-regard of individuals over sixty-five, they most likely will have to expend psychic energy deflecting the social stigma of being seen as pathetic because of their age alone. If they are ill or dependent on others, this task will be especially difficult.

Many years ago Alex Comfort called ageism "idiotic" and "anachronistic" and predicted that "the old to come will not acquiesce in it."[33] Perhaps the aging baby boomers will fulfill Comfort's expectation, but the large increase in the numbers of elderly people will not in itself eradicate ageism or internalized ageism. Gatherings comparable to the consciousness-raising meetings held by feminists in the late 1960s and 1970s are a needed antidote to both forms of oppression. Virtual gatherings like aging blogs could also play a part in this effort.[34]

More dramatic epidemics, such as economic collapses, AIDS, and violence against women, demand our attention, but the powerful, pervasive, and often-ignored bias of ageism kills the spirit and thus requires careful analysis and conscious behavioral change.

NOTES

1. Deborah C. Rupp, Stephen J. Vodanovich, and Marcus Crede, "The Multidimensional Nature of Ageism: Construct Validity and Group Difference," *Journal of Social Psychology* 145, no. 3 (2005): 338.

2. Robert Butler, "Ageism: Another Form of Bigotry," *Gerontologist* 9 (1969): 243.

3. Alex Comfort, *A Good Age* (New York: Crown, 1976), 35.

4. Gerald Falk and Ursula Adler Falk, *Ageism: On Being Old in an Alienated Society* (Springfield, IL: Charles C. Thomas, 1997), 31. Mary Lee Hummert, "Stereotypes of the Elderly and Patronizing Speech," in *Interpersonal Communication in Older Adulthood*, ed. Mary Lee Hummert et al. (Thousand Oaks, CA: Sage, 1994).

5. Falk and Falk, *Ageism*, 31. Hummert, "Stereotypes of the Elderly and Patronizing Speech."

6. In the 1970s older people did have a fairly visible organization to represent them: the Gray Panthers. It was begun by Maggie Kuhn, who convened a group of five friends, all of whom were retiring from national religious and social work organizations. They identified common problems faced by retirees—loss of income, loss of contact with associates, and loss of one of our society's most distinguishing social roles, one's job. They also discovered a new kind of freedom in their retirement—the freedom to speak personally and passionately about what they believed in, such as their collective opposition to the Vietnam War. First calling themselves the Consultation of Older and Younger Adults for Social Change, they were later named the Gray Panthers. They still exist but are not as visible; see their Web site: http://www.graypanthers.org.

7. Robert L. Kane and Rosalie A. Kane, "Ageism in Healthcare and Long-Term Care," *Generations* 29, no. 3 (2005): 52.

8. Kathryn R. Remmes and Becca R. Levy, "Medical Students," in *Encyclopedia of Ageism*, ed. Erdman B. Palmore, Laurence Branch, and Diana K. Harris (New York: Haworth, 2005), 218.

9. Kane and Kane, "Ageism in Healthcare and Long-Term Care," 53.

10. Mary Meigs, *Beyond Recall*, ed. Lise Weil (Vancouver: Talon Books, 2005).

11. Falk and Falk, *Ageism*, 50.

12. Christine Overall, *Aging, Death, and Human Longevity: A Philosophical Inquiry* (Berkeley: University of California Press, 2003), 95.

13. Kane and Kane, "Ageism in Healthcare and Long-Term Care," 53.

14. Overall, *Aging, Death, and Human Longevity*, 58

15. For a good analysis of elderspeak see John Leland, "In 'Sweetie' and 'Dear,' a Hurt Beyond Insult for the Elderly," *New York Times,* October 7, 2008.

16. Diana K. Harris, "Nursing Homes," in *Encyclopedia of Ageism*, ed. Palmore, Branch, and Harris, 236.

17. Nancy Folbre, "When a Commodity Is Not Exactly a Commodity," *Science* 319 (March 28, 2008): 170.

18. I thank gerontologist Elizabeth Johns for this point.

19. Falk and Falk, *Ageism*, 39.

20. Overall, *Aging, Death, and Human Longevity*, 69. Old women and men who choose suicide cannot tell us if their age made them feel unworthy or a drain on family members, but perhaps some left suicide notes that would shed light on this question, or interviews with surviving relations could tease out a connection.

21. Nancy J. Osgood, "Suicide," in *Encyclopedia of Ageism,* ed. Palmore, Branch, and Harris, 311.

22. Betty Friedan, *The Fountain of Age* (New York: Simon & Schuster, 1993), 542.

23. Sally Gadow, "Death and Age: A Natural Connection?" *Generations* (Spring 1987): 18.

24. Joseph Sacco, "Incapacitated, Alone, and Treated to Death," *New York Times*, October 7, 2008.

25. Jane Gross, "The Right to Know, Then to Say 'No,'" *New York Times*, The New Old Age (blog), posted October 21, 2008, http://newoldage.blogs.nytimes.com/.

26. Friedan, *The Fountain of Age*, 561.

27. Nancy Manahan and Becky Bohan, *Living Consciously, Dying Gracefully* (Edina, MN: Beaver's Pond Press, 2007). The book has won several honors, including the Midwest Independent Publishers Association award for best book in its health category, 2008, and the award for best book in women's literature given by Women in Writing, 2008.

28. Overall, *Aging, Death, and Human Longevity*, 228.

29. See, for example, Toni M. Calasanti and Kathleen F. Slevin, eds., *Age Matters: Realigning Feminist Thinking*, (New York: Routledge, 2006); Leni Marshall, ed., *National Women's Studies Association Journal* 18, no. 1 (2006), the aging and ageism issue; and my *Learning to Be Old: Gender, Culture, and Aging* (Lanham, MD: Rowman & Littlefield, 2003; rev. ed. 2009). See also the numerous writings of Ruth Ray, Carroll Estes, Martha Holstein, Kathleen Woodward, Meredith Minkler, and Margaret Gullette, among others. Because few memoirs describe the end of life, Diana Athill's *Somewhere Towards the End* is especially valuable (New York: W. W. Norton, 2009).

30. Laurie Russell Hatch, "Gender and Ageism," *Generations* 29, no. 3 (2005): 21.

31. Kane and Kane, "Ageism in Healthcare and Long-Term Care," 51.

32. Erdman B. Palmore, Preface, in *Encyclopedia of Ageism*, ed. Palmore, Branch, and Harris, xvii.

33. Alex Comfort, "Age Prejudice in America," *Social Policy* 7, no. 3 (1976): 8.

34. In addition to The New Old Age, some other blogs on aging (from a list compiled by Harry R. Moody at the AARP Office of Academic Affairs, "Teaching Gerontology," October 15, 2008) are: Aging as Exile, from Steve Dahlberg, at http://news.aarp.org/UM/T.asp?A910.52851.6987.21.406874; Changing Aging, from Bill Thomas, founder of the Eden Alternative at http://news.aarp.org/UM/T.asp?A910.52851.6987.22.406874; Time Goes By: What It's Really Like to Get Older, at http://news.aarp.org/UM/T.asp?A910.52851.6987.23.406874; and The Future of Aging, from AAHSA (American Association of Homes and Services for the Aging), at http://news.aarp.org/UM/T.asp?A910.52851.6987.24.406874.

Physician-Assisted Suicide

Why Both Sides Are Wrong

IRA BYOCK

For the past three decades, the debate over whether physicians should be legally able to write lethal prescriptions has been the dominant medium through which American society has wrestled with what to do when someone who is seriously ill is suffering. In state after state, lawyers and legislative champions act as warriors for right-to-die and right-to-life organizations. In each camp, meetings are held, bills and citizen initiatives drafted, lawsuits developed, rallies organized and, of course, checks written. The arguments are all too familiar and, by now, feel stale. Although little has changed since Oregon became the first state to sanction the practice, year after year legislative time and attention are conscripted to participate in the fight.

A dispassionate observer might conclude that endless rounds of legal wrangling have rendered this debate pointless. Not for those doing battle; the sense of being so right when the other side is so wrong is addictive. Like compulsive gamblers, each side ardently believes that this time they can prevail. As a former partisan (for the con side), I have come to a different conclusion. In the debate over physician-assisted suicide, both sides are wrong.

The debate was not always pointless. In the 1980s the issue of physician-assisted suicide helped call attention to the plight of dying Americans—problems we still desperately need to address. Now, however, the fracas has become the focus, distracting us from tangible solutions that are well within our reach. Like rescuers called to the scene of a burning building, the media and public stand captivated by a fistfight on the front lawn, either watching wide-eyed or cheering for their side.

Before explaining the fallacies of each side, it is worth acknowledging that the most vehement opponents in this debate agree that a genuine public health crisis surrounds the way many Americans die.

Crisis Defined

The Institute of Medicine has delineated serious deficiencies in clinical education and training, common errors of omission and commission in medical practices, as well as systemic legal, organizational, and economic barriers that result in needless suffering.

Prevailing patterns of practice and health services inadvertently contribute to people who are ill feeling overwhelmed.[1] Even those with higher educations, who are assertive and effective in other realms of life, find themselves bewildered by the maze of specialists, often with conflicting opinions and approaches, and inconsistent, often changing, rules and restrictions regarding services and payments.[2] Adding insult to illness and injury, health insurance, Medicare, and Medicaid routinely pauperize people for being seriously ill and not dying quickly enough—along the way, circumstances frequently pauperize patients' families.[3]

American families with aging parents commonly struggle to find alternatives. Many middle-aged adults with children simply cannot stop working (sometimes two jobs) to care for their frail aging or ill parents. Many of the 78 million baby boomers live a significant distance from their parents. Similarly, their own young adult children have often moved in pursuit of education, careers, and their own families.

Assisted-living facilities are in short supply and too expensive for many people. Nursing homes likewise can easily bankrupt a couple, leaving a surviving spouse with very few assets. A dying man who feels that he is a financial drain on his family may come to experience himself and his life as a burden to others. I am a palliative-care physician, and it is not uncommon for patients in such situations to tell me that they would rather die than enter a nursing home.

Public surveys consistently find that large majorities of respondents say they want to spend their last days at home, in comfort, surrounded by people they know and love. In fact, at present, nearly 50 percent of Americans die in hospitals and 25 to 30 percent in nursing homes.[4] Nearly 20 percent of Americans spend their last days in an intensive care unit,[5] often sedated or with their arms and hands physically restrained to prevent them from dislodging endotracheal tubes, intravenous lines, or urinary catheters. Dying is inherently hard, but it does not need to be *this* hard.

Some causes of this crisis are easy to identify. Inadequate medical education and deficiencies in long-term care are two instructive examples.

Inadequate Medical Education

Despite significant improvements in the last decade, most newly minted physicians have not been adequately taught to assess and treat cancer pain, know little about hospice care, and would not know where to begin in counseling people with advanced illness.[6] Consider the context: in medical schools across the country, students are required to take classes and rotations in obstetrics amounting to 150 hours or more of training, much as they were in the 1950s. Yet today few doctors in the United States deliver babies in their practices and every physician who does has completed postgraduate residency training in obstetrics or family medicine. In contrast, the large majority of physicians participate in the care of people who are chronically or acutely ill, yet required medical school curricula remain scant in topics such as communication, pain assessment and management, ethics of decision making, and guidance for people facing life's end.

People who are living with advanced illness are often understandably worried about the future, what will become of them and their families, and may even question whether life is still worth living. These are not psychiatric conditions, merely difficult, normal aspects of human life. Physicians should be able to respond therapeutically to these concerns, and the basic counseling skills required to do so must be taught and tested as the core medical school curricula. To be clear, these skills are not the sole purview of psychiatrists and palliative-care specialists, or even internists, geriatricians, and family physicians who care for older adults. The ability to provide basic counseling to people who are facing the end of life can be considered among the core skills for every physician who cares for seriously ill patients of any age. That principle applies to pediatricians, surgeons, intensivists, emergency medical physicians, and oncologists, as well as gynecologists, infectious disease specialists, neurologists, gastroenterologists, cardiologists, pulmonologists, and all the surgical subspecialties. Given the broad relevance of such counseling skills in clinical practice, it is

reasonable and prudent for such training to be part of required undergraduate medical education.

Deficiencies in Long-Term Care

Adult children with elderly parents are frequently dismayed by the nursing
home conditions they and their mothers and fathers experience. Many
express a sense of shame at being unable to care for their mother or father at
home and of having to put them in a nursing home, yet they do not know
what else to do. In public opinion surveys, being a burden on one's family is
consistently the first or second most common reason people cite for wanting
to have the option of assisted suicide. Currently, frail ill or elderly people may
fairly conclude that they have become a burden to their families.

By any measure, America's long-term care system is broken.[7] In calling
attention to this situation, I am not criticizing the professionals and staff
who work in nursing homes. Quite the contrary, they are among the most
committed caregivers I know; many of them are unsung heroes in our communities. Rather, I am calling attention to the facts: short staffing is endemic,
a sad truth that has been repeatedly documented in academic and government studies. It doesn't matter how well-trained, caring, and compassionate
a facility's staff is, if there is one nurse for thirty or more residents and one
aide for fifteen people and no one to answer the bell when a person needs to
get to the bathroom or is lying in a wet bed. In 2002 a large federal study concluded that 90 percent of the nation's nursing homes have too few workers
to take proper care of patients. A 2000 Commonwealth Fund study estimated that 30 percent of nursing home residents are malnourished because
they do not receive enough help in eating from aides, who must assist as
many as fifteen patients at mealtime.[8]

These findings have all been reported in academic journals, government
reports, and newspapers, but little has changed. Budget cuts have made services for frail elders, seriously ill people of any age, and family caregivers ever
more meager.

Cultural Underpinnings of This Crisis

While problems of medical education, dysfunctional financing, rules, regulations, and patterns of practice all are components of this calamity, this crisis

is fundamentally cultural. Our collective psychological avoidance of illness, physical dependence, dying, death, and grief have enabled woeful social deficiencies to persist despite sound data and common personal experiences of unsatisfactory and sometimes frankly awful outcomes.

As a culture we are fixated on youth, beauty, vitality, and independence. Frailty and dependence on others seem somehow undignified. Americans want to die with our boots or our makeup on. We are focused on remaining active and independent and psychologically—and too often literally—tend to avoid anything that threatens to remind us of physical dependence, dying, and death. The things we avoid include ill and old people. It's easy to do.

A high proportion of elders live alone, including nearly a quarter of all men and half of all women over the age of seventy-five.[9] Contemporary America is so mobile and fast paced that without a car, or the ability to drive, a person's world rapidly shrinks. Seriously ill or simply frail, elderly people often describe feeling isolated. Gradually add the accumulated effects of failing eyesight and balance, shortness of breath and pain from osteoporosis or arthritic hips, and it's easy to see how living alone is isolating. Elders living alone are at high risk for falls and unwitnessed acute health problems that can result in needless suffering.

Given the sense of isolation—and of being old and in the way—and the difficulties with medical treatment and long-term care, it is not surprising that some people who become seriously ill and dependent on others decide that they would be better off dead. Today, a seriously ill or debilitated person's decision to commit suicide may be entirely rational. From a social perspective that makes it seem all the more tragic. A responsive community would enable people to retain a sense of self-worth through the very end of life. Public policy should be directed at supporting the social structures and processes that enable our communities to respond in comprehensive, caring ways to those who are facing the end of life.

Why the Proponents of Legalizing Physician-Assisted Suicide Are Wrong

One need not invoke philosophical or moral arguments to conclude that in this social context it is not sound public policy to give physicians authority to write lethal prescriptions.

Proponents of assisted suicide are wrong because their proposals would change little and solve nothing. As they are quick to point out, since the opportunity became legal, very few people in Oregon have died by lethal prescriptions. Despite early claims of dramatic improvements, pain treatment for dying Oregonians is as deficient as ever,[10] and the proportion of hospital deaths and frequency of hospice use, while better than some regions, looks a lot like it does in neighboring states where physician-assisted suicide is illegal.[11] If the Oregon experience has proven anything, it is that legalized physician-assisted suicide is largely irrelevant.

Were Oregon's law to be adopted nationwide tomorrow, basic education of doctors and nurses would still be seriously deficient; medical and social services would still be woefully inadequate; Medicare, Medicaid, and insurance payments would still incentivize doctors and hospitals to provide aggressive treatments, while inhibiting access to palliative care and hospice services; and staffing in many nursing homes would still not provide a sufficient level of care for the people who reside there.

Instead, making lethal prescriptions legal might subtly reduce pressure on the medical profession, the health system, Congress, and state legislatures to address the shameful deficiencies in care and support for the most ill, elderly, and vulnerable among us. But even if legalizing physician-assisted suicide did no harm, it would do little good.

Why Opponents of Legalizing Physician-Assisted Suicide Are Wrong

At least the proponents of legalizing physician-assisted suicide have expressed a response to the suffering of dying people. Self-proclaimed "pro-life" organizations, which have been the most vigorous opposition to assisted suicide, are wrong for telling us only what they are against. The failure of the pro-life movement to articulate an alternative to hastening death for people who are suffering as they die makes their statements sound callous. If every human life matters, we need to respond in life-affirming ways.

The Catholic Church and other faith-based pro-life groups have been right to oppose legalizing physician-assisted suicide. Being against physician-assisted suicide is half a stance. In saying no to allowing licensed physicians to preempt death, what should society say to a man who is suffering from advanced emphysema, prostate cancer, and osteoporosis, is weak, in pain, short of breath, and feels like a burden—physically and financially—to his family?

Pope John Paul II's pronouncement that withdrawing tube feedings from people in a persistent vegetative state (PVS) is tantamount to euthanasia left unanswered critical questions. How should people in comas or persistent vegetative states be allowed to die? What happens when a tube-fed patient in PVS develops pneumonia from aspirating nutrient solution? Must the person be hospitalized to receive intravenous antibiotics for the infection? Must she have a tube inserted into her windpipe and submit to mechanical ventilation? If so, for how long? And with what imposed discomfort? Moral guidance on these common contemporary medical dilemmas seems a requisite part of a complete pro-life stance.

In the context of the contemporary crisis that surrounds dying, a comprehensive life-affirming moral position would include a call to individuals and communities of faith to act on their fundamental responsibilities to care for people who are dying and support their families during caregiving and in grief.

In the national discourse, religious denominations and pro-life groups have missed important opportunities to proactively refocus conversation *from* whether it is permissible to assist someone in suicide *to* how we can care well for each and every person through the end of life.

Doing so would require demonstrating in practice what enlightened care looks like. Faith leaders, congregations, faith-based medical centers and social services organizations would all need to be involved. Substantial, possibly unprecedented commitments of time and money would need to be invested in large-scale initiatives in health care, independent and assisted living, long-term care, and community-based social support.

If all this seems expensive, it is. However, proactive clinical and social programs and residential, community-based strategies developed in recent decades may well save our health-care system money. Most importantly, such approaches would preserve the dignity and quality of life for frail elders and terminally ill Americans, as well as the families who care for them. If it seems unlikely that religious denominations would invest this level of resources, consider the many millions of dollars and untold collective hours of work already spent on the political battles to prevent physician-assisted suicide from becoming legal. In contrast, the time and money invested in building enlightened models of living and caring would seem a bargain.

A complete stance would also require a vigorous response by pro-life organizations to evidence that thousands of elderly Americans in nursing homes are malnourished because there are too few aides to help them at mealtimes. Religious groups could mount both public policy initiatives and programs in faith-based long-term care and assisted-living facilities that demonstrate the feasibility of enlightened models of care. This would provide a powerfully positive, coherent message for our culture.

For example, a faith community might launch a national initiative for local congregations to "adopt" needy nursing homes, supplementing institutions' meager resources with donations and volunteers to visit with and assist every resident who needs more help. One denomination might invite or even challenge others to join in the effort.

In addition, denominations with faith-based medical systems could commit to higher standards of care, greater availability of specialized palliative care, and transparent reporting of measures of patient pain, continuity of care, place of death, and patient and family satisfaction with care.

Constructive Public and Social Policy in Unprecedented Times

The challenge to society as a whole is of unprecedented, historic proportion. A demographic flood of elderly and chronically ill Americans has already exposed serious fractures in our nation's health-care and social systems. Soon the gathering tide will overwhelm American communities and families. As stark as the current situation is, these may be the good old days. Budget deficits show no sign of abating and cuts in health care and social services seem destined to continue. It is sobering to think that the nursing homes of tomorrow may make the nursing homes of today seem luxurious.

But this dark future is not inevitable. This is one social crisis for which solutions are apparent. In order to address the root problems underlying this crisis, society must awaken from the persistent legislative state of the assisted suicide debate. Doing so would require a willingness to jettison anger in favor of working together to correct the component deficiencies that cause dying people and their families to suffer.

A collective citizen-consumer effort could insist that nursing homes recruit and retain sufficient numbers of qualified people to care well for our grandparents and parents, if necessary through laws and regulations that double or even triple current levels of staffing of nurses and aides in long-term care. Paying a living wage to nurses and aides will not require more money than our health-care system currently wastes on unnecessary hospitalizations and unwanted or futile treatments. Americans of all religions, political leanings, and walks of life could volunteer to keep company with frail elders and extend help with eating to those who need it. We could monitor specific elements of long-term care, documenting any deficiencies we see, asking for them to be corrected and, if they are not, filing formal complaints, or even lawsuits.

We could promote legislation to mandate that every health insurance and long-term care insurance policy sold in our states include adequate insurance coverage for hospice and palliative care.

We could hold deans and curriculum committees of America's medical schools accountable for adequately training doctors. When medical educators complain that they have only four years to teach all that doctors need to know, with our voices and our votes we could collectively say, "Fine, take five years or whatever it requires, but stop graduating doctors who have not been trained to treat our pain or care well for people as they age and die!" A reasonable benchmark would be a proportion of curriculum equal to that devoted to pregnancy, childbirth, and neonatal care, including a mandatory clinical rotation in hospice and palliative care equal in length to that required for obstetrics.

Similarly, we could insist that our state medical boards require physicians to pass tests in basic pain management as a condition for receiving a license to practice. Standardized examinations have been developed and could be applied. This requirement could be implemented in a manner that is budget neutral and not unduly burdensome for physicians.

I realize policy proposals of this nature would likely be as contentious within academic and organized medicine as calls for legalizing physician-assisted suicide. The difference is that these citizen-consumer initiatives would dramatically improve care and transform the way people die.

Conclusion

It is often said that the moral worth of a civilization can be gauged by the manner in which it treats its most vulnerable members. The history of civilization in the third millennium is being written. All of us have work to do. Legislators must address issues of aging, dying, and caregiving with careful deliberation and fierce determination. In our respective roles as health-care providers, educators, leaders of faith communities, and members of workplace communities and neighborhoods, we must commit to meeting the needs and respecting the inherent worth of our patients, students, clients, coworkers, congregants, friends, and neighbors.

People of good will and intentions will continue to disagree about whether or not physician-assisted suicide should be legalized. But while disagreeing on that single issue of public policy, there is so much we could accomplish together to substantially improve care, social support, and quality of life for people who are dying and the families who love them.

In the current and future crisis that surrounds the way we die, solutions will not be found in the battles over physician-assisted suicide, but can be reached by taking the social and cultural high road of building common ground above and beyond the fray. By our words and, far more importantly, by our actions we can demonstrate how a civilized society cares well for its members through the end of life.

NOTES

1. Stephen P. Kiernan, *Last Rights: Rescuing the End of Life from the Medical System* (New York: St. Martin's/Griffin, 2006).

2. Jan Hoffman, "Awash in Information, Patients Face a Lonely, Uncertain Road," *New York Times*, August 14, 2005; Denise Grady, "Cancer Patients, Lost in a Maze of Uneven Care," *New York Times*, July 29, 2007.

3. K. E. Covinsky, L. Goldman, E. F. Cook, et al., "The Impact of Serious Illness on Patients' Families: SUPPORT Investigators' Study to Understand Prognoses and Preferences for Outcomes and Risks of Treatment," *Journal of the American Medical Association* 272, no. 23 (December 21, 1994):1839–1844.

4. Centers for Disease Control and Prevention National Center for Health Statistics, http://www.cdc.gov/nchs/data/dvs/MortFinal2004_Worktable309.pdf (accessed May 5, 2008); J. Flory, Y. X. Yinong, I. Gurol, N. Levinsky, A. Ash, and E. Emanuel, "Place of Death: U.S. Trends since 1980," *Health Affairs* (Millwood) 23, no. 3 (May–June 2004): 194–200.

5. D. C. Angus, A. E. Barnato, W. T. Linde-Zwirble et al., "Use of Intensive Care at the End of Life in the United States: An Epidemiologic Study," *Critical Care Medicine* 32, no. 3 (March 2004): 638–643.

6. J. A. Billings and S. Block, "Palliative Care in Undergraduate Medical Education: Status Report and Future Directions," *Journal of the American Medical Association* 278, no. 9 (September 3, 1997): 733–738.

7. U.S. House of Representatives, Committee on Government Reform, Special Investigations Division, "Abuse of Residents Is a Major Problem in U.S. Nursing

Homes," prepared for Rep. Henry A. Waxman, July 30, 2001; R. Butler and L. Wright, "Caregiving in America: International Longevity Center Schmieding Center for Senior Health and Education," 2006, www.ilcusa.org; Sarah Greene Burger, Jeanie Kayser-Jones, and Julie Prince, "Malnutrition and Dehydration in Nursing Homes: Key Issues in Prevention and Treatment," National Citizens' Coalition for Nursing Home Reform, Commonwealth Fund, July 2000.

8. R. Tanner, "Providers Issue Brief: Nursing Home Staffing Standards: Year End Report—2002," *Issue Brief Health Policy Track Service* (December 31, 2002): I–II; T. E. Trapps, "Violations Mount as Long-Term Care Facilities Have a Hard Time Finding and Keeping Good Help," *Los Angeles Times*, July 31, 2001; J. Kayser-Jones, "Malnutrition, Dehydration, and Starvation in the Midst of Plenty: The Political Impact of Qualitative Inquiry," *Qualitative Health Research* 12, no. 10 (December 2002): 1391–1405.

9. U.S. Department of Health and Human Services, Administration on Aging, "A Profile of Older Americans: 2007," http://www.aoa.gov/prof/statistics/profile/2007/2007profile.pdf (accessed April 14, 2008).

10. E. K. Fromme, V. P. Tilden, L. L. Drach, and S. W. Tolle, "Increased Family Reports of Pain or Distress in Dying Oregonians: 1996 to 2002," *Journal of Palliative Medicine* 7, no. 3 (June 2004): 431–442.

11. *Dartmouth Atlas*, 2008, http://www.dartmouthatlas.org/atlases/2008_Chronic_Care_Atlas.pdf (accessed April 14, 2008).

End of days

MARGE PIERCY

Almost always with cats, the end
comes creeping over the two of you—
she stops eating, his back legs
no longer support him, she leans
to your hand and purrs but cannot
rise—sometimes a whimper of pain
although they are stoic. They see
death clearly through hooded eyes.

Then there is the long weepy
trip to the vet, the carrier no
longer necessary, the last time
in your lap. The injection is quick.
Simply they stop breathing
in your arms. You bring them
home to bury in the flower garden,
planting a bush over a deep grave.

That is how I would like to cease,
held in a lover's arms and quickly
fading to black like an old fashioned
movie embrace. I hate the white
silent scream of hospitals, the whine
of pain like air conditioning's hum.

I want to click the off switch.
And if I can no longer choose

I want someone who loves me
there, not a doctor with forty patients
and his morality to keep me sort
of, kind of alive or sort of undead.
Why are we more rational and kinder
to our pets than with ourselves or our
parents? Death is not the worst
thing; denying it can be.

ABOUT THE EDITORS AND
CONTRIBUTORS

Before she retired, **Nan Bauer-Maglin** was Professor of English, Borough of Manhattan Community College, CUNY for twenty-seven years and then was Academic Director of The CUNY Baccalaureate Program for nine years. In retirement, her many commitments include: part-time Director of Special Projects at John Jay College, CUNY; a volunteer at the Global Action on Aging, NGO, the United Nations; recruiting for ReServe, whose mission is to connect retired professionals with nonprofits and civic institutions; and opening a retirement consulting business with a colleague. She co-edited *Women Confronting Retirement: A Nontraditional Guide*; *"Bad Girls/Good Girls": Women, Sex, and Power in the Nineties*; and *Women and Stepfamilies: Voices of Anger and Love* and edited *Cut Loose: (Mostly) Older Women Talk about the End of (Mostly) Long-term Relationships*.

Donna Perry has taught literature, writing, and women's studies courses at William Paterson University since 1982. A Professor of English, she interviewed fifteen authors for her collection, *Backtalk: Women Writers Speak Out*; co-edited (with Nan Bauer Maglin) *"Bad Girls/Good Girls": Women, Sex, and Power in the Nineties*; and has published on feminist criticism and pedagogy, contemporary women writers, and composition theory and practice. Recent projects include a memoir about growing up Catholic (See "Saint Mary of Egypt, Who Had Been a Sinner" in *Fourth Genre: Explorations in Nonfiction*, 2 [2000] for a sample) and a study of Louisa May Alcott's *Little Women* as cultural phenomenon. She was Fulbright Senior Lecturer in American Studies at the University of Rome in 2004.

Nancy Barnes is a cultural anthropologist on the faculty of Lang College. Her ethnographic research has centered on the small public high schools in New York City. She has worked with high school-to-college transition programs for years, most recently at The New School's Institute for Urban

Education. She also teaches in the Graduate Liberal Studies Program at Wesleyan University and leads workshops in Burma. Nancy lives in New Haven, where she is writing a book of essays about the pleasures of a teaching life.

June Bingham was an author and playwright. She published biographies of Reinhold Niebuhr and U Thant and co-authored books on health with two different psychiatrists. Her plays have been produced off-Broadway and in several states. At the time of her death on August 21, 2007, she had three living children, ten grandchildren, and fourteen great grandchildren, plus two in utero. Her late first husband, Jonathan Bingham, was a member of Congress for eighteen years; her second husband, Robert Bowen Birge, cofounded the Living Pulpit, www.pulpit.org.

Ira Byock is a practicing physician and Director of Palliative Medicine at Dartmouth-Hitchcock Medical Center and a Professor at Dartmouth Medical School in Lebanon, New Hampshire. Dr. Byock has been involved in hospice and palliative care since 1978 and has written widely on the ethics and practice of end-of-life care for academic journals and for the general public. His first book, *Dying Well* (1997), has become a standard in the field. He is a past president (1997) of the American Academy of Hospice and Palliative Medicine. From 1996 to 2006, he directed Promoting Excellence in End-of-Life Care, a national program of the Robert Wood Johnson Foundation.

Margaret Cruikshank is the author of *Learning to Be Old: Gender, Culture and Aging* (2009) and the editor of *Fierce with Reality: An Anthology of Literature on Aging* (2007). Feminist gerontology and critical gerontology are her special interests. She is a lecturer in women's studies at the University of Maine, where she is also a faculty associate of the Center on Aging. In 2007 she was a Fulbright Senior Scholar at the Centre on Aging of the University of Victoria, British Columbia.

Sara M. Evans, Regents Professor Emerita at the University of Minnesota, was born in a Methodist parsonage in rural South Carolina in 1943. Active in the civil rights, antiwar, and feminist movements since the 1960s, she spent her career teaching and writing the history of women in the United States. Her books include *Personal Politics: The Roots of Women's Liberation in the Civil Rights Movement and the New Left* (1979), *Born for Liberty: A History of Women in America* (1989), and *Tidal Wave: How Women Changed America at Century's End* (2003).

Candace Cummins Gauthier received a PhD in philosophy from the University of North Carolina at Chapel Hill in 1986. She has been teaching in the Department of Philosophy and Religion at the University of North Carolina—Wilmington since then. Dr. Gauthier teaches courses in ethics, medical ethics, media ethics, and research ethics. She serves on the Ethics Committee at the New Hanover Regional Medical Center in Wilmington. She also leads regular discussions of issues and cases in medical ethics for the Internal Medicine Residency Program at the medical center. Dr. Gauthier has numerous publications in medical ethics and media ethics, including a coauthored textbook, *Evidence-Based Medical Ethics*.

Natalie R. Hannon served as the Director of Training at a hospital in New York City for over ten years. She was also a member of the hospital's ethics committee. She has her doctorate in sociology from Fordham University and a certificate in bioethics and the humanities from a joint program between Columbia University and Montefiore Hospital (Bronx, NY). She teaches bioethics at Lehman College of the City University of New York and is the coauthor of a textbook on death and dying for nursing students.

Dr. Mary Jumbelic is currently the Chief Medical Examiner for Onondaga County in Syracuse, New York. She also serves as Clinical Associate Professor and Director of Postmortem Services for the State University of New York Upstate Medical University. In addition, she serves as an adjunct faculty member to Lemoyne College and Syracuse University, where she teaches forensic pathology to undergraduate students. Her special interests include injury prevention and mass fatality incidents. She has published extensively, including a seminal article for *JAMA* in 1990 describing the hazards of toddlers drowning in five-gallon buckets. She serves on the federal Disaster Mortuary Operational Response Team and has been deployed for large-scale crises such as the attack on the World Trade Center in 2001, the Andaman Sea tsunami, and Hurricane Katrina, as well as numerous plane crashes resulting in hundreds of fatalities. She lives with her husband, who is also a physician (an ophthalmologist), and has three growing sons, along with innumerable pets.

Stephen P. Kiernan has written for the *Boston Globe* and other publications, and for fourteen years wrote for the *Burlington Free Press* as a columnist, editorial writer, and investigative reporter. He was educated at Middlebury College, with master's degrees from Johns Hopkins University and the University of Iowa's Writers Workshop, and his numerous awards include the George Polk Award for medical reporting, the Joseph Brechner Center's Freedom of Information Award, and two-time finalist honors for the Gerald Loeb Award for Financial Journalism. He lives with his two sons in Vermont, and can be reached at stephenpkiernan.com.

Jean Levitan, PhD, is a professor in the Department of Public Health at William Paterson University of New Jersey, having joined the faculty in 1978. She teaches at the undergraduate level, offering courses in human sexuality, current health issues, women's health, and reproductive rights. She is co-author of the undergraduate textbook *Healthy Sexuality*, published by Wadsworth (2005). Apart from her professional life, she cherishes her roles as mother, wife, sister, daughter, and friend.

Cherylynn MacGregor received her BA in psychology and anthropology, her MA in anthropology, and her PhD in public health. She has retired from the University of Houston-Downtown, where she was a professor for fifteen years, teaching "Cultural Anthropology," "Health, Medicine, and Culture," and "Death and Dying." She has also taught "Victimology" and "Death Notification" at the Houston Police Academy, along with giving a seminar for Parents of Murdered Children.

Dr. Philip Nitschke (PhD, MD) is Director of the Australian nonprofit end-of-life choices organization Exit International. In 1996, Dr. Nitschke became the first doctor in the world to administer a legal, lethal voluntary injection under the Rights of the Terminally Ill Act of the Northern Territory of Australia—a law overturned eight months later. Based in Sydney, Australia, he travels internationally conducting workshops about practical end-of-life methods. Dr. Nitschke is the coauthor (with Dr. Fiona Stewart) of two books, *The Peaceful Pill eHandbook* (Exit International US, 2008—www.peacefulpill-handbook.com) and *Killing Me Softly: Voluntary Euthanasia and the Road to the Peaceful Pill* (Penguin, 2005).

Carol K. Oyster, PhD, is Professor of Psychology and Women's, Gender, and Sexuality Studies at the University of Wisconsin–La Crosse. A social psychologist by training, her interests have varied widely over the course of her career. She has written on a wide range of topics, including research design, group dynamics, women and retirement, suicide and law enforcement, emotions in children, and women and firearms. As the occupant of a recently empty nest, she devotes her spare time to her pets, quilting, knitting, target practice, hunting, and the unending quest for just the right color to paint the entry hall.

Susan Perlstein is an innovator, educator, social worker, administrator, and artist. She has written extensively on creativity and late-life learning. Thirty years ago, Ms. Perlstein founded Elders Share the Arts (ESTA), a New York City community-based arts organization that affirms the time-honored role of elders as the bearers of history and culture by using the power of the arts to transmit their stories in diverse communities. In 2001 widespread interest in ESTA's work led to the establishment of the National Center for Creative Aging (NCCA), a national organization dedicated to fostering an understanding of the vital relationship between creative expression and the quality of life of older people. NCCA serves as a networking, educational, advocacy, and policy center for the emerging field of "creative aging."

Marge Piercy is the author of seventeen novels including *Gone to Soldiers*; *He, She and It*; *Woman on the Edge of Time*; and recently, *Sex Wars*. She has authored seventeen volumes of poetry, most recently *The Crooked Inheritance*, and the memoir *Sleeping with Cats*. Born in center-city Detroit, educated at the University of Michigan, and the recipient of four honorary doctorates, she has been active in antiwar and women's movements. A popular speaker on college campuses, she has been a featured writer on Bill Moyers's PBS specials, Garrison Keillor's *Prairie Home Companion*, Terri Gross's *Fresh Air*, the *Today Show*, and many radio programs nationwide. Her work has been translated into sixteen languages.

Alan Pope is Associate Professor and Acting Chair of the Psychology Department at the University of West Georgia. He received his PhD in clinical existential-phenomenological psychology at Duquesne University following advanced graduate studies in computer science and artificial intelligence. He also has been a longtime student of Tibetan Buddhism. Among the graduate seminars he currently teaches are Buddhist Psychology, Psychology of Loss, and Explorations into Creativity. His research generally aims to elucidate the processes of psycho-spiritual transformation resulting from involuntary suffering and from disciplined spiritual and creative practice. He is the author of *From Child to Elder: Personal Transformation in Becoming an Orphan at Midlife*.

Ruthann Robson is still alive ten years after being diagnosed with a rare cancer. Her work in creative nonfiction has been recognized by a 2007 fellowship in Nonfiction Literature from the New York Foundation for the Arts, a 2006 Djerassi Residence Artists residency, a Creative Nonfiction (magazine) award, and publication in the Best of Creative Nonfiction (W. W. Norton, 2004). She is Professor of Law and Distinguished University Professor at the City University of New York, where she teaches Constitutional Law and Law and Sexuality. More of her work is available at www.ruthannrobson.com.

Mimi Schwartz is the author of five books, most recently *Good Neighbors, Bad Times—Echoes of My Father's German Village*, 2008; paperback, 2009

(University of Nebraska Press). Other books include *Thoughts from a Queen-Sized Bed* and *Writing True: The Art and Craft of Creative Nonfiction* (with Sondra Perl). Her short work has appeared in *The Missouri Review, Creative Nonfiction, Fourth Genre, Calyx,* the *New York Times, Tikkun, Jewish Week,* the *Writer's Chronicle, Florida Review, Brevity, River Teeth,* and *Writer's Digest,* among other publications. She is Professor Emerita of Richard Stockton College of New Jersey.

Dr. Fiona Stewart (PhD, MPol and Law) is a public health sociologist and Executive Director of Exit International. With Philip Nitschke, she is coauthor of *The Peaceful Pill eHandbook* (Exit International US, 2008, www.peacefulpillhandbook.com) and *Killing Me Softly: Voluntary Euthanasia and the Road to the Peaceful Pill* (Penguin, 2005). She is based in Sydney, Australia.

Kathryn Temple, JD, PhD, has taught English at Georgetown University since 1994. She specializes in the British eighteenth century and in cultural studies of law. She has published a number of essays on these topics and in 2002 a book, *Scandal Nation: Law and Authorship in Britain, 1750–1832.* Currently, she is writing about how the English legal system became a public relations project. Her husband, Jim Slevin, to whom her essay here is dedicated, died in 2006. She lives in Northern Virginia with her daughter, Lucy, an artist and math whiz, who never fails to brighten her day.

Kathryn L. Tucker, a graduate of Georgetown University Law School, is Director of Legal Affairs for Compassion and Choices, a national nonprofit public interest organization dedicated to improving end-of-life care and expanding and protecting the rights of the terminally ill. Ms. Tucker practiced law with the Seattle-based law firm Perkins Coie prior to moving to Compassion and Choices. She has served as an adjunct professor of law at the University of Washington, Seattle University, and Lewis and Clark Schools of Law for many years, teaching in the areas of law, medicine, and ethics, with a focus on the end of life. Ms. Tucker served as lead counsel representing patients and physicians in two landmark federal cases decided by the United States Supreme Court, asserting that mentally competent terminally ill patients have a constitutional right to choose aid in dying. She is recognized as a national leader in spearheading creative and effective efforts to promote improved care for seriously ill and dying patients and has been principal author of various state legislative measures to ensure physician education in pain management and provision of information to terminally ill patients about their end-of-life care options.

INDEX